Manual of
Cardiac Surgery

Bradley J. Harlan, MD

Chief, Section of Thoracic and Cardiovascular Surgery, Sutter Memorial Hospital,
Sacramento, California; Assistant Clinical Professor of Surgery, University of California
Davis Medical School, Sacramento, California; Formerly: Associate Professor of Surgery,
Oregon Health Sciences University, Portland, Oregon

Manual of

Springer-Verlag
New York Berlin Heidelberg London Paris
Tokyo Hong Kong Barcelona Budapest

Albert Starr, MD

Professor of Surgery, Oregon Health Sciences University, Portland Oregon;
Director, Heart Institute at St. Vincent Hospital, Portland, Oregon

Fredric M. Harwin, BFA, MS

Harwin Studios, Portland, Oregon

Cardiac Surgery

Second Edition

With 363 Color Illustrations

With Contributions by Alain Carpentier, MD
Professor of Cardiac Surgery, Hôpital Broussais, University of Paris, Paris, France

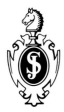

Bradley J. Harlan, MD
5301 F Street, Suite 312
Sacramento, California 95819
USA

Albert Starr, MD
Starr-Wood Cardiac Group, P.C.
9155 SW Barnes Rd., Suite 240
Portland, Oregon 97225-6629
USA

Fredric M. Harwin
Harwin Studios
9101 SW 15th Avenue
Portland, OR 97219
USA

Library of Congress Cataloging-in-Publication Data
Harlan, Bradley, J.
    Manual of cardiac surgery / Bradley J. Harlan, Albert Starr,
Fredric Harwin. — 2nd ed.
        p.   cm.
    Includes bibliographical references and index.
    ISBN 0-387-94220-3. — ISBN 3-540-94220-3
    1. Heart—Surgery. I. Starr, Albert, 1926– . II. Harwin,
Fredric M.   III. Title.
    [DNLM: 1. Heart Surgery—methods.   2. Heart Diseases—surgery.
WG 169 H283m 1994]
RD598.H32   1994
617.4′12—dc20
DNLM/DLC
for Library of Congress   93-47190
                                                                   CIP

Printed on acid-free paper.

Production managed by Jim Harbison and Natalie Johnson;
    manufacturing supervised by Jacqui Ashri.
Typeset by Bytheway Typesetting Services, Norwich, NY.
Printed and bound by Walsworth Publishing Co., Marceline, MO.
Printed in the United States of America.

9 8 7 6 5 4 3 2 1

ISBN 0-387-94220-3 Springer-Verlag New York Berlin Heidelberg
ISBN 3-540-94220-3 Springer-Verlag Berlin Heidelberg New York

To our wives, Sharon, Victoria, and Sara
and to our familes,
whose love and support
made this book possible

Preface

The second edition of the *Manual of Cardiac Surgery* has the same goal as the first edition: to be detailed as possible regarding the process of cardiac surgery, from coverage of basic surgical technique to careful description of every essential step of each operation. Carefully conceived and superbly executed full-color illustrations are the primary vehicle for conveying this information.

The techniques chosen are those developed over three decades of clinical practice and resident training at the Oregon Health Sciences University and St. Vincent Hospital, Portland, Oregon, and Sutter Memorial Hospital, Sacramento, California. These techniques have served us well.

The first author moved from the Oregon Health Sciences University to Sutter Memorial Hospital in Sacramento in 1981. During the ensuing decade some of the techniques used by the first two authors have evolved in different directions. Where this is the case, the text indicates where the technique shown is used at the present time.

The text authors are proud to have the illustrator, Mr. Fredric Harwin, as coauthor. Mr. Harwin has been a significant contributor to the basic concepts and intellectual substance of the book. His art is a powerful instrument of education.

It is hoped that this second edition will have broad appeal to all persons caring for cardiac surgical patients. If it increases knowledge and understanding of cardiac surgery and thereby improves patient care, it will have met its main objective.

Bradley J. Harlan, MD
Albert Starr, MD

A medical illustrator must understand the philosophies and techniques of the scientist as well as those of the artist. For the second edition of *Manual of Cardiac Surgery* I worked with Dr. Harlan and Dr. Starr to create illustrations that allow the reader to visualize the surgical field as the surgeon sees it. For each illustration, I drew upon direct observation, operative photographs, fresh specimens, and, most importantly, extensive consultations with my surgeon co-authors. The sequence of creation was, first, discussion of desired illustrations, then a rough sketch, consultation with the surgeons, finished pencil drawing, another consultation, then finally the color rendering. These color renderings were then checked against actual surgery for accuracy in representation of tissues, instrumentation, tissue responses to manipulation, and consistency of representation.

Close communication between artist and surgeon is essential to produce illustrations that are both anatomically and surgically correct and artistically viable. Such communication was present during the preparation of this book to convey not only the fundamentals of the operations, but also their most subtle details.

Fredric M. Harwin

Acknowledgments

We wish to thank our colleagues who directly and indirectly inspired many concepts of this book and provided support and stimulation during its creation: from Sacramento, Edward A. Smeloff, George E. Miller Jr, Paul B. Kelly, Jr, Forrest L. Junod, Kenneth A. Ross, Kuppe G. Shankar, Douglas R. Schuch, Michael T. Ingram, and Eric A. Peper; and from Portland, James A. Wood, Richard D. Chapman, Aftab Ahmad, H. Storm Floten, Jeffrey Swanson, Hugh L. Gately, Duane S. Bietz, Hagop Hovaguimian, and Anthony P. Furnary.

Valuable review and modification of the manuscript was provided by A. Glen Brooksby, Charles F. Collins, Jeffrey Leon, and Cornelius G. Wesseling for the chapter, "Anesthesia for Cardiac Surgery," and by Pat Brady and Gregory Meiling for the chapter "Conduct of Cardiopulmonary Bypass." We would like to thank Rodd Ambroson and Jeanne Koelling for their assistance with the production of illustrations. The creation of the illustrations was enhanced by the excellent photographs of our operations taken by Norman Meder. Gratitude is extended to Dee Sanchez, who helped greatly with the logistics required when a book is written and illustrated by authors living in different cities. We wish to thank Dr. Richard H. Egdahl for initiating the first edition of this project.

Finally, our thanks to Springer-Verlag, their superb staff, and our editor, William Day. We consider ourselves very fortunate to be beneficiaries of Springer-Verlag's longstanding expertise in the field of color reproduction and their strong commitment to quality.

Contents

1

Preoperative Preparation

Most steps in preoperative preparation of the patient for cardiac surgery are standardized and self-explanatory regardless of the operation planned, the preoperative state of the patient, or preoperative medications. Some facets of preoperative preparation, however, do involve preoperative medication management. This chapter covers routine preoperative preparation and the management of preoperative medications.

Routine Preparation

Autologous Blood Donation

The advent of acquired immune deficiency syndrome (AIDS) has provided further stimulation to the ongoing efforts to avoid the use of homologous blood products in patients undergoing cardiac surgery. California law requires that patients be informed of the risks and alternatives of homologous blood transfusion, including the alternative of autologous donation. Separate documentation of informed consent is required, and the law provides for penalties to physicians who do not follow its provisions.

Predonated autologous blood can reduce the use of homologous blood transfusion. In properly selected patients, autologous donation is associated with a low incidence of complications (less than 1%) and can lower the use of homologous blood to 27% of those donating autologous blood.[12,16]

Admission Orders

Routine admission orders include care of the patient, preoperative diagnostic assessment, preparation of blood products, and management of medications. Cardiac status determines the sodium content of the patient's diet. Most patients are given a solid meal the night before surgery. Activity is unrestricted unless otherwise indicated by cardiac status. Routine diagnostic procedures relating to blood values, chest x-ray, and electrocardiogram are performed. For adult patients, blood is typed and cross-matched for 2 units of whole blood and 2 units of packed cells. Additional blood products, such as platelets or fresh frozen plasma, are ordered if indicated by the patient's clotting status or if a particularly long time on cardiopulmonary bypass is expected. One unit of whole blood and two units of packed cells are usually prepared for children and infants.

Infection Control

Control of infection in cardiac surgery patients requires coordination of efforts during the preoperative, operative, and postoperative periods. Preoperative infection control involves diagnosis and treatment of any abnormal amount or type of bacteria the patient may harbor and the administration of prophylactic antibiotics.

Careful physical examination may reveal a skin infection. Oral hygiene should be checked; carious teeth should be treated prior to elective surgery, especially when a valve replacement is planned. When teeth were an obvious source of subacute bacterial endocarditis, we have had them extracted prior to valve replacement. Specimens from the nasopharynx of patients with chronic sinusitis may need to be cultured. Sputum of patients with chronic bronchitis may be cultured. Pathogenic bacteria should be eradicated prior to surgery. Also, bacteriuria should be treated.

Since infection following cardiac surgery, particularly on a valvular prosthesis, can be disastrous, all measures to reduce its incidence are taken. Certainly the most important factors relating to prevention of postoperative infection are meticulous sterile technique, gentle handling of tissue, and expeditious perfomance of the operation. Prophylactic antibiotics are also of value and are given to all patients undergoing cardiac surgery.

In adults we administer cephazolin, 1–2 g intravenously, on arrival in the operating room. This antibiotic is continued intravenously in the postoperative period at 1–2 g every 8 hours for 2 to 3 days, or longer if central lines remain in place. The same temporal regimen is used in infants and children, with the dosage adjusted appropriately.

Respiratory Management

The respiratory system of each patient should be carefully assessed by the history and physical exam. A history of smoking or chronic productive cough indicates an increased probability of respiratory problems in the postoperative period. The presence or extent of pulmonary disease can be quantitated by pulmonary function tests and analysis of arterial blood gases with the patient breathing room air. Knowledge of preoperative room-air blood gases will help indicate the level of respiratory function to be expected in the postoperative period.

Preoperative preparation includes encouraging patients who smoke to stop. Chronic productive cough may be improved by a period of intensive, in-hospital respiratory therapy.

Medication Management

Digitalis

Digitalis results in direct improvement of the contractile state of the myocardium. The inotropic effect appears to be related to a cellular membrane effect resulting in an increase in cellular calcium.[11,17]

Although it was our previous practice, we no longer withhold digitalis from patients who have been on long-term therapy. It is also no longer our practice to administer a subdigitalizing dose to those patients who are not on digitalis.

Beta-Blockers

Beta-adrenergic blocking agents decrease myocardial oxygen demand by decreasing heart rate, blood pressure, and myocardial contractility. This decrease in demand can bring the oxygen requirement down to a level that can be supplied by the limited coronary blood flow, thereby decreasing or eliminating angina and other ischemic cardiac events. Propranolol was the first beta-blocker released in the United States. Atenolol, metoprolol, nadolol, pindolol, and timolol have also been released.[5,7,13]

For most patients our general policy is to administer beta-blockers up to the night before surgery or up to the time of surgery. The dose is sometimes tapered, but only if there is no change in the anginal pattern. Patients who have unstable angina or have had a recent pattern of unstable angina should have beta-blockers continued up to the time of surgery without alteration of dosage. The continuation of propranolol and the other beta-blockers up to the time of surgery makes the preoperative period and the induction of anesthesia smoother and is not associated with depressed myocardial performance postoperatively.[1,8,15,18]

Calcium-Channel Blockers

The calcium-channel blockers, diltiazem, nifedipine, and verapamil, have become an important class of drugs in the management of angina pectoris.[3,6,10,19,20] These drugs are also continued up to the time of surgery.

Anticoagulants

Management of anticoagulants prior to cardiac surgery must balance the risk of thromboembolism following withdrawal against the risk of increased operative bleeding if substantial effects are still present at the time of surgery. Sodium warfarin (Coumadin) is the most commonly used oral anticoagulant. Warfarin depresses the synthesis of prothrombin by the liver. This action can be potentiated by a number of drugs, especially the barbiturates.[9] The effect of sodium warfarin can be counteracted or reversed by vitamin K.

Our practice is to withhold sodium warfarin beginning 1 week prior to scheduled surgery, allowing the prothrombin time to drift back to normal. Patients at particular risk of thromboembolism can be placed on heparin during normalization of their prothrombin time. We do not administer vitamin K. If rapid reversal of the anticoagulated state is required, component therapy with fresh frozen plasma is used.

Aspirin

Aspirin inhibits platelet aggregation by blocking biosynthesis of prostaglandin synthetase.[4] This apparently inhibits the release of endogenous adenosine diphosphate from platelets, thus preventing normal platelet aggregation and platelet plug formation.[2] The effect of aspirin persists for the life of the platelet. Since the half-life of platelets is five to ten days, it is desirable to withhold aspirin from patients for a week prior to surgery, although this is not possible in many patients today because of the large number requiring urgent or emergency surgery.

Preoperative use of aspirin is reported to result in increased postoperative bleeding if taken within 7 days of surgery.[14] Platelets can be administered to patients who have serious postoperative bleeding that may be secondary to aspirin, in spite of a normal platelet count.

Patient and Family Preparation

Preoperative communication among the surgeon, the patient, and the patient's family is an essential part of preoperative preparation. This communication educates the patient about the risks and expected benefits of surgery and informs the surgeon about the patient's drive, ambition, fears, and expectations, all of which are important factors in overall patient management.

The patient and family are informed of events that will occur during and after surgery and told of visiting hours and procedures. The environment of the Intensive Care Unit is explained to the patient, so that the surroundings will be familiar after recovery from anesthesia. This can diminish the anxiety that may result from a strange environment. Further instruction can include postoperative respiratory management. Breathing exercises are best explained by a respiratory therapist, who emphasizes their importance in preventing or treating potential postoperative respiratory problems.

If the patient and family are properly informed about what to expect during the postoperative period, their cooperative understanding facilitates a smoother postoperative experience.

References

1. Boudoulas J, Snyder GL, Lewis RP, Kates RD, Karayanacos PE, Vasko JS: Safety and rationale for continuation of propranolol therapy during coronary bypass operation. Ann Thorac Surg 26:222,1978.
2. Champion LAA, Schwartz AD, Luddy RE, Schindler S: The effects of four commonly used drugs on platelet function. J Pediat 89:653,1976.
3. Chew CYC, Brown BG, Singh BN, Wong MM, Pierce C, Petersen R: Effects of verapamil on coronary hemodynamic function and vasomobility relative to its mechanism of antianginal action. Am J Cardiol 51:699,1983.
4. Crook D, Collins AJ: Comparison of effects of aspirin and indomethacin on human platelet prostaglandin synthetase. Ann Rheumatic Dis 36:459,1977.
5. Frishman WH: Beta-adrenoceptor antagonists: new drugs and new indications. N Engl J Med 305:500,1981.
6. Frishman WH, Charlap S, Goldberger J, Kimmel B, Stroh J, Dorsa F, Allen L, Strom J: Comparison of diltiazem and nifedipine for both angina pectoris and systemic hypertension. Am J Cardiol 56:41H,1985.
7. Harris FJ, Low RI, Paumer L, Amsterdam EA, Mason DT: Antianginal efficacy and improved exercise performance with timolol. Am J Cardiol 51:13,1983.
8. Jones EL, Kaplan JA, Dorney ER, King SB III, Douglas JS Jr, Hatcher CR Jr: Propranolol therapy in patients undergoing myocardial revascularization. Am J Cardiol 38:696,1976.
9. Koch-Weser J, Sellers EM: Medical progress: drug interactions with coumarin anticoagulants. N Engl J Med 285:487, 547,1971.
10. Krikler DM, Rowland E: Clinical value of calcium antagonists in treatment of cardiovascular disorders. J Am Coll Cardiol 1:355,1983.
11. Langer GA: The intrinsic control of myocardial contraction—ionic factors. N Engl J Med 285:1065,1971.
12. Love TR, Hendren WG, O'Keefe DD, Daggett WM: Transfusion of predonated blood in elective cardiac surgery. Ann Thorac Surg 43:508,1987.
13. Manyari DE, Kostuk WJ, Carruthers SG, Johnston DJ, Purves P: Pindolol and propranolol in patients with angina pectoris and normal or near-normal ventricular function. Am J Cardiol 51:427,1983.
14. Michelson EL, Morganroth J, Torrosian M, MacVaugh H III: Relation of preoperative use of aspirin to increased mediastinal blood loss after coronary artery bypass surgery. J Thorac Cardiovasc Surg 76:694,1978.
15. Olinger GN, Bonchek LI, Keelan MH, Tresch DD, Siegel R, Bamarah V, Tristani FE: Unstable angina: the case for operation. Am J Cardiol 42:634,1978.
16. Owings DV, Kruskall MS, Thurer RL, Donovan LM: Autologous blood donations prior to elective cardiac surgery. JAMA 262:1963,1989.
17. Schwartz A, Allen JC, Harigaya S: Possible involvement of cardiac Na^+, K^+-adenosine triphosphate in the mechanism of action of cardiac glycosides. J Pharmacol Exp Ther 168:31,1969.
18. Slogoff S, Keats AS, Ott E: Preoperative propranolol therapy and aortocoronary bypass operation. JAMA 240:1487,1978.
19. Vetrovec GW, Parker VE, Cole S, Procacci PM, Tabatznik B, Terry R: Nifedipine gastrointestinal therapeutic system in stable angina pectoris. Am J Med 83:24,1987.
20. White HD, Polak JF, Wynne J, Holman BL, Antman EM, Nesto RW: Addition of nifedipine to maximal nitrate and beta-adrenoreceptor blocker therapy in coronary disease. Am J Cardiol 55:1303,1985.

Anesthesia for Cardiac Surgery

Anesthesia for cardiac surgery is often more demanding than anesthesia for other types of surgery. Almost all patients have hemodynamic abnormalities that must be managed properly during induction and maintenance of anesthesia in order to avoid myocardial injury or injury to other organs.

With cardiopulmonary bypass, a profound alteration of normal physiology requires close cooperation and careful communication among the anesthesiologist, the cardiopulmonary perfusionist, and the surgeon. Many patients undergoing cardiac surgery must be extensively monitored with a variety of sophisticated equipment and techniques. Cardiac anesthesia necessitates a broad range of techniques and a thorough knowledge of the alterations in cardiac physiology caused by anesthesia.

This chapter describes our methods of intraoperative monitoring and the physiologic basis for these methods. Drugs used before and during anesthesia and their advantages for the cardiac patient are discussed. Our techniques of anesthetic induction and maintenance are described as they relate to different patient groups and physiologic states.

Monitoring

Electrocardiogram

The electrocardiogram is a valuable indicator not only of cardiac rate and rhythm but also of myocardial ischemia and the level of myocardial oxygen consumption. Standard limb leads are placed on all patients shortly after arriving in the operating room. Limb lead II is usually monitored, since its axis parallels the electrical axis of the heart and the P wave is easily seen. A V5 lead is placed on patients with coronary artery disease or severe valvular disease. This lead is more sensitive than the limb leads in the detection of ischemia of the anterior wall of the left ventricle.[8,9]

Systemic Arterial Pressure

A blood pressure cuff, with doppler probe, monitors arm blood pressure. In addition, an arterial pressure line is placed prior to induction of anesthesia. Arterial pressure is usually monitored by an indwelling radial artery catheter, occasionally by a femoral artery catheter. The arterial line is placed before induction in adults and after induction in infants and children. The pressure is displayed digitally and in wave form on large monitoring screens. If possible, the radial artery catheter is placed percutaneously. If percutaneous place-ment is not possible, cutdown on the artery and direct placement of the catheter are performed. Cutdown is often necessary in the infant. If an umbil-ical artery catheter is already in place in the neonate, it is used.

Pulmonary Arterial Pressure

Pulmonary arterial pressure and occasionally wedge pressure are monitored by a Swan-Ganz catheter in almost all adult patients. The Swan-Ganz cathe-ter is usually placed percutaneously via the right internal jugular vein. To diminish the likelihood of pulmonary artery perforation, the catheter is not kept in a wedge position, but advanced to the wedge position as needed. Pulmonary artery wedge pressure is an accurate reflection of left atrial pres-sure. In the absence of mitral stenosis, left atrial pressure is an accurate reflection of left ventricular diastolic pressure. In most patients the Swan-Ganz catheter can therefore be used to monitor left ventricular filling pressure during induction, the prebypass period, and the postbypass period. With the use of a thermodilution catheter, cardiac output and systemic vascular resistance can also be measured.

Systemic Venous Pressure

Systemic venous pressure is monitored in adults from the sideport of the Swan-Ganz catheter sheath, placed in the internal jugular vein. In infants and children, a dual-lumen catheter is placed percutaneously in the right internal jugular vein. In infants cutdown on the internal jugular vein is occa-sionally required. The dual-lumen catheter can be used for both monitoring and infusion.

Pulse Oximetry

Arterial oxygen saturation is monitored from a digit on the hand or foot. Pulse oximetry measures the adequacy of oxygenation and can show the presence of right-to-left shunting of blood.

Capnography

Measurement of the end tidal carbon dioxide level verifies placement of the endotracheal tube in the trachea and measures the adequacy of ventilation.

Temperature

Nasopharyngeal temperature probes are used in all patients. In infants rectal temperature is monitored as well.

Premedication

Premedication in adults is usually a benzodiazapine and/or a narcotic. An antisialagogue is rarely used.

Myocardial Protection: The Anesthesiologist's Role

Determinants of Myocardial Oxygen Supply and Demand

Myocardial necrosis and ventricular arrhythmias can occur during the precar-diopulmonary bypass period. Isom and colleagues,[7] in their 1975 report, found enzymatic evidence of myocardial necrosis occurring before bypass in 92% of patients undergoing coronary artery surgery. Moore and colleagues[14] found progressive improvement in survival following bypass surgery for left main coronary stenosis after adoption of anesthetic techniques that prevented both myocardial ischemia and depressed myocardial performance during the induction and bypass periods. In spite of the newer, safer anesthetic agents and the widespread use of beta-blockers, calcium-channel blocking drugs, and nitrates, Slogoff and Keats, in their 1989 report,[21] found a 30% incidence of new ST segment depression occurring from anesthetic induction to start of cardiopulmonary bypass. We have not experienced such a high incidence of new ST segment depression.

Myocardial necrosis and ventricular arrhythmias may result from an abnormal myocardial oxygen supply/demand ratio, caused either by a fall in oxygen supply secondary to hypotension or hypoxia, or by an increase in myocardial oxygen demand that cannot be met by an increase in oxygen supply. Such an increase in oxygen demand is usually due to increases in heart rate and blood pressure.

Determination of oxygen demand of the myocardium is multifactorial.[22] Development of tension and the contractile state of the myocardium are the primary determinants of myocardial oxygen consumption. Other factors, including basal myocardial oxygen consumption, activation energy, and external work, also contribute to myocardial oxygen consumption, but to a relatively minor extent. Development of tension in the myocardium is reflected by hemodynamic correlates of heart rate and aortic blood pressure. These hemodynamic parameters can be used to determine the level of myocardial oxygen demand.[10,17]

The product of the heart rate and the systolic blood pressure (the rate-pressure product) is a sensitive measure of the myocardial oxygen demand in patients without gross left ventricular dysfunction.[10,17,28] Rate-pressure products below 12,000 appear to reflect myocardial oxygen demands which can be met, even in the presence of severe coronary artery disease.[9] In other words, if the heart rate is kept below 90 and the systolic pressure is kept below 130 mm Hg, the level of oxygen demand is probably safe. A delicate balance must be achieved between hypertension (which increases demand) and hypotension (which decreases supply). There are three periods when the supply/demand balance may be upset, resulting in myocardial ischemia or necrosis: preinduction, induction, and prebypass.

Preinduction

The period immediately after entry into the operating room and the period of placement of the venous and arterial lines can be stressful to the patient, resulting in increased heart rate and blood pressure. Monitoring should be started immediately, using cuff blood pressure, electrocardiogram, and pulse oximetry. Oxygen, local anesthetics, and judicious intravenous sedation are usually sufficient to prevent hypertension and tachycardia. Tachycardia should be treated with more sedation or incremental doses of esmolol. Increased blood pressure should be treated with more sedation, nitroglycerin, or nitroprusside.

Induction

In cardiac surgery the basic anesthesia principles of avoidance of hypotension and hypoxia must be followed, since they are critical to the level of myocardial oxygen supply. Myocardial oxygen demand may increase during the period of induction, particularly during intubation.[2] Patients with coronary disease seem to be more prone to increase in rate-pressure product during intubation than are patients with valvular disease.[2] Adjustments in anesthetic induction, as well as the use of vasodilators, esmolol, calcium-channel blockers, and an additional anesthetic agent, may be required in order to treat increased myocardial oxygen demand that may occur during induction and intubation.

Prebypass

Skin incision and sternotomy may stimulate an increase in heart rate and blood pressure, which will require treatment either by increasing the depth of anesthesia or by using vasoactive agents. The anesthesiologist should know the determinants of myocardial oxygen supply and demand and how these may be affected by anesthetic techniques, anesthetic agents, and other factors. Close attention to these variables will make myocardial ischemia or necrosis in the precardiopulmonary bypass period much less likely.

Anesthetic Agents

Opioids

Cardiovascular response to large doses of intravenous morphine was described by Lowenstein and co-workers[12] in 1969. Following this report, the use of morphine for cardiac anesthesia became widespread during the 1970s. Although in the strictest sense morphine causes analgesia rather than anesthesia, since it may not cause hypnosis or amnesia, small amounts of other drugs such as diazepam, nitrous oxide, or halothane can be used to achieve complete anesthesia.

Morphine is advantageous for use in cardiac patients for a number of reasons. It is not a myocardial depressant. It does not cause ventricular irritability. High concentrations of inspired oxygen can be used if required. Since morphine has a prolonged effect and gradual reversal, there is no risk of sudden awakening; the transition from the operating room to the recovery room is smooth, and significant postoperative analgesia is provided. However, use of high-dose morphine can have disadvantages. Hypertension, hypotension, and venodilation can occur. Amnesia can be incomplete. For these reasons the search has continued for opioids that result in better hemodynamic stability.

In 1978 Stanley and Webster[23] reported the use of fentanyl, a new synthetic narcotic, for mitral valve replacement. Fentanyl decreased heart rate and arterial blood pressure but did not significantly change stroke volume, cardiac output, central venous pressure, or peripheral arterial resistance. In 1980 the use of fentanyl for cardiac anesthesia was approved by the Food and Drug Administration, and soon fentanyl largely supplanted morphine anesthesia.

Sufentanil[20] is a newer synthetic opioid that is more potent than fentanyl and also results in excellent hemodynamic stability. Although some studies[4,13] have suggested that sufentanil is superior to fentanyl, other studies[6,24,26] have not shown any differences between the two drugs.

Opioid anesthesia, using either fentanyl or sufentanil, is our usual choice for cardiac anesthesia for adults, children, and infants. The opioid is sometimes augmented with a benzodiazepine, such as midazolam or lorazepam, although this should be done with caution.[25] Opioid anesthesia can also be augmented with an inhalational agent.

Inhalational Agents

Enflurane and isoflurane are our inhalational agents of choice in adults, and halothane is the agent of choice in children. The use of isoflurane in the presence of coronary artery disease is controversial,[3] with some studies suggesting that it causes coronary vasodilatation and a coronary steal syndrome.[19] Other studies[11,18] have not documented myocardial ischemia with the use of isoflurane, as long as hypotension is avoided.

Ketamine

Ketamine is an intravenous or intramuscular agent with rapid onset, producing profound analgesia and a cataleptic state. Ketamine is unique among anesthetic agents because it stimulates the cardiovascular system, causing increases in blood pressure, heart rate, and cardiac output.[27] This property makes ketamine a useful drug in patients with severe cyanosis and acidosis or an acutely depressed cardiac output, such as in acute tamponade.

Paralyzing Agents

Pancuronium and vecuronium are nondepolarizing neuromuscular blocking agents that have little effect on the circulatory system and do not cause the hypotension that can occur with curare. Pancuronium occasionally causes an increase in heart rate and blood pressure, making it the agent of choice for most children as well as adults with mitral or aortic regurgitation. Vecuronium does not cause an increase in heart rate and blood pressure.[16]

Vasodilators

Nitroprusside is a vasodilator acting directly on the smooth muscle in the arterioles and veins. It is our drug of choice in the management of hypertension occurring before, during, or after anesthesia. It is also used to improve postoperative cardiac performance by lowering afterload.

Anesthetic Methods

Noncyanotic Neonates and Infants

Halothane is usually used for those patients arriving in the operating room without a peripheral intravenous line. In patients who are hemodynamically unstable or in marked congestive heart failure, ketamine is used. Succinylcholine is used for intubation. Following intubation, lines are placed. The anesthetic is then augmented and maintained with fentanyl or sufentanil.[1,5,15] If the patient arrives in the operating room with a peripheral intravenous line, induction is with fentanyl or sufentanil or with sodium pentathol as well as muscle relaxants. Maintenance is with fentanyl or sufentanil.

Cyanotic Neonates and Infants

Anesthetic agents are chosen which maintain systemic vascular resistance and do not lower pulmonary vascular resistance. For these reasons, inhalational agents are usually avoided. Ketamine with a muscle relaxant is usually used for induction, and fentanyl or sufentanil for maintenance.

Children Undergoing Elective Open Cardiac Procedures

Older children are usually premedicated, resulting in a less stressful preinduction and induction period. A peripheral intravenous line is placed if it is not stressful for the patient and induction is with fentanyl or sufentanil and a muscle relaxant. Sodium pentothal is sometimes used. Fentanyl or sufentanil is used for maintenance.

Adults

Premedication is usually lorazepam or midazolam. Induction and maintenance are with fentanyl or sufentanil, supplemented by benzodiazepines, morphine, and inhalational agent as needed.

References

1. Anand KJS, Hickey PR: Halothane-morphine compared with high-dose sufentanil for anesthesia and postoperative analgesia in neonatal cardiac surgery. N Engl J Med 326:1,1992.
2. Bassell GM, Lin YT, Oka Y, Becker RM, Frater RWM: Circulatory response to tracheal intubation in patients with coronary artery disease and valvular disease. Bull NY Acad Med 54:842,1978.
3. Becker LC: Is isoflurane dangerous for the patient with coronary artery disease? Anesthesiology 66:259,1987.
4. deLange S, Boscoe MJ, Stanley TH, Pace N: Comparison of Sufentanil-Oxygen and Fentanyl-Oxygen for coronary artery surgery. Anesthesiology 56:112,1982.
5. Hickey PR, Hansen DD, Wessel DL, Lang P, Jonas RA: Pulmonary and systemic hemodynamic responses to fentanyl in infants. Anesth Analg 64:483,1985.
6. Howie MB, McSweeney TD, Lingam RP, Maschke SP: A comparison of fentanyl-oxygen and sufentanil-oxygen for cardiac anesthesia. Anesth Analg 64:877,1985.
7. Isom OW, Spencer FC, Feigenbaum H, Cunningham J, Roe C: Prebypass myocardial damage in patients undergoing coronary revascularization: an unrecognized vulnerable period (abstr). Circulation 51(Suppl II):II-119,1975.
8. Kaplan JA (ed): Cardiac Anesthesia. New York, San Francisco, London, Grune & Stratton, 1979.
9. Kaplan JA, King SB: The precordial electrocardiographic lead (V5) in patients who have coronary artery disease. Anesthesiology 45:570,1976.
10. Kitamura K, Jorgensen CR, Gobel F, Taylor HL, Wang Y: Hemodynamic correlates of myocardial oxygen consumption during upright exercise. J Appl Physiol 32:516,1972.
11. Leung JM, Goehner P, O'Kelly BF, Hollenberg M, Pineda N, Cason BA, Mangano DT: Isoflurane anesthesia and myocardial ischemia: comparative risk versus sufentanil anesthesia in patients undergoing coronary artery bypass graft surgery. Anesthesiology 74:838,1991.
12. Lowenstein E, Hallowel P, Levin FH, Daggett WM, Austen WG, Laver MB: Cardiovascular response to large doses of intravenous morphine in man. N Engl J Med 281:1389,1969.
13. Mathews HML, Furness G, Carson IW, Orr IA, Lyons SM, Clarke RSJ: Comparison of sufentanil-oxygen and fentanyl-oxygen anesthesia for coronary artery bypass grafting. Br J Anaesth 60:530,1988.
14. Moore CH, Lombardo TR, Allums JA, Gordon FT: Left main coronary artery stenosis: hemodynamic monitoring to reduce mortality. Ann Thorac Surg 26: 445,1978.
15. Moore RA, Yang SS, McNicholas KW, Gallagher JD, Clark DL: Hemodynamic and anesthetic effects of sufentanil as the sole anesthetic for pediatric cardiovascular surgery. Anesthesiology 62:725,1985.
16. Morris RB, Cahalan MK, Miller RD, Wilkinson PL, Quasha AL, Robinson SL: The cardiovascular effects of vecuronium (ORG NC45) and pancuronium in patients undergoing coronary artery bypass grafting. Anesthesiology 58:438,1983.
17. Nelson RR, Gobel RL, Jorgennsen CR, Wang K, Wang Y, Taylor HL: Hemodynamic predictors of myocardial oxygen consumption during static and dynamic exercise. Circulation 50:1179,1974.
18. O'Young J, Mastrocostopoulos G, Hilgenberg A, Palacios I, Kyritsis A, Lappas DG: Myocardial circulatory and metabolic effects of isoflurane and sufentanil during coronary artery surgery. Anesthesiology 66:653,1987.
19. Reiz S, Balfors E, Sorensen MB, Ariola S, Friedman A, Truedsson H: Isoflurane—a powerful coronary vasodilator in patients with coronary artery disease. Anesthesiology 59:91,1983.
20. Rosow CE: Sufentanil citrate: a new opioid for use in anesthesia. Pharmacotherapy 4:11,1984.
21. Slogoff S, Keats AS: Randomized trial of primary anesthetic agents on outcome of coronary artery bypass operations. Anesthesiology 70:179,1989.
22. Sonnenblick EK, Ross J Jr, Braunwald E: Oxygen consumption of the heart: newer concepts of its multifactorial determination. Am J Cardiol 22:328,1968.
23. Stanley TH, Webster LR: Anesthetic requirements and cardiovascular effects of

fentanyl-oxygen and fentanyl-diazepam-oxygen anesthesia in man. Anesth Analg 57:411,1978.

24. Thomson IR, Hudson RJ, Rosenbloom M, Meatherall RC: A randomized double-blind comparison of fentanyl and sufentanil anaesthesia for coronary artery surgery. Can J Anaesth 34:227,1987.

25. Tomicheck RC, Rosow CE, Philbin DM, Moss J, Teplick RS, Schneider RC: Diazepam-fentanyl interaction—hemodynamic and hormonal effects in coronary artery surgery. Anesth Analg 62:881,1983.

26. Turman KJ, McCarthy RJ, Speiss BD, DaValle M, Dabir R, Ivankovich AD: Does choice of anesthetic agent significantly affect outcome after coronary artery surgery? Anesthesiology 70:189,1989.

27. Tweed WA, Minuck M, Mymin D: Circulatory responses to ketamine anesthesia. Anesthesiology 37:613,1972.

28. Wilkinson PL, Moyers JR, Ports T, Chatterjee K, Ullyot DJ, Hamilton WK: Rate pressure product and myocardial oxygen consumption during surgery for coronary artery bypass. Circulation 58(Suppl II):II-84,1978.

3

Basic Surgical Technique

The physical aspect of surgery is at least as important as the intellectual aspect. The surgeon who knows what to do and when to do it is obviously ineffective, in fact dangerous, if he or she cannot physically do it. Although technical excellence is obviously admired and valued, the basics of surgical technique (which are essential components of technical excellence) are absent from many standard surgical textbooks.

The multiple coordinated and precise movements that result in technical excellence require not only a steady hand and smooth motion, but also knowledge of the most atraumatic and efficient motions to accomplish a specific physical action.

Knowledge of the fundamentals of how surgical instruments are held and moved is essential to accomplish smooth surgical movements. Surgery is also an art, requiring a continuing ability to create and accommodate. Nevertheless, the basics are required before the art is possible.

This chapter describes some of these fundamentals as they relate to the techniques of dissection and suturing as well as describing the mental and physical preparation that enhances surgical technique.

Dissection

Most cardiac operations do not involve a lot of tissue dissection. Some, such as repair of a patent ductus arteriosus, consist predominantly of tissue dissection. In other procedures, such as reoperation, tissue dissection may be the most challenging and potentially dangerous portion of the entire operation. Fundamentals of tissue dissection are therefore important for the cardiac surgeon.

Scissor Dissection

Most tissue dissection in cardiac surgery is accomplished sharply with scissors. The majority of dissection involves freeing blood vessels for clamping or suturing. This can usually be accomplished by cutting the connective tissue that attaches to the adventitia of the vessel. The assistant's retraction of the tissue layer over the vessel stretches and tenses this connective tissue, displaying its numerous tiny fibers. These fibers can be cut with the tips of the scissors, the scissors being held at right angles to the tissue being cut. The scissors should be held with the thumb and ring finger in the rings and the index finger extended down the handle to provide stabilization and balance (Fig. 3–1).

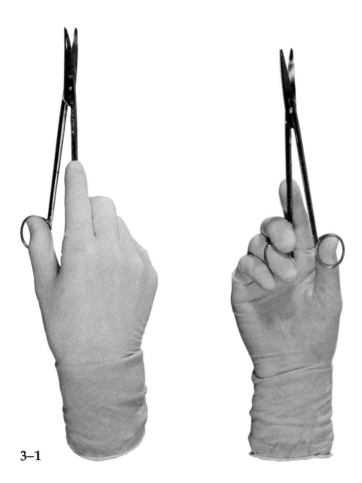

3–1

Scalpel Dissection

The scalpel can be superior to scissors for dissection in close quarters and for cutting through tissue that is particularly adherent to other tissue, such as mediastinal tissue which may be stuck to the back of the sternum at reoperation.

The scalpel is also used for incision of epicardium and exposure of coronary arteries. Gentle stroking or "painting" of the tissue overlying the coronary artery frees the artery wall for precise incision. Once the epicardium is incised, the strands of tissue connecting the epicardium and the coronary artery can also be divided by "shaving" the surface of the artery, exposing the artery and separating the epicardium and subepicardial fat so that the latter is not included in the suture line.

Suturing

Almost all cardiac operations involve suturing, passing a needle and suture material through tissue and often through material such as valve sewing rings or grafts. A coronary artery operation can involve 200 or more such passes of needle and suture material. The accuracy, smoothness, and efficiency with which suturing is accomplished are the major determinants of the success or failure of most cardiac operations. For this reason the way a needle is placed in the needle holder, the way the needle holder is held in the hand, and the motions of the hand, wrist, arm—indeed the entire body—are fundamental to cardiac surgery.

The surgeon should know which sutures are most feasible in the many physical situations occurring during an operation. The ability to select the most efficient motion required and the ability to execute that motion smoothly are far more important than speed of motion. In fact, the best surgeons do not make fast moves—they make *efficient* moves.

In this section we shall outline the basics of suturing as we perceive them and describe how they relate to some of the commonly occurring suture lines in cardiac surgery. It is hoped that this discussion not only will be informative but will also stimulate the surgeons reading this to analyze more exhaustively their own basic motions.

Forehand Suture

The forehand suture, resulting from supination of the wrist, is certainly the most common suture in surgery. The needle usually passes down into the tissue and then up out of the tissue with the needle tip ending at or above the plane at which it entered the tissue. This is accomplished by movement of the wrist from a position of end pronation through the motion of supination.

The needle holder is best held as shown in Figure 3–2. The distal phalanx of the thumb is placed partially in the upper ring so the thumb can exert both an outer and an inner force on the upper handle and thereby on the holder ratchets. The distal phalanx of the ring finger is in the lower ring in a position of flexion, providing an inward force on the ring toward the palm. The tip of the middle finger is over the junction of the ring and lower handle, also providing inward force toward the palm.

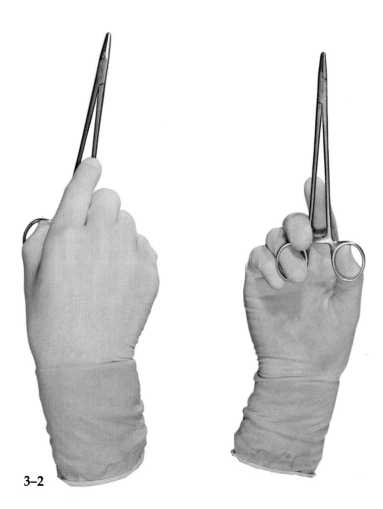

3–2

The stability of the needle holder is provided by forces opposite to those of the ring and middle fingers. These outward forces come from the little finger and the index finger. The tip and distal joint of the little finger push out against the lower portion of the lower ring. The tip of the index finger pushes out against the midportion of the lower handle (the handle attached to the lower ring). The lower handle is thereby fixed and stabilized by two outside forces (the index finger and the little finger) pushing outward and two inside forces (the ring and middle fingers) pushing in.

The forces on both handles result in a stable lower handle against which the upper handle moves. The opening of the jaws of the needle holder is thereby caused by upward movement of the thumb, which moves the lower jaw down. Closure of the jaws results from downward movement of the thumb, causing upward movement of the lower jaw against the relatively immobile upper jaw.

Supination of the wrist can result in many different planes of movement of the needle, depending on the position of the wrist, elbow, and body.

Level Forehand Suture
The forehand suture generally moves from right to left for the right-hander (Fig. 3–3). The plane of the needle is usually parallel to the coronal plane of the surgeon's body, and the level of the suture is at or near the level of the surgeon's elbow. This is a common suture used when joining two structures that are on the same plane, such as vein to coronary artery. The needle tip usually ends at the same level as it began. The needle front is then gripped

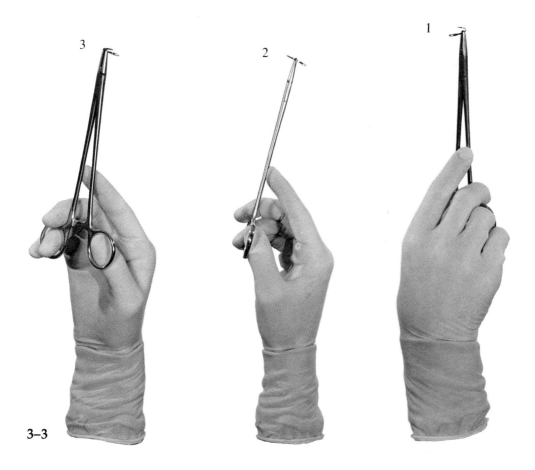

3–3

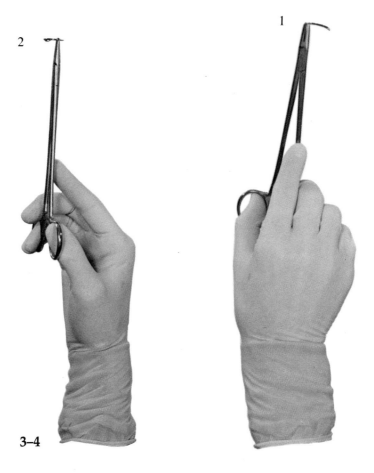

3–4

and brought smoothly through the tissue (Fig. 3–4). A level forehand suture can also be taken left to right if the shoulder is extended with the elbow away from the body and the body rotated so the right shoulder is in front of the left.

Forehand-Up Suture
The forehand-up suture results in the needle tip ending higher than it began. This is a relatively simple suture to accomplish and often does not require full pronation of the wrist prior to supination. The forehand-up suture is useful during aortic valve replacement for the half of the left coronary cusp near the noncoronary cusp commissure (Fig. 3–5) and for the half of the noncoronary cusp near the right cusp commissure. The forehand-up suture can be used during mitral valve replacement in the posterior medial quadrant, with the needle moving through the anulus from the ventricular to the atrial side.

Forehand-Down Suture
The forehand-down suture moves the needle tip to a level lower than that at which it started. This can end with the needle tip away from the surgeon, by keeping the elbow in toward the body and extending the wrist (Fig. 3–6). This suture can be used during aortic valve replacement on the noncoronary cusp near the left coronary cusp commissure and on the left coronary cusp near the right coronary cusp commissure. It is useful in mitral valve replacement on the posterolateral portion of the anulus, moving the needle from the atrial to the ventricular side.

A forehand-down suture can also end with the needle tip toward the surgeon, by moving the elbow away from the body and pronating the wrist so

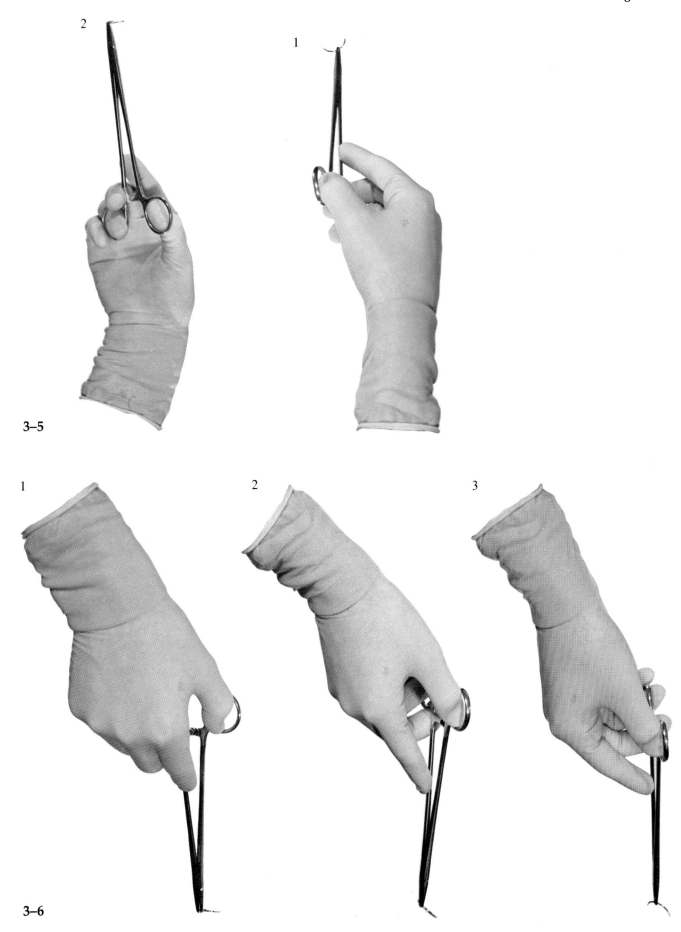

2

1

3–5

1

2

3

3–6

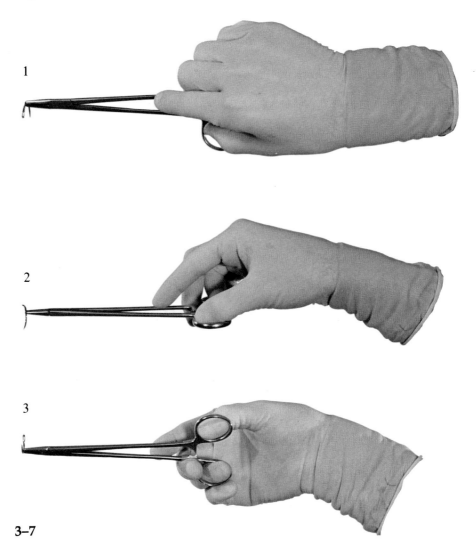

1

2

3

3–7

the needle tip goes away from, then down, then toward the surgeon (Fig. 3–7). This suture is useful in aortic valve replacement on the right coronary cusp near the noncoronary cusp commissure. It can be used during mitral valve replacement on the anterolateral quadrant and occasionally on the anteromedial quadrant.

Backhand Suture

The forehand suture becomes more difficult as the wrist is progressively extended or the elbow positioned extremely tightly in toward the body or markedly out in front of the body. The backhand suture, using pronation of the wrist, can be a smooth and easily accomplished suture in situations where the forehand suture is difficult or not feasible.

The needle holder is held the same way as for a forehand suture. The movement of the needle during a backhand suture is determined by the position of the needle in the jaws, the degree of flexion and abduction of the wrist, the amount of pronation of the wrist, and the amount of rotation and abduction of the arm.

Level Backhand Suture

The needle tip stays in the same plane (Fig. 3–8). The level suture can be

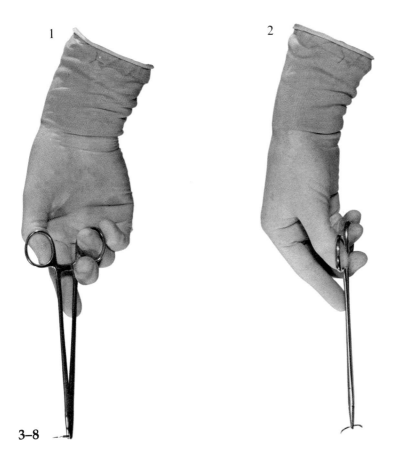

3–8

useful on the side of the right atrium and in closing an aortotomy on the right side of the aorta.

Backhand-Up Suture
The needle tip moves from a lower to a higher plane during the backhand-up suture (Fig. 3–9). This suture is particularly useful during mitral valve replacement—on the posteromedial quadrant, moving the needle through the anulus from the atrial to ventricular side, and on the anterolateral quadrant under the aortic curtain, moving the needle through the anulus from the ventricular to the atrial side. It can also be useful during aortic valve replacement of the left coronary cusp near the right commissure.

Backhand-Down Suture
The needle tip moves from a higher to a lower plane during the backhand-down suture. This can be a relatively simple half-pronation of the wrist, resulting in a down-and-away motion of the needle, and can be used during aortic valve replacement on the noncoronary cusp near the right commissure. The backhand-down suture can also involve full pronation of the wrist, with abduction and rotation of the arm resulting in needle tip movement away from, down, and back toward the surgeon (Fig. 3–10). This suture is particulary useful on the anteromedial portion of the mitral anulus and on the aortic valve right coronary cusp near the left coronary cusp commissure.

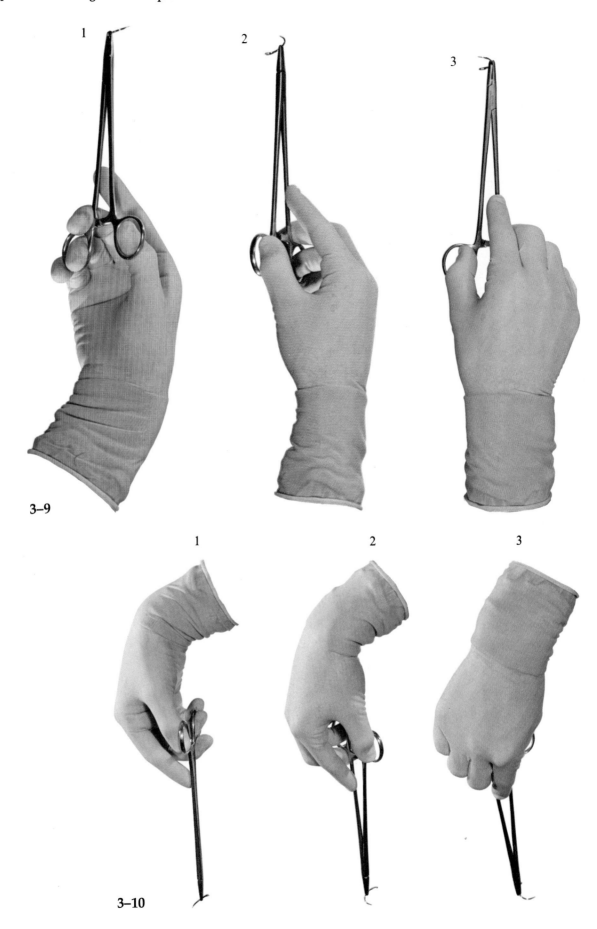

3–9

3–10

Additional Factors Affecting Technical Performance

Factors other than motions of the body also obviously affect surgical performance. Understanding and control of these factors enhances a surgeon's performance.

Mental State

Equanimity is the desired state in surgery as in all other fields of medicine. Situations arise in cardiac surgery that strain even the most controlled surgeon. Management of such situations requires a level of self-discipline that can create a calm operating-room environment, resulting in the best performance of all individuals involved.

Practice

The concert musician and the great athlete, even at the peak of their skills, realize the fundamental importance of practice; surgeons should do no less. Practice is obviously of most importance to a surgeon during the most intense period of learning—the residency. It should be utilized whenever necessary after residency to maintain or attain the highest level of technical skill.

Drugs

Two commonly used drugs—nicotine and caffeine—impair steadiness of the hands. Cardiac surgeons have a multitude of other reasons to avoid nicotine. Consumption of caffeine should be properly controlled or eliminated so it does not interfere with a surgeon's precision and accuracy.

Left-Handedness

The world often appears to be ruled by right-handers. This has little importance if an individual's instruments and that upon which he or she works are symmetric. The left-handed tennis player or baseball batter has little problem; the tennis racket and the baseball bat are the same on both sides, and the tennis court and the baseball diamond are symmetric.

The difficulty of the left-handed surgeon using right-handed instruments is somewhat akin to that of the left-handed golfer using right-handed clubs. In addition to difficulties with instruments, left-handed surgeons usually must learn operations as they are approached by right-handers—an approach that can be difficult without considerable translation.

The left-hander may partially overcome the difficulties with instruments by obtaining some left-handed instruments. The approach to operations can be handled by attempting mirror imaging of the right-handed approach, which may involve doing some operations from the left side of the patient.

A more comprehensive adaptation is to become right-handed as well as left-handed. The left-hander who becomes ambidextrous not only has added versatility but is likely to gain insight into surgical technique that a right-hander may never have.

Illumination

The deep cavities in which cardiac surgery is often performed frequently are difficult to illuminate by the standard overhead fixtures. The new illumination systems utilizing fiberoptic lighting, usually with a head mounting, beautifully overcome this problem and provide excellent illumination for every type of operation.

Magnification

The increasing frequency with which cardiac surgeons operate on very small structures, such as coronary arteries and infant hearts, has emphasized the importance of visual acuity. Magnification is an important component of good visual acuity. Accurate and comfortable magnification can be obtained with custom-fitted prescription loupes. Strength of magnification, focal length, and size of visual field can be selected. The most commonly selected strengths of magnification range between $2\frac{1}{2}\times$ and $3\frac{1}{2}\times$.

Preparation for Cardiopulmonary Bypass

4

Sternotomy, exposure of the heart, and cannulation are usually simple and safe steps beginning an operation. However, in the case of repeat operation, they can be formidable tasks. This chapter describes our routine steps in preparation for cardiopulmonary bypass and includes techniques used for reoperation.

Skin Preparation and Draping

Skin is sterilely prepared with povidone-iodine. Cloth drapes are placed as shown in Figure 4–1. The "bird cage," which is placed over the patient's head, maintains the anesthesiologist's access to the endotracheal tube and also provides a sterile platform for the surgeon's use at the upper part of the surgical field.

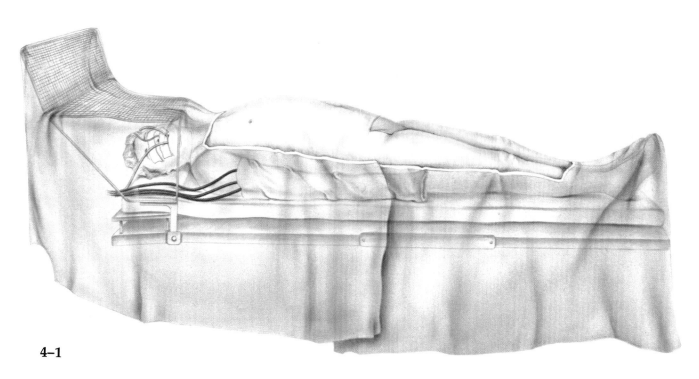

4–1

Median Sternotomy

Almost all of our primary and secondary cardiac procedures are performed through a median sternotomy. This thoracic incision provides the best overall access to the heart chambers, results in the least respiratory impairment, and results in the least discomfort for the patient.

Skin Incision

The skin incision is made in the midline from below the sternal notch to the linea alba below the xiphoid process (Fig. 4–2).

Division of Sternum and Manubrium

The midline of the manubrium and sternum is marked by coagulating the periosteum. The xiphoid process is cut in the midline, and the retrosternal space is bluntly dissected with the finger. A retractor is placed at the upper part of the incision, and the sternum is divided from xiphoid to manubrium with a saw (Fig. 4–3). Sternal periosteum is electrocoagulated and hemostasis of the marrow achieved with bone wax. Orthopedic stockinette wound towels are placed and the sternal retractor inserted and opened.

Heart Exposure

The pericardium is incised in an inverted-T fashion. The longitudinal incision is carried to the base of the innominate artery. The thymus and mediastinal

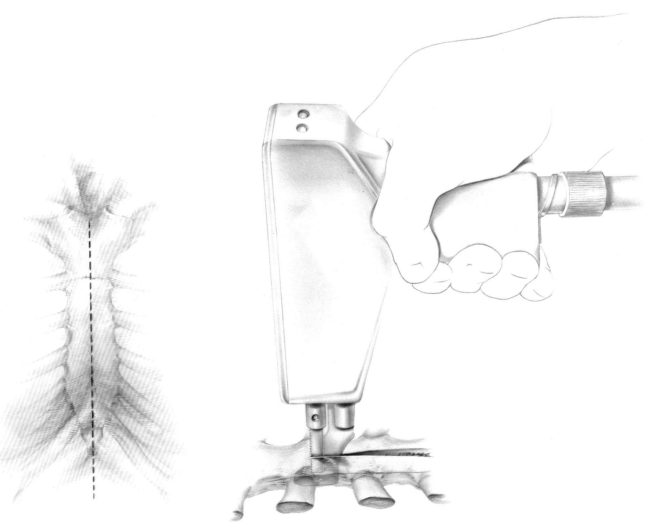

4–2   4–3

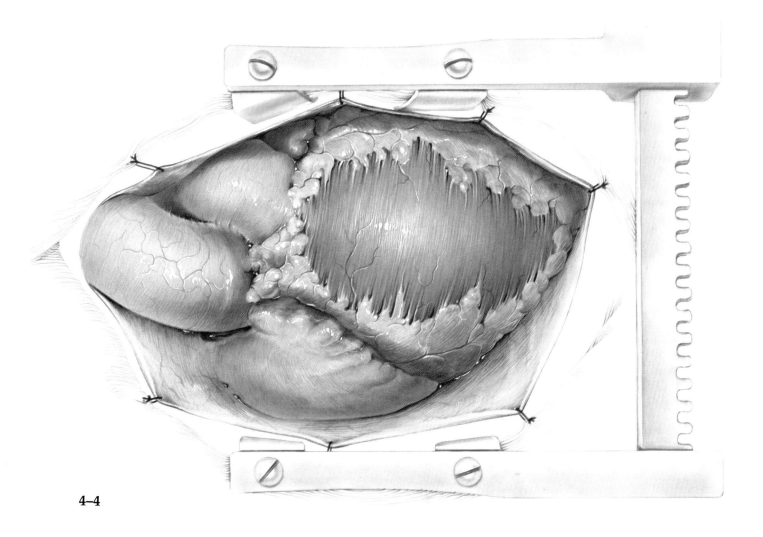

4–4

fat overlying the upper portion of the pericardium are divided, taking care to avoid injury to the innominate vein. The pericardium is sutured to the wound towels, elevating the heart for better exposure (Fig. 4–4).

Repeat Sternotomy

The presence of adhesions from a previous cardiac operation performed through a median sternotomy makes repeat sternotomy a potentially dangerous procedure. Assessment of the chest x-ray can help determine the proximity of the right ventricle, right atrium, or aorta to the posterior table of the manubrium and sternum. In selected patients, a computerized tomographic (CT) scan of the chest can more accurately show the relationship of the cardiac structures to the retrosternal area. Careful progression of the repeat sternotomy with assessment of risk at each step will decrease the incidence of severe problems. If proper assessment is made and groin cannulation instituted whenever indicated, fatal hemorrhage is extremely rare. Preparations for institution of femorofemoral bypass are made in every case of repeat sternotomy, with both groins prepared and draped into the surgical field. In instances where the risk is judged to be high, the femoral vessels are exposed and prepared for cannulation with the administration of heparin prior to sternotomy. In those patients considered to be at highest risk, femoral cannulation is performed prior to sternotomy. The sternal wires or Dacron sutures are divided. These can be left in place so that the sternal saw abuts against

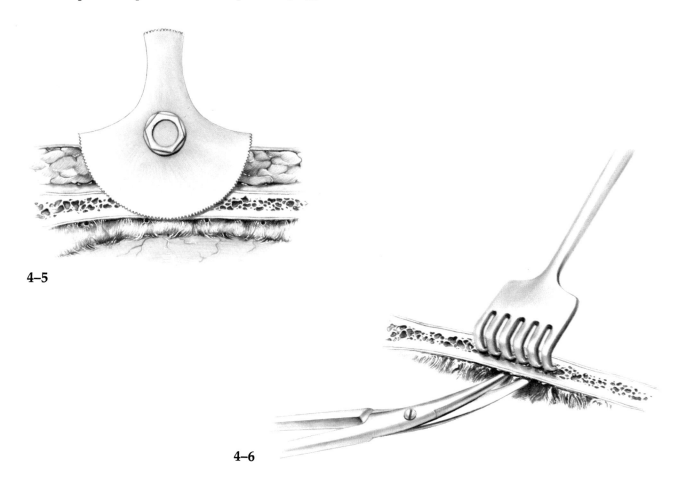

4–5

4–6

them as it cuts through the posterior table. The fascial closure at the lower part of the sternum is reopened and the retrosternal area is assessed. Inability to easily open a plane alerts the surgeon to the presence of marked retrosternal adhesions to the heart or great vessels. In such an instance, cannulation of the femoral artery and vein and institution of partial bypass may be indicated.

The sternum and manubrium are divided with a vibrating saw (Fig. 4-5), taking care to cut just into or slightly beyond the posterior table of the sternum. Once the sternum has been divided, rake retractors can be placed and the retrosternal tissue cut free (Fig. 4-6). The heart must be freed from the sternum before placement of the sternal retractor; wide opening of the sternum before freeing the heart can tear the right ventricle or right atrium.

Dissection of the heart proceeds after retraction of the sternum. A relatively free plane of dissection can usually be found at the diaphragmatic surface of the heart. This plane can serve to identify structures and provide for an orderly and smooth dissection. The dissection usually proceeds around the right atrium, over the right ventricle, and over the aorta and pulmonary artery (Fig. 4-7).

Proper conduct of repeat sternotomy will decrease the incidence of hemorrhage and diminish its severity should it occur. Any serious bleeding encountered during sternotomy or dissection of the heart should be controlled by pressure and bypass instituted as simply as possible. Coronary suckers can return blood from the field to the oxygenator. Bleeding that cannot be controlled with standard bypass may require profound hypothermia and periods of very low flow or circulatory arrest.

Repeat sternotomy can be performed safely using these precautions. Macmanus and colleagues[1] reported 100 consecutive patients undergoing repeat

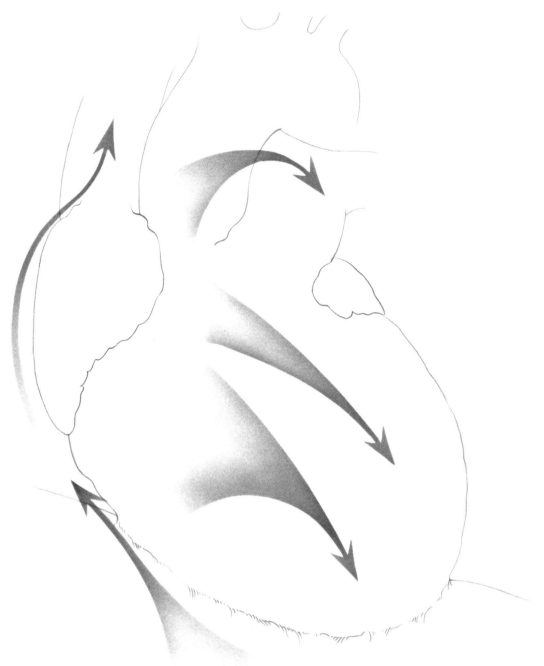

4–7

sternotomy. Although operative hemorrhage occurred in 8 patients, it was controlled in 7; the 1 patient with uncontrolled hemorrhage accounted for the only operative death in the series.

Cannulation

Arterial Cannulation

Ascending Aorta Cannulation
The arterial cannula is usually placed in the ascending aorta. Femoral cannulation is used for some patients undergoing repeat operation and for resection

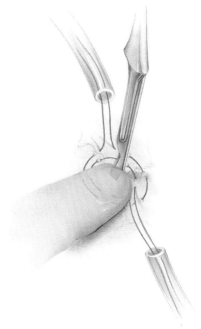

4–8

of the ascending aorta whenever cannulation of the ascending aorta is not feasible. A purse-string suture is placed in the ascending aorta. A stab incision is made (Fig. 4-8). This can be dilated with a graduated dilator (Fig. 4-9). The aortic cannula is inserted (Fig. 4-10). The aortic cannula is then filled with blood, and bubbles are tapped free from the inside. The arterial infusion line and arterial cannula are then connected as the clamp is released from the arterial cannula, excluding all air during connection (Fig. 4-11).

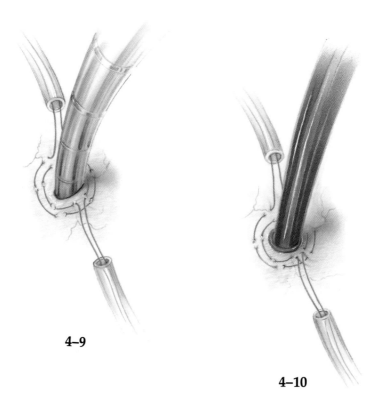

4–9

4–10

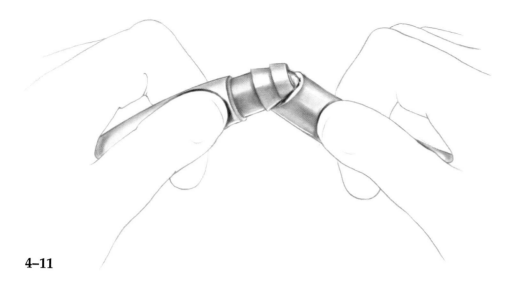

4–11

Femoral Artery Cannulation

The common femoral artery is dissected and encircled with tapes for femoral cannulation. Vascular clamps are placed and a transverse arteriotomy is made (Fig. 4–12). The femoral cannula is then inserted and secured (Fig. 4–13).

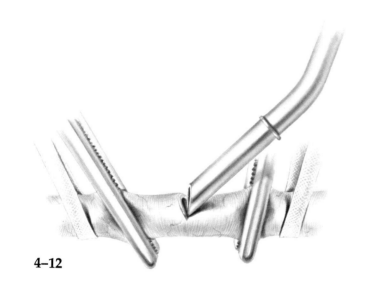

4–12

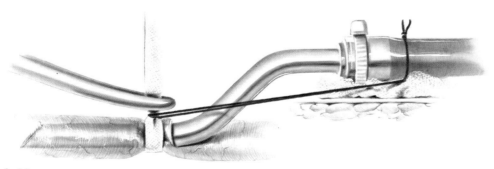

4–13

Venous Cannulation

Right atrial cannulation with a single two-stage cannula is used for patients undergoing coronary artery bypass or aortic valve procedures. Both cavae are cannulated for patients undergoing mitral valve procedures and for repair of most congenital defects.

The right atrial cannula or the inferior vena cava cannula can be placed through the right atrial appendage. The appendage is clamped and a purse-

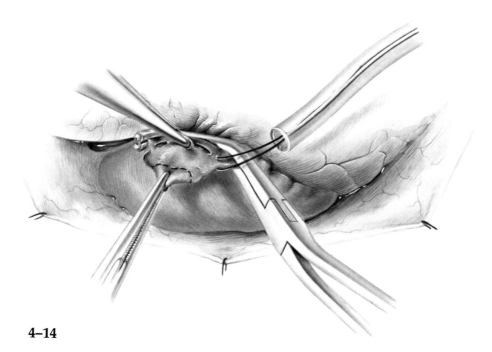

4–14

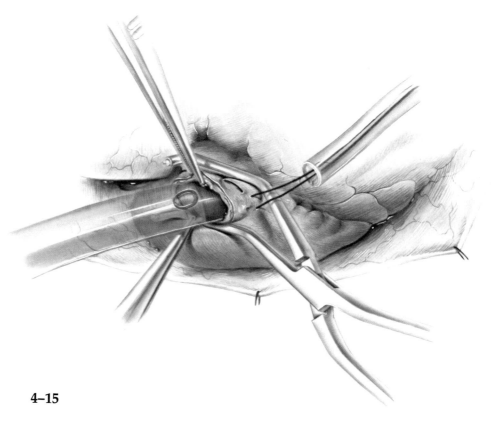

4–15

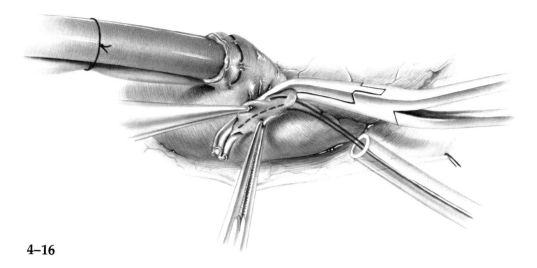

4–16

string suture placed. The tip of the appendage is excised (Fig. 4–14) and the trabeculae are cut. One edge of the appendage wall is held by the assistant and one is held by the surgeon. The assistant then opens the clamp as the surgeon inserts the cannula (Fig. 4–15). The cannula is positioned, the tourniquet is tightened, and the tourniquet and cannula are tied together.

The superior vena cava cannula is inserted through a second purse-string suture placed in a portion of atrial wall excluded within a partial occluding clamp. An incision is made (Fig. 4–16), and the cannula is inserted in the same manner as in the inferior vena cava.

Repeat atrial cannulation, in an atrium that has had the appendage obliterated and that has a thickened, slippery wall, frequently requires the "no-clamp" technique. A purse-string suture is placed and the midportion placed in an Allis clamp. Traction is then put on the Allis clamp and the clamp on the suture ends; this allows an incision to be made within the purse-string suture with control of bleeding. A knife is used to incise the atrium (Fig. 4–17) without placing a partial occluding clamp on the atrium. The cannula is then inserted and the purse-string suture is snugged.

Caval tapes can be placed before or after caval cannulation. The superior vena cava is encircled by incising the pericardial tissue medial to the superior vena cava over the right pulmonary artery. This opens the plane behind the

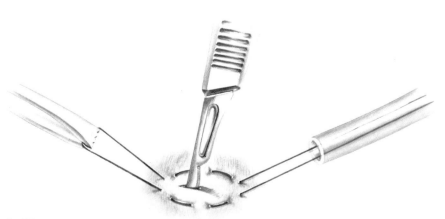

4–17

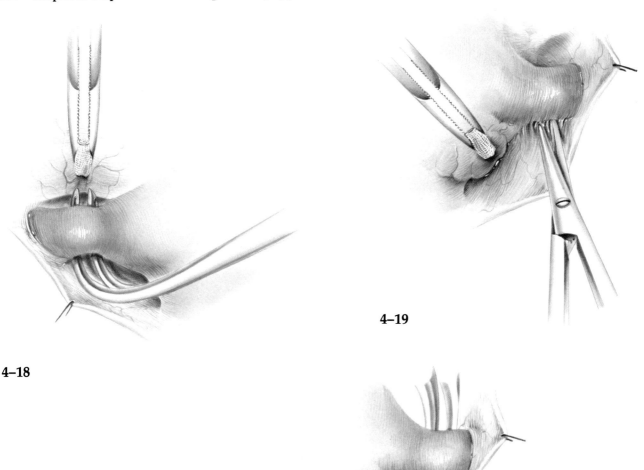

4–19

4–18

4–20

superior vena cava. A right-angle clamp or Semb clamp is then placed behind the cava (Fig. 4–18) and a tape is brought through.

A plane behind the inferior vena cava is opened by incising the pericardial tissue lateral to the cava, below the inferior border of the right inferior pulmonary vein (Fig. 4–19). A clamp is then placed around the back of the inferior vena cava and a tape is brought through (Fig. 4–20).

Reference

1. Macmanus Q, Okies JE, Phillips SJ, Starr A: Surgical considerations in patients undergoing repeat median sternotomy. J Thorac Cardiovasc Surg 69:138,1975.

5

Conduct of Cardiopulmonary Bypass

The first successful use of mechanically supported circulation and respiration during open cardiac surgery, by Gibbon[18] in 1953, opened the door for the explosive growth in heart surgery that has occurred during the past four decades. Equipment and techniques for cardiopulmonary bypass are exceptionally safe, and now there is almost no risk associated with properly performed cardiopulmonary bypass.

This chapter presents our basic techniques of conducting cardiopulmonary bypass and the fundamental rationale underlying the choice of these techniques. More detailed coverage of the physiology, conduct, and equipment of cardiopulmonary bypass is available elsewhere.[2,40,51,52]

Standard Bypass

Standard cardiopulmonary bypass is used for all operations in children and adults and for most infants over 10 kg. Standard bypass usually consists of flows between 1.8 and 2.4 L/min/m^2 body surface area, moderate hypothermia of 26°–30°C, and moderate hemodilution with the hematocrit between 20 and 30.

Priming of Oxygenator and Circuit Preparation

Our standard oxygenator is a hollow-fiber membrane oxygenator. The volume and composition of the priming solution used for adults are shown in Tables 5–1 and 5–2. The alterations in prime with anemia or renal insufficiency are indicated. The volume and composition of the priming solution for infants and children are shown in Table 5–3. The bypass hematocrit can

Table 5–1. Adult Prime (Sacramento)

Normosol-R	1300 ml
Plasmanate	500 ml

1. If the bypass hematocrit will be less than 20, add packed red cells or whole blood and subtract an equal volume from the Normosol. One unit of packed cells requires 1000 U heparin and 250 mg CaCl. These amounts are doubled for whole blood.
2. If renal insufficiency is present, add 12.5 g mannitol.

Table 5–2. Adult Prime (Portland)

Lactated Ringer's solution	500 ml
10% mannitol	500 ml
NaHCO$_3$	15 ml

1. If the bypass hematocrit will be less than 20, add packed red cells or whole blood and subtract an equal volume from the lactated Ringer's solution.

Table 5–3. Pediatric Prime (Sacramento and Portland)

Normosol-R	500 ml (400 ml if less than 12 kg)
Plasmanate	250 ml

1. Mannitol is added to all pediatric primes in the dose of 0.5 g/kg.
2. If bypass hematocrit will be less than 19, replace Normosol with whole blood or packed cells and 20 mEq of NaHCO$_3$. Heparin and CaCl are added in the same doses as for adults.

be estimated by relating the circulating blood volume of the patient to the total priming volume of the bypass circuit.

Our pump tubing is a medical-grade polyvinyl chloride. Standard tubing for adults is $\frac{3}{8}$ inch arterial, $\frac{1}{2}$ inch venous, and $\frac{1}{4}$ inch suction; for children $\frac{3}{8}$ inch arterial and venous; and for infants $\frac{1}{4}$ inch throughout.

The pump console consists of five roller pumps, one for the aortic line, one for the cardioplegia line, one for the vent line, and two for suction lines. The oxygenator is removed from its sterile pack and placed on a mounting arm with the venous inlet approximately 18 inches below the heart, in order to optimize venous drainage. Tubing is connected to the oxygenator and placed in the pumpheads. The arterial pumphead is adjusted to prevent red cell trauma and hemolysis. A nonocclusive setting is produced by pumping the prime solution through the arterial line to a height of 12 inches above the pumphead. The pumphead is then adjusted to permit a fluid fall of 1 inch in 1 minute.

The circuit is flushed with 100% carbon dioxide before the prime solution is added. The prime solution is then circulated through the circuit while air is removed from the arterial filter and lines. Prime solution is circulated for 3 or 4 minutes to ensure oxygenation and warming. The prime solution is warmed to 30°–34°C at this time. Infusion of hypothermic solution at the beginning of bypass may cause cardiac dilatation or fibrillation.

A cardiotomy reservoir is used for collection of the blood returning from the pericardium. This blood is filtered through a microporous filter of 15 microns. Filtration of cardiotomy sucker return is important in removal of particulate matter.[21,32,33]

Heparin and Protamine Management

The initial heparin dose is 300 U/kg. The dose is displayed in clear view of the operating room team. The surgeon injects the heparin directly into the right atrium or the anesthesiologist injects it into a central line prior to cannulation. An activated coagulation time (ACT) is performed 5 minutes after heparin administration.[1,16] A value over 400 seconds is required before bypass is started. ACTs are performed at regular intervals of 20 minutes during bypass, and additional heparin is administered to maintain an ACT over 400 seconds.

Protamine is administered by the anesthesiologist. The dose is 1.0 to 1.5 times the original heparin dose. If additional heparin is administered during bypass, additional protamine is sometimes given. Protamine can cause vasodilatation and hypotension, which can be corrected by volume infusion.[20,25]

Rarely, protamine can cause a severe allergic reaction, which usually occurs in patients who have had previous exposure, such as patients receiving protamine-containing insulin.[57]

Parameters of Satisfactory Bypass

Flow

The patient's height and weight are used to calculate body surface area. Pump flows are usually between 1.5 $L/min/m^2$ (low flow) and 2.5 $L/min/m^2$ (high flow).[46] Flow rates for children are often increased to 3.5 $L/min/m^2$ during normothermia, since children have a higher metabolic rate. Flow is nonpulsatile. High flow is usually maintained at normothermia and during cooling and rewarming. Low flow is satisfactory during hypothermia, since body oxygen consumption at 30°C is half that at 37°C.[22] Low flow also decreases bronchial flow and noncoronary collateral flow and can thereby facilitate operations.

Determination of satisfactory perfusion requires evaluation of arterial blood pressure, arterial blood gases, acid-base status, venous blood pO_2 or oxygen saturation, systemic vascular resistance, and urine output. Monitoring venous blood oxygen tension can also be useful. Mean arterial blood pressure is usually maintained between 50 and 80 mm Hg. Hypertension is usually treated with nitroprusside. Hypotension is usually treated with neosynephrine. Satisfactory perfusion is possible at mean arterial pressures that are lower than normal. Cerebral autoregulation maintains adequate flow to the brain over a wide range of flows and pressures,[9,45] even in patients with cerebrovascular disease.[26] We generally maintain normal or slightly high mean arterial pressures in patients with known cerebrovascular or renal disease.

Arterial Blood Gases and Acid-Base Balance

The management of acid-base balance during cardiopulmonary bypass remains controversial.[5,30,31,37,53] Two methods are used: (1) pH stat, in which the pH is maintained at 7.4 at the patient's core temperature, by adding carbon dioxide to the pump oxygenator, maintaining a temperature-corrected pCO_2 of 35–40 mm Hg[54]; and (2) alpha stat, in which the pH is kept at 7.4 and the pCO_2 is kept at 40 mm Hg when measured at 37°C.[38,39,41,42] With deepening levels of hypothermia, the environment becomes more alkaline.[44]

The pH stat method impairs cerebral autoregulation, resulting in abnormally high cerebral blood flow.[34,36,47] This may be detrimental by causing more microemboli to the brain. However, alpha stat acid-base regulation maintains cerebral autoregulation.[47] For these and other hypothetical reasons, we use the alpha stat method.

Arterial blood gases are measured approximately 15 minutes after initiation of bypass. We use an in-line arterial blood gas monitor. The in-line monitor is checked against the initial arterial blood gases for correlation. Arterial blood gases are then measured every hour or more often if needed. If an in-line arterial monitor is not used, arterial blood gases are determined every 20 minutes and recorded on the perfusion record.

An in-line venous line oximeter is also used.[49] Venous blood saturation is one of the best parameters for determining adequate perfusion. The venous saturation is maintained at 80% or higher during hypothermia and at 65–70% during normothermia.

The membrane oxygenator is ventilated with 100% O_2 and compressed air, run through a blender so the patient's pO_2 and pCO_2 can be controlled independently. We maintain the pO_2 between 100 and 200 mm Hg and the pCO_2 between 35 and 40 mm Hg at all times during bypass. Any substantial drop in the patient's pH is adjusted accordingly with $NaHCO_3$, or by an increase in the perfusion flow, since metabolic acidosis is a sign of deficient perfusion.

Hematocrit

The hematocrit is measured at the same time as arterial blood gases. Blood is added to the circuit if the hematocrit falls below 20. The addition of crystalloid to the circuit should be monitored so that severe hemodilution is avoided. Any marked drop in hematocrit should raise the suspicion of blood loss, such as into a leg incision or into the pleural cavities.

Potassium

Serum potassium is measured at the same time as arterial blood gases and hematocrit. Potassium frequently must be added to the circulating blood to maintain a normal serum potassium level. It is not unusual to add 20 mEq to the prime solution and to give up to 40 mEq or more during a standard adult pump run. Increases in potassium can usually be managed with diuretics.

Urine Output

The urine output is a good reflection of systemic perfusion. Urine output during bypass is usually more than 3 ml/kg/h. If it falls below 1 ml/kg/h, the flow rate or arterial pressure should be raised. If this does not result in improvement in urine output, furosemide or mannitol or renal-dose dopamine (2–3 μg/kg/min) should be administered.

Discontinuation of Bypass

At the completion of the open operative procedure, steps are taken to remove air from the aorta and cardiac chambers. Air is removed from the aorta with a needle as the clamp is removed. This needle may be connected to suction.[7] Air is removed from the left ventricle through the apex by a needle. The heart is defibrillated if necessary, although this is rarely required with present methods of cardioplegia. A current of 10 joules is usually sufficient for defibrillation. High currents should be avoided unless absolutely necessary, since they can injure the myocardium.[50] Systemic temperature is checked to confirm completion of rewarming. Ventilation of the lungs is begun.

Bypass is gradually discontinued by progressive retarding of venous drainage by the perfusionist or surgeon. If the caval cannulas are large, they can be slipped into the atrium to avoid caval obstruction. Bypass flows are decreased as the heart fills and systemic pressure rises. Cardiac function is assessed by measuring the wedge pressure and cardiac output by thermodilution as indicated. Depressed cardiac function may be improved by administration of calcium.[6] More severely depressed myocardial performance should be managed pharmacologically or mechanically, as covered in Chapter 8.

Following discontinuation of bypass, the atrial cannula or caval cannulas are removed. Protamine sulfate is administered. Blood from the oxygenator is infused through the arterial cannula. The arterial cannula is removed toward the end of protamine administration. After the protamine is given, an activated clotting time is determined to confirm adequate heparin reversal. If the ACT has not returned to the preoperative level and bleeding continues, additional protamine can be given.

Blood Conservation

The rapid growth of cardiac surgery, particularly coronary artery surgery, has placed increased demands on blood resources throughout the world. The risk of transmitting disease, particularly acquired immune deficiency syndrome (AIDS), by homologous blood transfusion is recognized and feared by almost all our patients. These factors have increased the importance of blood conservation.

It has been possible for years to perform cardiac surgery without the use of blood.[12] This is required for performance of cardiac surgery in certain religious groups which have rigid proscriptions against the use of blood. The benefits of surgery with the use of little or no bank blood can be extended to a large proportion of the general population through careful surgery and modern techniques of blood conservation. There are a number of methods for achieving blood conservation: (1) withdrawal of autologous blood prebypass with infusion postbypass, (2) infusion of all blood remaining in the oxygenator and lines at the completion of bypass, and (3) autotransfusion of shed mediastinal blood, in both the operating room and recovery room.

Withdrawal of fresh autologous blood prior to cardiopulmonary bypass and reinfusion after bypass has been suggested as a means of decreasing bank blood requirements; the technique has not been shown to decrease the total amount of postoperative bleeding. Although a number of methods for withdrawal and storage have been described,[11,35] the simplest and most effective technique appears to be withdrawal of heparinized blood from the caval cannula and preservation at room temperature.[28] The processing of blood prebypass to obtain platelet-rich plasma which is reinfused postbypass has been proposed as a method of reducing transfusion requirements.[14,19,27] A carefully conducted prospective randomized study by Hofer and colleagues[24] did not show any benefit of autologous platelet-rich plasma infusion.

Infusion of oxygenator contents after termination of cardiopulmonary bypass is an effective method of decreasing bank blood usage.[29] The volume given can be reduced by centrifugation and administration of the packed cells.

Autotransfusion of shed mediastinal blood can be performed in the operating room, recovery room, and intensive care unit utilizing properly filtered collection and infusion systems.[13,43] This blood lacks fibrinogen but contains significantly more platelets and clotting factors than does bank blood.

Cardiopulmonary Bypass in Neonates and Children

The technique of profound hypothermia and circulatory arrest reported in 1967 by the Kyoto University Group[23] and subsequently popularized by Barratt-Boyes[3,4] and others[10,56] was a major advance in the surgical treatment of congenital heart disease. This technique resulted in improved results in infants compared to the use of standard cardiopulmonary bypass and moderate hypothermia. Profound hypothermia and circulatory arrest became widely used during the 1970s.

However, reports began appearing documenting neurological sequelae using this technique, including postoperative seizures and choreoathetosis.[8,15] Additionally, animal experiments documented the neurological injury that could occur with this technique.[55] For these reasons, in the early 1980s, we adopted the use of profound hypothermia (18°C) and very low flow (0.25–0.5 L/min/m^2) for almost all neonates. Swain[48] has shown, in studies on sheep, that flow rates as low as 10 ml/kg/min preserve brain high-energy phosphates and intracellular pH. Fox[17] has shown, in a study on monkeys, that at 20°C and flow rates as low as 0.25 L/min/m^2 the brain remains well perfused and brain oxygen consumption is maintained. We use circulatory arrest only for short periods of less than 15 minutes when absolutely necessary for a completely dry operative field. Most repairs of congenital heart disease are possible without the use of any periods of circulatory arrest.

The prime for infants is shown in Table 5–2. The prime is composed so that the bypass hematocrit is about 24–28. The prime is circulated and oxygenated, and blood gases are checked to ensure correct acid-base balance. In many children weighing over 12 kg, the operation can be done without the use of additional blood. If blood is not used in the prime, 20 mEq of $NaHCO_3$ is added to the prime.

Surface cooling is not used. Nasopharyngeal and rectal temperatures are monitored. Cooling on cardiopulmonary bypass is accomplished with flows of about 2.4 L/min/m², using a hollow-fiber membrane oxygenator. The patient is cooled to a nasopharyngeal temperature of 18–20°C (Sacramento) or 22°C (Portland). Flow is then reduced to as low as 0.25–0.5 L/min/m² (Sacramento) or to 1.0–1.2 L/min/m² (Portland). Experimental studies have shown these low flows perfuse all areas of the brain adequately at profoundly hypothermic temperatures.[48] Rewarming is begun toward the end of the repair and completed after the aortic cross-clamp is released, increasing flows to 2.4 L/min/m². At the completion of the procedure, air removal and weaning from bypass are accomplished as previously described.

References

1. Aren C: Heparin and protamine during cardiac surgery. Perfusion 4:171,1989.
2. Austin JW, Harner DL: The Heart-Lung Machine and Related Technologies of Open Heart Surgery. Phoenix Medical Communication, 1990.
3. Barratt-Boyes BG, Neutze JM, Clarkson PM, Shardey GC, Brandt PWT: Repair of ventricular septal defect in the first two years of life using profound hypothermia-circulatory arrest techniques. Ann Surg 184:376,1976.
4. Barratt-Boyes BG, Simpson M, Neutze JM: Intracardiac surgery in neonates and infants using deep hypothermia with surface cooling and limited cardiopulmonary bypass. Circulation 43(Suppl I):I-25,1971.
5. Bashein G, Townes BD, Nessly ML, Bledsoe SW, Hornbein TF, Davis KB, Goldstein DE, Coppel DB: A randomized study of carbon dioxide management during hypothermic cardiopulmonary bypass. Anesthesiology 72:7,1990.
6. Bixler TJ, Flaherty JT, Gardner TJ, Bulkley BH, Schaff HV, Gott VL: Effects of calcium administration during post-ischemic reperfusion on myocardial contractility, stiffness, edema, and ultrastructure. Circulation 58(Suppl I):I-184,1978.
7. Brenner WI, Wallsh E, Spencer FC: Efficiency of aortic vents in the prevention of air embolism. Surg Forum 21:139,1970.
8. Brunberg J, Doty D, Reilly E: Choreoathetosis in infants following cardiac surgery with deep hypothermia and circulatory arrest. J Pediatrics 84:232,1974.
9. Brusino FG, Reves JG, Smith LR, Prough DS, Stump DA, McIntyre RW: The effect of age on cerebral blood flow during hypothermic cardiopulmonary bypass. J Thorac Cardiovasc Surg 97:541,1989.
10. Castaneda AR, Lamberti J, Sade RM, Williams RG, Nadas AS: Open-heart surgery during the first three months of life. J Thorac Cardiovasc Surg 68:719,1974.
11. Cohn LH, Fosberg AM, Anderson WP, Collins JJ: The effects of phlebotomy, hemodilution, and autologous transfusion on systemic oxygenation and whole blood utilization in open-heart surgery. Chest 68:283,1975.
12. Cooley DA, Crawford ES, Howell JF, Beall AC: Open heart surgery in Jehovah's Witnesses. Am J Cardiol 13:779,1964.
13. Cosgrove DM, Thurer RL, Lytle BW, Gill CG, Peter M, Loop FD: Blood conservation during myocardial revascularization. Ann Thorac Surg 28:184,1979.
14. DelRossi AJ, Cernaianu AC, Vertees RA, et al: Platelet-rich plasma reduces postoperative blood loss after cardiopulmonary bypass. J Thorac Cardiovasc Surg 100:281,1990.
15. Ehyai A, Fenchel G, Bender H Jr: Incidence and prognosis of seizures in infants after cardiac surgery with profound hypothermia and circulatory arrest. JAMA 252:3165,1984.
16. Esposito RA, Culliford AT, Colvin SB, Thomas SJ, Lackner H, Spencer FC: The role of the activated clotting time in heparin administration and neutralization for cardiopulmonary bypass. J Thorac Cardiovasc Surg 85:174,1983.
17. Fox LS, Blackstone EH, Kirklin JW, Bishop SP, Bergdahl LAL, Bradley EL: Relationship of brain blood flow and oxygen consumption to perfusion flow rate during profoundly hypothermic cardiopulmonary bypass. J Thorac Cardiovasc Surg 87:658,1984.

18. Gibbon JH Jr: Application of a mechanical heart and lung apparatus to cardiac surgery. Minn Med 37:171,1954.
19. Giordano GF, Rivers SL, Chung GKT, et al: Autologous platelet-rich plasma in cardiac surgery: effect on intraoperative and postoperative transfusion requirements. Ann Thorac Surg 46:416,1988.
20. Gourin A, Streisand RL, Greinder JK, Stuckey JH: Protamine sulfate administration and the cardiovascular system. J Thorac Cardiovasc Surg 62:193,1971.
21. Heimbecker R, Robert A, McKenzie FN: The extracorporeal pump filter—saint or sinner? Ann Thorac Surg 21:55,1976.
22. Hickey RF, Hoar PR: Whole body oxygen consumption during low-flow hypothermic cardiopulmonary bypass. J Thorac Cardiovasc Surg 86:903,1983.
23. Hikasa Y, Shirotani H, Satomura K, Muraoka R, Abe K, Tsushimi K, Yokota Y, Miki S, Kawai J, Mori A, Okamoto Y, Koie H, Ban T, Kanzaki Y, Yokoto M, Mori C, Kamiya T, Tamura T, Mishii A, Asawa Y: Open heart surgery in infants with an aid of hypothermic anesthesia. Arch Jpn Chir 36:495,1967.
24. Hofer BO, Vocelka CR, Gilles B, Tobe C, Sepulvada R, Verrier ED: Does autologous platelet rich plasma infusion reduce blood loss and product utilization after coronary artery surgery? A prospective, randomized, blinded study. J Thorac Cardiovasc Surg 105:1007,1993.
25. Horrow JC: Protamine: a review of its toxicity. Anesth Analg 64:348,1985.
26. Johnsson P, Algotsson L, Ryding E, Stahl E, Messeter K: Cardiopulmonary perfusion and cerebral blood flow in bilateral carotid artery disease. Ann Thorac Surg 51:579,1991.
27. Jones JW, McCoy TA, Rawitscher RE, Lindsley DA: Effects of intraoperative plasmapheresis on blood loss in cardiac surgery. Ann Thorac Surg 49:585,1990.
28. Kaplan JA, Cannarella C, Jones EL, Kutner MH, Hatcher CR, Dunbar RW: Autologous blood transfusion during cardiac surgery: a re-evaluation of three methods. J Thorac Cardiovasc Surg 74:4,1977.
29. Moran JM, Babka R, Silberman S, Rice PL, Pifarre R, Sullivan HJ, Montoya A: Immediate centrifugation of oxygenator contents after cardiopulmonary bypass: role in maximum blood conservation. J Thorac Cardiovasc Surg 76:510,1978.
30. Murkin JM, Farrar JK, Tweed WA, McKenzie FN, Guiraudon G: Cerebral autoregulation and flow/metabolism coupling during cardiopulmonary bypass: the influence of pCO_2. Anesth Analg 66:825,1987.
31. Murkin JM. Con: blood gases should not be corrected for temperature during hypothermic cardiopulmonary bypass: alpha-stat mode. J Cardiothorac Anesth 2:705,1988.
32. Okies JE, Goodnight SH, Litchford B, Connell RS, Starr A: Effects of infusion of cardiotomy suction blood during extracorporeal circulation for coronary artery bypass surgery. J Thorac Cardiovasc Surg 74:440,1977.
33. Page US, Bigelow JC, Carter CR, Swank RL: Emboli (debris) produced by bubble oxygenators: removal by filtration. Ann Thorac Surg 18:164,1974.
34. Patel RL, Turtle MRJ, Chambers DJ, Venn GE: Effect of differing acid-base regulation on cerebral blood flow autoregulation during cardiopulmonary bypass. Eur J Cardio-thorac Surg 6:302,1992.
35. Pliam MB, McGoon DC, Tarhan S: Failure of transfusion of autologous whole blood to reduce banked blood requirements in open-heart surgical patients. J Thorac Cardiovasc Surg 70:338,1975.
36. Prough DS, Rogers AT, Stump DA, Mills SA, Gravlef GP, Taylor C: Hypercarbia depresses cerebral oxygen consumption during cardiopulmonary bypass. Stroke 21:1162,1990.
37. Prough DS, Stump DA, Troost BT: P_aCO_2 management during cardiopulmonary bypass: intriguing physiologic rationale, convincing clinical data, evolving hypothesis? Anesthesiology 72:3,1990.
38. Rahn H, Reeves RB, Howell BJ: Hydrogen ion regulation, temperature, and evolution. Am Rev Respir Dis 112:165,1975.
39. Rahn H: Body temperature and acid-base regulation (review article). Pneumonologie 151:87,1974.
40. Reed CC, Kurusz M, Lawrence AE Jr: Safety and Techniques in Perfusion. Stafford, Texas, Quali-Med Inc., 1988.
41. Reeves RB: An imidazole alphastat hypothesis for vertebrate acid-base regulation:

tissue carbon dioxide content and body temperature in bullfrogs. Respir Physiol 14:219,1972.

42. Reeves RB: The interaction of body temperature and acid-base balance in ectothermic vertebrates. Annu Rev Physiol 39:559,1977.

43. Schaff HV, Hauer JM, Bell WR, Gardner TJ, Donahoo JS, Gott VL, Brawley RK: Autotransfusion of shed mediastinal blood after cardiac surgery. J Thorac Cardiovasc Surg 75:632,1978.

44. Severinghaus JW: Blood gas calculation. J Appl Physiol 21:1108,1966.

45. Soma Y, Hirotani T, Yozu R, Onoguchi K, Misumi T, Kawada K, Inoue T: A clinical study of cerebral circulation during extracorporeal circulation. J Thorac Cardiovasc Surg 97:187,1989.

46. Starr A: Oxygen consumption during cardiopulmonary bypass. J Thorac Cardiovasc Surg 38:46,1959.

47. Stephan H, Weyland A, Kazmaier S, Henze T, Menck S, Sonntag H: Acid-base management during hypothermic cardiopulmonary bypass does not affect cerebral metabolism but does affect blood flow and neurological outcome. Br J Anaesth 69:51,1992.

48. Swain JA, McDonald TJ, Griffith PK, Balaban RS, Clark RE, Ceckler T: Low-flow hypothermic cardiopulmonary bypass protects the brain. J Thorac Cardiovasc Surg 102:76,1991.

49. Swan H, Sanchez M, Tyndall M, Koch C: Quality of control of perfusion: monitoring venous blood oxygen tension to prevent hypoxic acidosis. J Thorac Cardiovasc Surg 99:868,1990.

50. Tacker WA Jr, Guinn GA, Geddes LA, Bourland JD, Korompai FL, Rubio PA: The electrical dose for direct ventricular defibrillation in man. J Thorac Cardiovasc Surg 75:224,1978.

51. Taylor KM: Cardiopulmonary Bypass. Baltimore, Chapman and Hall Ltd., 1990.

52. Tinker JH: Cardiopulmonary Bypass: Current Concepts and Controversies. Philadelphia, WB Saunders Co, 1989.

53. Tinker JH, Campos JH: Pro: blood gases should be corrected for temperature during cardiopulmonary bypass: pH-stat mode. J Cardiothorac Anesth 2:701,1988.

54. Tinker JH, Roberts SL: Management of cardiopulmonary bypass. *In* Kaplan JA (ed): Cardiac Anesthesia, 2nd ed. Philadelphia, Grune & Stratton, 1987, pp 895–926.

55. Treasure T, Naftel D, Conger K, Garcia JH, Kirklin JW, Blackstone EH: The effect of hypothermic circulatory arrest time on cerebral function, morphology, and biochemistry. J Thorac Cardiovasc Surg 86:761,1983.

56. Venugopal P, Olszowka J, Wagner H, Vlad P, Lambert E, Subramanian S: Early correction of congenital disease with surface-induced deep hypothermia and circulatory arrest. J Thorac Cardiovasc Surg 66:375,1973.

57. Weiler JM, Freiman P, Sharath MD, Metzger WJ, Smith JM, Richerson HB, Ballas ZK, Halverson PC, Shulan DJ, Matsuo S, Wilson RL: Serious adverse reactions to protamine sulfate: are alternatives needed? J Allergy Clin Immunol 75:297,1985.

6

Myocardial Preservation

As cardiac surgery has evolved, experience has markedly improved the technical performance of operations, diminishing technical factors as a major cause of mortality and morbidity. With increasing knowledge of the physiology of the postoperative cardiac patient and sophisticated monitoring technology, postoperative care is now scientific and effective. Refined techniques of cardiopulmonary bypass and improved oxygenators and other devices have markedly diminished the incidence of organ failure in the pulmonary, renal, gastrointestinal, and neurologic systems. Depressed postoperative myocardial performance has been decreased by the many advances in the operative management of the myocardium or the technique of myocardial preservation.

This chapter analyzes the methods of operative myocardial preservation that have been used: (1) coronary perfusion, (2) ischemic arrest, normothermic and modified by topical hypothermia, and (3) cardioplegic arrest. The history, experimental background, physiology, operative techniques, and clinical results of these methods are reviewed. The rationale underlying our choice of methods for myocardial preservation is discussed.

Operative (Mechanical) Coronary Perfusion

History

Mechanical coronary perfusion with oxygenated blood has been an established method of operative myocardial protection since the beginning of intracardiac surgery.[109] The first mitral valve replacement at the University of Oregon in 1960 utilized coronary perfusion in the fibrillating heart.[175] The first aortic valve replacement at the University of Oregon, performed September 20, 1961, utilized continuous coronary perfusion at moderate hypothermia in the beating heart.[176]

One of the remarkable early achievements in valvular surgery was the series of 100 aortic valve replacements without mortality reported by McGoon[133] in 1965. Continuous coronary perfusion with moderate hypothermia of 30°C was used. McGoon's perfusion techniques reveal several principles of safe and adequate perfusion that have been supported by the large amount of experimental and clinical data obtained since the time of his report: (1) Adequate perfusion of the left coronary system was achieved in six instances of early bifurcation of the left main coronary artery by separate cannulation of the left anterior descending and circumflex arteries. (2) Excessive flow and insufficient flow were prevented, with average flows of 190 ml/min in the left coronary system and 120 ml/min in the right coronary system. (3) Excessive perfusion pressure was avoided by measuring the pressure in the coronary line. (4) A beating heart was maintained in 85% of cases.

McGoon's excellent early results and the theoretical attractiveness of coronary perfusion made it the method of choice for myocardial preservation in many centers for many years. However, with increasing use it became apparent that the mere infusion of oxygenated blood into the closed aortic root, or into the coronary ostia by means of coronary cannulas, did not always prevent the occurrence of depressed postoperative myocardial function or death secondary to inadequate cardiac output.[4,145,165]

A large number of experiments have clarified the factors that relate to adequate coronary perfusion. These include the flow rate and the pressure, as well as the electrical and mechanical state of the myocardium. A comparison of the physiology of normal coronary circulation with the different physiologic states that may exist with operative perfusion helps explain the factors that can contribute to the myocardial necrosis sometimes encountered with operative coronary perfusion.

Normal Coronary Flow

Normally functioning myocardium is in a state of aerobic metabolism. Oxygen and energy substrates are continuously supplied by a blood flow that averages about 250 ml/min in the normal adult heart. The blood is oxygenated by a superb membrane oxygenator—the lungs—and has a normal hematocrit. The flow responds to changes in coronary resistance and occurs almost entirely during diastole. Maximum pressure in the coronary system usually does not exceed 150 mm Hg. Normal coronary flow is therefore evenly distributed throughout the myocardium, is not injurious to the coronary arteries or myocardium, is rapidly responsive to changes in blood pressure and myocardial resistance, and contains no blood elements injurious to microcirculation or myocardium.

Factors Affecting Operative Coronary Perfusion

The objective of operative coronary perfusion is maintenance of aerobic metabolism throughout the myocardium without physical injury to the coronary arteries or myocardium. Four factors influence the degree to which this objective is achievable: (1) the perfusion factor, (2) the coronary anatomy factor, (3) the myocardial factor, and (4) the operation factor.

The Perfusion System Factor

The perfusion system usually used for mechanical coronary perfusion consists of a bubble oxygenator, roller pumps, plastic tubing, and coronary cannulas. The bubble oxygenator can cause deleterious alteration of the blood, resulting in denatured protein,[117] microaggregates of platelets and fibrin,[6] and microemboli of air, all of which can impair flow in the microcirculation. The flow is regulated by the roller pumps, is constant (occurring in systole and diastole), and is not responsive to changes in coronary resistance.

Such steady-state flow can be injurious by being excessive.[47] It can be metabolically injurious by being insufficient. The pressure in the system can rise well over pressures normally present in the coronary system, since the flow is not responsive to increases in coronary vascular resistance. This markedly increased pressure can cause mechanical injury to the coronary vasculature and myocardium. The coronary cannulas can injure the coronary arteries. Acute injury resulting in dissection can occur.[64] Late manifestations of coronary cannula injury can present as coronary ostial stenosis, which has been reported in up to 3.5% of cases.[141]

The Coronary Anatomy Factor

Anatomic variations in the coronary arteries and the presence of coronary artery disease affect the adequacy of operative coronary perfusion. Cannulation of the coronary ostia, required for coronary perfusion in the open aortic root, should be occlusive and should not impinge on any branches of the coronary arteries. A short left main coronary artery, which occurs in 25% of patients with isolated aortic stenosis,[144] can lead to preferential flow into the circumflex artery, with resulting ischemia in that region of the myocardium supplied by the left anterior descending artery. Murphy[144] found that perioperative myocardial infarction following coronary perfusion occurred in 27% of patients with a short left main coronary artery, compared with 7% in patients with a normal-sized left main coronary artery.

The right coronary artery also may present difficulties in cannulation. The location and size of the right coronary orifice can be such that continuous cannulation is extremely difficult. Inability to maintain continuous perfusion in the right coronary artery can cause deleterious changes in the right ventricle and posterior ventricular septum. The presence of coronary artery disease increases the incidence of ischemic injury if techniques of providing flow distal to coronary stenoses are not used.[127] Macmanus and colleagues[127] reported a low perioperative infarction rate following adoption of a method of perfusion through vein grafts as well as through the coronary ostia during combined aortic valve replacement and coronary bypass.

The Myocardial Factor

Coronary flow is affected by myocardial hypertrophy and ventricular fibrillation. Ventricular hypertrophy causes increased coronary resistance, which can result in subendocardial underperfusion at pressures that do not cause subepicardial or midmyocardial underperfusion.[2,29,91] The increased coronary vascular resistance that occurs with ventricular hypertrophy has been clinically studied by Sapsford[165] and Isom.[98] Ventricular fibrillation causes maldistribution of coronary flow away from the subendocardial muscle by the strength of fibrillation.[95] Ventricular fibrillation also results in a higher oxygen requirement by the myocardium than that existing in the nonworking beating heart. Ventricular fibrillation can cause marked underperfusion of the subendocardium in the hypertrophied heart.[95]

The Operation Factor

Although continuous coronary perfusion has been shown to be superior to intermittent perfusion,[98,119] continuous perfusion may be unwise or impossible because of more important factors involved in the conduct of the operation. A study by Isom and colleagues[98] of coronary perfusion during aortic valve replacement showed that perfusion was intermittently suspended in half the patients for more than 50% of the total time that the aortic root was open.

Technical conditions often require temporary suspension of coronary perfusion as well as fibrillation of the myocardium. Excision and debridement of a severely calcified aortic valve in a beating heart is often imprecise, dangerous, and prone to loss of calcium fragments into the left ventricular cavity, with the danger of subsequent systemic embolism. Accurate, atraumatic placement of sutures in portions of the aortic anulus may be impossible in the beating heart. Precise seating of the valve may be prevented by the presence of the coronary cannulas and the tonic condition of the aortic anulus.

Mitral valve replacement is hampered at several critical steps by a perfused, beating heart. Accurate, safe excision of the valve becomes more difficult. Safe, atraumatic placement of sutures in the beating heart is less likely. Seating of the valve and tying of the sutures are more difficult.

Most intraventricular surgery for the repair of congenital defects is difficult or impossible in the beating heart. Exposure is difficult. Placing sutures in the delicate tissue is hazardous when the heart is beating, since the sutures may tear through the moving muscle and endocardium.

The conditions present during human cardiac operations often differ considerably from the ideal conditions present in most animal experiments. Although such experiments show normal ventricular function after coronary perfusion for as long as 4 hours,[67] the studies are usually in the normal canine heart, through the closed aortic root, in a continuously perfused and beating heart, which is not undergoing any manipulations. The differences between the experimental and the clinical situations must be considered as the clinical results achieved with mechanical coronary perfusion are reviewed.

Clinical Results

Sapsford and colleagues[165] studied 31 patients who had continuous coronary perfusion with mild hypothermia during isolated aortic valve replacement. These patients were part of a group randomized in order to compare continuous coronary perfusion with ischemic arrest modified by topical hypothermia. There was one death in the coronary perfusion group, and the incidence of myocardial infarction was 16%. Enzymatic indicators of myocardial necrosis were positive in 69% of patients undergoing continuous coronary perfusion. Karp,[108] in a separate report, described 22 patients who underwent continuous coronary perfusion. They found a perioperative infarction rate of 9% and a requirement for inotropic support in 18%. Mulder[142] described 40 patients with continuous coronary perfusion at 32°C with 2 deaths (neither of which was cardiac related) and a postoperative requirement for inotropic support in 3%. Mulder did not give the incidence of myocardial infarction.

Appelbaum and colleagues[4] reported on 35 patients undergoing mitral valve replacement with coronary perfusion on an intermittent basis. Fifteen-minute periods of ischemia were interrupted by 3-minute periods of coronary perfusion with a beating heart. They noted 6% mortality, all of which was secondary to inadequate postoperative cardiac performance. Of all patients, 50% required inotropic support in the postoperative period.

Conclusions

Mechanical coronary perfusion demands careful monitoring to insure adequate coronary flow and pressure; the myocardium should be maintained in a continuously beating, continuously perfused state. In spite of adherence to these principles, myocardial necrosis may occur. We prefer cold cardioplegic arrest to mechanical coronary perfusion and do not use coronary perfusion.

Normothermic Ischemic Arrest

Technical limitations and poor operating conditions of coronary perfusion made ischemic arrest attractive to many surgeons. Ischemic arrest became the basis of a number of methods of operative myocardial management. Although normothermic or unmodified ischemia has been used, most current methods modify the conditions of the ischemic myocardium.

History

During the 1960s, Cooley and his associates were the main proponents of normothermic or unmodified ischemic arrest, but they have since adopted cold cardioplegic arrest. Examination of their results with normothermic ischemic arrest and their reasons for abandoning it demonstrates the limitations of that method and adds to our basic understanding of the biology of myocardial ischemia.

Bloodwell[18] reported in 1969 on a large series of patients operated on by Cooley and colleagues using normothermic ischemic arrest: 636 patients undergoing ischemic arrest for valve replacement in 1966 and 1967 were compared with 353 undergoing valve replacement using coronary perfusion in 1965. In terms of operative mortality (7.6% for isolated aortic valve replacement and 11.4% for isolated mitral valve replacement), the results with ischemic arrest were similar or superior to those achieved with coronary perfusion.

The skill and speed of their surgery was demonstrated by the short average ischemic time of 38 minutes. Few surgeons are able to complete most valve replacements in less than 40 minutes. A temporal limitation of normothermic ischemia is suggested by Cooley's results in patients undergoing double valve replacement. This group, with longer periods of ischemia, had an operative mortality of 43%, which suggests that the longer ischemic periods caused irreversible changes in the myocardium in a substantial portion of the patients.

Another limitation of normothermic ischemic arrest was described by Cooley[45] in 1972 when he reported the occurrence of ischemic contracture of the heart and named it "stone heart." This invariably fatal condition, characterized by a spastic contracture of the myocardium, occurred in patients with advanced left ventricular hypertrophy. Postmortem histologic examination revealed myocardial necrosis with hypercontracted cardiac muscle fibers.[12] The occurrence of some preoperative myocardial necrosis was indicated by the extensive interstitial myocardial fibrosis present in most hearts. Normothermic ischemic arrest appeared to be a poor method of operative management for the hypertrophied heart.

In 1972 Cooley and colleagues[194] adopted total body hypothermia to 30°C, with some application of topical hypothermia as well, for all patients undergoing aortic valve replacement. No instance of stone heart occurred with this method. They subsequently adopted cold cardioplegic arrest.

Experimental Background

A broad experimental background contributes to our knowledge of normothermic ischemia. Experiments have been conducted by surgeons interested in ischemia as it relates to the conduct and success of cardiac surgery, cardiologists studying acute myocardial infarction, and cellular pathologists seeking to define the subcellular pathophysiology of ischemia and the mechanisms of cell death. These experiments have increased our knowledge of the metabolic and structural changes occurring during ischemia and of the relation of such changes to the development of irreversibility or lethal cell injury.

Metabolic Changes of Ischemia

Cessation of myocardial blood flow initiates a series of metabolic events within the cell. The cellular pO_2 drops to less than 5 mm Hg within seconds, and the oxidative phosphorylation occurring in the mitochondria stops.[113] Anaerobic glycolysis is initiated in the cytosol through activation of the enzyme phosphorylase, which breaks down glycogen. The glucose-6-phosphate thus produced is converted through intermediary steps to pyruvate, which is metabolized to lactate, and adenosine triphosphate (ATP) is produced. ATP production by anaerobic metabolism is usually insufficient to supply cellular energy requirements, so existing cellular energy stores are utilized. This breakdown of high-energy phosphates results in a fall in creatine phosphate followed by a fall in ATP.

Enzymes essential to the glycolytic pathway are adversely affected by the products of anaerobic metabolism and the depletion of high-energy phosphates. Increasing cellular lactate decreases the cellular pH. This increasing acidosis adversely affects enzymes essential to the glycolytic pathway. The fall in the level of cellular high-energy phosphates also limits glycolysis, since high-energy phosphates are necessary for early steps in the glycolytic pathway. As the cellular acidosis progresses and the depletion of high-energy phosphates continues, the point of cellular irreversibility or cell death approaches.

The metabolic state of the ischemic myocardial cell that can resume normal function after blood flow is restored is not sharply different from that of the cell that is irreversibly injured and will progress to necrosis in spite of restoration of blood flow. The metabolic correlates of a clearly reversible state are known, however, as are the correlates of a clearly irreversible state. These metabolic correlates include intracellular pH and the level of high-energy phosphates. Indirect methods of measuring cellular acidosis by measuring tissue pCO_2 have been utilized by Gott and associates.[74] They have shown that a high tissue pCO_2 correlates with absence of functional recovery of the myocardium.

Apstein and co-workers[5] studied the effect of global ischemia of different degrees of severity in the isolated working rat heart. The amount of calculated tissue lactate accumulation correlated with the occurrence of irreversible ischemic injury: the severely ischemic groups that failed to recover with reperfusion accumulated three to five times as much lactate as the moderately ischemic groups that recovered completely. Cellular acidosis, reflected by high tissue pCO_2 and lactate level, is therefore associated with development of the irreversible state.

Depletion of cellular high-energy phosphates also correlates well with irreversibility. Kubler[113] has shown that an irreversible state occurs when the myocardial ATP content falls to about 50% of normal. Hearse,[86] studying ischemic contracture of the myocardium, found that contracture began when ATP levels reached about 55%–60% of the preischemic levels and was complete when the ATP concentration reached about 20% of preischemic levels. Glycogen was about 25% of preischemic levels when contracture began. Preischemic depletion of glycogen or inhibition of anaerobic ATP production accelerated the onset of contracture. Depletion of ATP below 50% of its normal level is therefore associated with irreversibility or lethal cell injury.

The specific metabolic event or events that herald the onset of cellular irreversibility are not known. It is known, however, that as the irreversible state is reached, or shortly after it is reached, several things happen. Glycolysis is inhibited or blocked through substrate depletion, accumulation of intermediary metabolites, acidosis, and cofactor loss. Increasing cellular acidity not only affects glycolysis, but causes protein denaturation, with resultant structural, enzymatic, and nuclear changes. There is progressive loss of cell volume regulation with ionic shifts, increase in membrane permeability, and increase in cellular water content. Mitochondrial failure occurs. The loss of ability to synthesize ATP by mitochondria in ischemic cells, even in a favorable medium, correlates with the loss of cell viability.[183]

Subcellular Morphologic Changes of Ischemia
Jennings and co-workers[101,102] have carefully studied the subcellular morphologic changes that occur during myocardial ischemia. They studied the posterior papillary muscle in dogs that had temporary occlusion of the circumflex coronary artery for variable time periods. Figure 6–1 shows normal subcellular morphology. Ultrastructural changes of acute ischemia were correlated with the later development of necrosis in groups of dogs with similar ischemic times. Changes in organelles at a stage of reversibility include slight swelling of the mitochondria, dilated sarcoplasmic reticulum, expanded cell sap, and clumped chromatin in the nucleus (Fig. 6–2). No irreversible changes were seen following periods of ischemia up to 18 minutes. The structure of irreversibly injured cells following 60 minutes of ischemia showed absence of glycogen, margination of nuclear chromatin, marked mitochondrial swelling

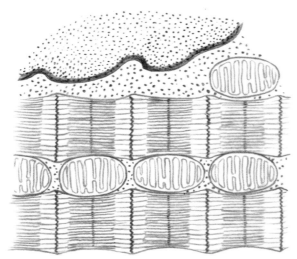

Figure 6–1 Normal subcellular morphology: the mitochondria have tightly packed cristae; chromatin in evenly distributed within the nucleus; glycogen granules are plentiful.

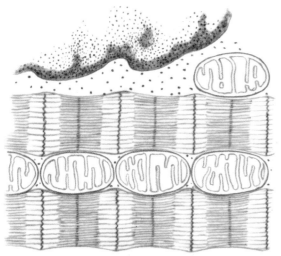

Figure 6–2 Reversible stage of ischemia: there is slight swelling of the mitochondria; there is clumping of chromatin in the nucleus; glycogen granules are becoming depleted.

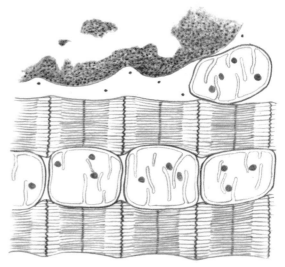

Figure 6–3 Irreversible stage of ischemia: mitochondria show marked swelling with disruption and fragmentation of cristae and development of amorphous densities in the matrix; there is margination of chromatin; glycogen granules are depleted.

with disruption and fragmentation of cristae, decrease in mitochondrial matrix density, and development of amorphous densities in the mitochondrial matrix (Fig. 6–3). Other investigators have described similar findings regarding the ultrastructural changes of irreversibility or lethal cell injury.[33,177,183]

Temporal Limits of Normothermic Ischemic Arrest

"Tolerance" of the myocardium to ischemia is therefore related to maintenance of a reversible state in most or all myocardial cells during the period of ischemia. Duration of the period of reversibility in normothermic ischemia varies from cell to cell. There is a time zone during which the irreversible state is reached by all cells; an irreversible state is reached sooner by subendocardial cells than by subepicardial cells,[30,101] and is reached sooner by cells in hypertrophied hearts than by those in normal hearts.[100,118] The proper use of ischemia during cardiac operations requires its termination before any cells have become irreversibly injured.

The period of reversibility during normothermic ischemia appears to vary somewhat from species to species. The rat heart begins to develop ischemic contracture shortly after 10 minutes, with completion of contracture by 20 minutes, and shows no recovery after 30 minutes of ischemia.[86] In 1962 Gott described myocardial rigor mortis or "stone heart" following normothermic arrest in the dog.[75] Rigor began at 50 minutes and ended at around 80 minutes. Most studies have shown recovery of function in the dog heart following 30 minutes of ischemia[30,191] with consistent depression at 45 minutes and severe depression or no recovery at 60 minutes.[126,140]

The human heart may have a longer period of reversibility during normothermic ischemia than does the dog heart. Recovery of function following more than 60 minutes of normothermic arrest is known to occur in the human.[18] However, caution is necessary in advancing the proposition that the human heart is less susceptible to ischemic injury, because 5 of 13 patients developing "stone heart" reported by Cooley and associates[45] had ischemic arrest times of less than 40 minutes, and one ischemic time was as brief as 22 minutes.

The absolutely safe duration of normothermic ischemic arrest is therefore brief, probably less than 20 minutes. For this reason, normothermic ischemic arrest is not a planned component of the procedure in any of our operations.

Ischemia Modified by Topical Hypothermia

History

Shumway and Lower[173] described their experimental studies of topical hypothermia in 1959. Although no specific measurements of left ventricular function were made, 4 of 5 dogs with 60 minutes of ischemia survived, as did some dogs with ischemia for 90 minutes. This became the basis of clinical use of profound local hypothermia by Shumway's group. Two large clinical series have been reported by his group, in 1964 by Hurley[97] and in 1973 by Griepp.[78] Reports by other surgeons[42,96,151] have confirmed the clinical effectiveness of this method of myocardial preservation. A prospective randomized study of isolated aortic valve replacement[165] and a retrospective study of isolated mitral valve replacement[4] showed no difference in postoperative cardiac function when coronary perfusion and topical hypothermia were compared.

Physiology and Experimental Background

Hypothermia causes a general lowering of metabolic rate and a subsequent decrease in myocardial energy demand. The lowering of energy consumption results in a longer period of ischemia before irreversible or lethal changes occur in the myocardial cell. Fuhrman and co-workers[71] studied the metabolism of rat heart slices subjected to different levels of hypothermia. They found that oxygen consumption bore a linear log relationship to temperature; in other words, for every 10°C decrease in temperature, oxygen consumption was halved. Buckberg and colleagues[27] have shown a similar decrease in oxygen consumption with decreasing temperature.

Most studies of topical hypothermia in the dog have shown some depression of myocardial contractility following 60 minutes of ischemia.[10,43,148] Canine studies of late ventricular function and morphology are conflicting. Schraut[167] showed no long-term morphologic injury or functional impairment following 60 minutes of ischemic arrest with topical hypothermia. Brody[22] showed some functional depression and some subendocardial fibrosis following a similar period of ischemia with topical hypothermia.

Operative Techniques

Most methods of profound topical hypothermia combine systemic hypothermia with epicardial topical hypothermia, by means of either continuous pericardial infusion of chilled saline[78] or pericardial packing with ice slush.[10] Endocardial hypothermia by bathing the ventricular cavity has also been described.[55]

The efficiency of myocardial cooling varies with the technique. Topical cooling is by convection. The effectiveness and rate are therefore determined by the temperature of the solution, the heart surface area exposed to the cold solution, the thickness of the myocardium, and factors inducing rewarming, such as noncoronary collateral myocardial blood flow and bronchial return to the left ventricle. Stiles and co-workers[178] have reported minimal effect of epicardial topical hypothermia on myocardial septal temperatures. However, myocardial temperatures as low as 10°–15°C have been reported within 5–15 minutes following copious epicardial and endocardial irrigation.[55,193] It is reasonable to assume that regardless of the technique used, topical hypothermia usually results in variable rates of myocardial cooling and regional variations in temperature of the myocardium.

Clinical Results

Series of aortic valve replacements using topical hypothermia have been performed without mortality.[108,165] However, the low or absent operative mortality that can be achieved using various techniques of myocardial preservation makes operative mortality an unsatisfactory variable for comparing them. More sensitive indicators of myocardial damage, such as early and late postoperative hemodynamics, electrocardiographic changes, and enzymatic changes, have been analyzed. In a careful study comparing continuous coronary perfusion and topical hypothermia in two randomized groups of patients undergoing isolated aortic valve replacement, Sapsford and co-workers[165] found no difference between the groups in terms of postoperative hemodynamics, myocardial metabolism, incidence of electrocardiographic myocardial infarction (13%), or enzymatic changes indicative of myocardial necrosis (69%). Aortic cross-clamp times were up to 74 minutes in the cold ischemic group. Cardiopulmonary bypass time was significantly shorter in the cold ischemic arrest group. They concluded that "cold ischemic arrest seems preferable for isolated aortic valve replacement when the cross-clamping time can be kept less than 68 minutes and the myocardial temperature between 22° and 24°C."

Neither the aortic cross-clamp time within which all myocardial cells remain in reversible state nor the safe ischemic time achievable with topical hypothermia is known. There are reports of ischemic times up to 2 hours without evidence of depressed postoperative myocardial function,[42,78,151,160] and Griepp[78] has stated that his group found no correlation between longer aortic cross-clamp times and operative mortality. However, Rossiter[160] found that myocardial infarction defined by new Q waves or operative myocardial death, following combined aortic valve replacement and coronary bypass, occurred in all patients (5/5) with aortic cross-clamp times greater than 70 minutes.

Conclusions

Ischemia modified by profound topical hypothermia that does not exceed 70 minutes is probably similar to coronary perfusion in the extent to which it preserves myocardial function. Whereas myocardial injury following coronary perfusion is usually related to inadequate perfusion, myocardial injury following topical hypothermia is probably related to inadequate hypothermia. The rate of onset, depth, and thoroughness of myocardial hypothermia achieved by topical hypothermia are all variable. This can result in hypothermia that is insufficient to maintain all myocardial cells in a condition of reversibility for the duration of the ischemic times required for all cardiac procedures. For these reasons, we employ systemic and topical hypothermia alone only for short periods of ischemia, such as the performance of a single distal coronary anastomosis when the intermittent clamping technique is used for coronary artery bypass. Otherwise, topical hypothermia is used only as necessary as an adjunct to cold cardioplegic arrest.

Cold Cardioplegic Arrest

History

The effect of electrolytes on the electrical activity of the heart was described by Ringer[153] in 1883. Hooker,[94] in 1929 described cardiac arrest produced by hyperkalemia. In 1955 Melrose[135] described potassium arrest using concentrations of potassium citrate varying from 9 to 245 mEq/L. His experiments were performed in intact adult dogs, as well as in isolated hearts of rabbits, a guinea pig, a kitten, and a puppy. Results in terms of objective measurement of ventricular function were not given, nor were the specific effects of the various concentrations reported. Neither the temperature of the injectate nor the temperature of the myocardium during the period of ischemia was reported. Melrose showed, however, that the heart could be arrested with hyperkalemic solutions and recover some function following periods of ischemia of 15 to 55 minutes. Although Melrose acknowledged that a great deal of work remained to be done, he believed his method offered an opportunity for useful surgery on the motionless heart.

Following Melrose's report of his experimental work, the technique of potassium cardioplegia was soon adopted for clinical use. Effler[53] reported in 1957 the clinical use of potassium citrate arrest. The potassium citrate was dissolved in heparinized blood and injected into the root of the aorta after the aorta was cross-clamped. The concentration of potassium was 245 mEq/L. The temperature of the injectate was not given. Effler's series included 51 patients, and operative mortality was 41%.

In 1959 Sealy[168] reported cardioplegia using a solution containing potassium, magnesium, and neostigmine. His series included 31 patients, with an operative mortality of 20%. Clinical use of potassium cardioplegia in the United States ended for the most part in 1960 with the report of McFarland[131] describing myocardial necrosis following the use of potassium citrate in heparinized blood with a potassium concentration of 245 mEq/L. McFarland observed a distinctive type of necrosis, with absence of both hemorrhage and congestion, usually occurring in the central portion of the myocardium.

Investigation of cardioplegic solutions was continued in Germany by Bretschneider,[21] who studied a low-sodium, mildly hyperkalemic (7 mEq/L), calcium-free, procaine solution, and by Kirsch,[112] who studied a hyperosmolar, high-magnesium (159 mEq/L), procaine solution, without sodium, potassium, or calcium. These solutions came into clinical use in Europe during the 1960s.

The report by Gay and Ebert[72] in 1973, describing their studies of potassium cardioplegia using the isolated dog heart, stimulated a resurgence of interest in cardioplegia by American surgeons. Gay and Ebert found that potassium crystalloid cardioplegia, at a potassium concentration of 24 mEq/L, increased recovery after 60 minutes of ischemia. Subsequent studies by Tyers and Todd[185,186] supported the effectiveness of moderately hyperkalemic potassium cardioplegia and demonstrated the deleterious effects of the markedly hyper-

Table 6-1. Cardioplegic Solutions: Clinical Use

	BRETSCHNEIDER #3 (21)	ROE (155)	SUTTER MEMORIAL, SACRAMENTO	ST VINCENT, PORTLAND
Basic Solution	–	D5W	Blood + Normosol R®	Blood + Ringer's solution
Hct	0	0	10–15	18–23
K+ (mEq/liter)	7	20	15	20
Na+ (mEq/liter)	12	27	147	145
Mg++ (mEq/liter)	4	6	2.5	2
HCO_3 (mEq/liter)	–	–	18	25
Glucose (mg%)	–	5	0.5	0.2
Procaine (mg%)	0.2	–	–	–
Lidocaine (mg%)	–	–	0.01	–
Other	Mannitol (43.5 g/liter)	THAM (2 mEq/liter)	Acetate (27 mEq/liter) Gluconate (23 mEq/liter)	–
pH	5.5–7.0	7.6	7.4	7.4

kalemic hyperosmolar Melrose solution. Subsequent experimental studies have confirmed the effectiveness of cold potassium arrest in maintaining normal cellular metabolism, structure, and function after at least 2 hours of ischemia.[57,69,116] Clinical studies in the 1970s reported excellent clinical results.[44,144,152] During the 1980s and early 1990s, hundreds of studies of cardioplegia were published[132] as well as several books on the subject.[34,56,84,154] Because of its superb operating conditions and its effectiveness in preserving myocardial function, cold cardioplegic arrest has become the most commonly used method of operative myocardial preservation.

Components

Cardioplegic solutions vary in terms of temperature, arresting agent, pH, osmolality, presence of red blood cells, and other factors. This creates an almost infinite variety of possible combinations and has led to the differing compositions of solutions used throughout the world. Table 6–1 shows the components of a number of cardioplegic solutions. The separate biologic effects of these components have been intensely investigated, and the resulting studies form the basis for rational choice of solution composition and temperature. The following review outlines our present state of knowledge of the biologic effects of the different components.

Hypothermia

Cold cardioplegic solutions are markedly hypothermic, usually around 4°C. A number of experiments have demonstrated that perfusion hypothermia is the most important factor causing lowering of cellular energy requirements during ischemia, and thus normal recovery after ischemia.[13,36,54,57,83,111]

Perfusion hypothermia has been studied using cold blood[15,52,74,77] or crystalloid solutions[188] without any arresting agents. Satisfactory recovery was found in the dog heart after 60 minutes of ischemia. Studies have analyzed the effect of arrest alone, perfusion hypothermia alone, and the two in combination.

Arrest with potassium[83] or procaine[166] at normothermia is only slightly better than unmodified normothermic ischemic arrest. Perfusion hypothermia without an arresting agent is far more effective than normothermic potassium or procaine arrest.[83,88,166] Perfusion hypothermia without an arresting agent causes electromechanical arrest when the myocardial temperature is lowered to below 16°C.[188] The effects of an arresting agent and hypothermia are additive and result in better postischemic ventricular function than when either is used alone.[83,88,166] Consumption of cellular energy stores decreases with progressive levels of myocardial hypothermia.[187] The lower the myocardial temperature of the arrested heart, the better the postischemic myocardial performance.[83,111]

The most common solution temperature is around 4°C. Tyers[187] has presented studies in isolated rat hearts which suggest that 10°–15°C is better than 4°C. Our studies in isolated rat hearts[83] and the studies of others[171,172] do not support the theory of hypothermic injury at 4°C. Several studies[13,57,67,111] in animal hearts have substantiated the excellent results achieved with a solution at 4°C. Excellent clinical results using a 4°–5°C solution have been reported.[1,152] Since the main effect of cold cardioplegia is obtained by profound myocardial hypothermia, we obtain it in the most efficient manner by using a solution of 4°C.

Arresting Agent

Most cardioplegic solutions contain potassium as the arresting agent. Potassium arrests the heart by depolarization of the membrane. Magnesium is also used as an arresting agent.[84]

The membrane-stabilizing agents procaine and xylocaine are also used as arresting agents.[17] They arrest the heart by preventing the propagation of an electrical stimulus. Lidocaine can be additive to the effect of potassium.[114] Lidocaine used clinically significantly reduces the incidence of ventricular fibrillation following release of the cross-clamp.[63] We have used lidocaine in our solution at Sutter/Sacramento for over 10 years and have had to defibrillate following release of the cross-clamp in less than 5% of patients.

Animal studies of the calcium-channel blockers diltiazem,[8,174,190] nifedipine,[37,40,104,128,129] and verapamil have been performed. Most of these studies have shown an additive effect to that of potassium. However, clinical use of diltiazem has been associated with negative inotropic effects and prolonged periods of electromechanical arrest.[11,38] These effects have limited the clinical adoption of calcium-channel blockers as additives to cardioplegic solutions.

pH

The marked deleterious effect on anaerobic metabolism caused by cellular acidosis[113] supports the use of a solution with a pH of 7.4 or above. This has been substantiated by animal experiments that have shown poor postischemic recovery following use of acidic cardioplegic solutions.[89] Most cardioplegic solutions have bicarbonate,[1] THAM,[155] or blood as the buffer. Blood is a more powerful buffer than either bicarbonate or THAM.

Osmolality

Extremes of osmolality are harmful. Tyers[186] has demonstrated the deleterious effect of the markedly hyperosmolar (450 mosmol) Melrose solution. Postischemic ventricular performance with the hyperosmolar (450 mosmol) Kirsch solution is poor as compared with the effect of solutions with osmolality between 300 and 320 mosmol.[107] Hypoosmolar solutions (272 mosmol) cause myocardial edema.[65] Isoosmolar[187] and slightly hyperosmolar[1] solutions have given excellent clinical results. It appears that solutions should be at least isoosmolar and, if hyperosmolar, should not exceed 380 mosmol. If moderate hyperosmolarity is present in a crystalloid solution, onconicity provided by protein appears to be unnecessary.[65]

Calcium

Excellent clinical results have been achieved with crystalloid solutions containing calcium[184] as well as with calcium-free solutions.[155] Proponents of solutions containing calcium have supported its use by citing the "calcium paradox," a syndrome described in the isolated rat heart following normothermic, aerobic perfusion with a calcium-free solution followed by perfusion with a calcium-containing solution.[195] This perfusion sequence results in an irreversible loss of electrical and mechanical activity of the heart.[87] This syndrome appears to be modified by profound hypothermia,[92] which may explain the good clinical results achieved with calcium-free solutions. Nevertheless, the presence of calcium has not been shown to be harmful, and calcium may well be beneficial.[105,106]

Glucose

Glucose is theoretically beneficial because it may provide substrate during anaerobic metabolism,[85] and it also can provide osmolality.[65]

Oxygen

Studies have shown that oxygenated crystalloid cardioplegia is superior to aerated cardioplegia when long aortic clamp times are studied. Bodenhamer and co-workers[19] subjected dogs to 4 hours of arrest and found oxygenated cardioplegia was superior to aerated cardioplegia. Guyton[81] found that in a small group of patients undergoing coronary artery bypass, those patients with a clamp time over 28 minutes had lower creatine kinase MB isoenzyme release if oxygenated crystalloid cardioplegia was used. Daggett and colleagues,[48] whose group performed the early laboratory studies of oxygenated crystalloid cardioplegia, subsequently adopted for clinical use an oxygenated dilute blood cardioplegic solution with a hematocrit of 5. As will be discussed in the following section, there are a number of reasons to consider blood superior to crystalloid as the vehicle for intermittent delivery of oxygen during cardioplegic arrest.

Blood

Cold oxygenated blood with potassium as the arresting agent was described in the 1970s[9,68,69,115] and has stimulated a large amount of laboratory and clinical investigation.[7,59] Earlier concerns about the rheology of blood at profoundly hypothermic temperatures and the complexity of the equipment necessary for administration of cold blood cardioplegia have not been substantiated. Cold blood cardioplegia actually has better rheology than crystalloid cardioplegia.[90] The medical device companies have responded with a number of devices that make the administration of all types of cardioplegia simple, safe, and predictable.

The oxygen availability of cold blood cardioplegia is affected by the profound hypothermia. With increasing hypothermia, the oxygen dissociation curve moves to the left, making less of the hemoglobin-bound oxygen available.[93,169] At 10°C approximately 38% of the hemoglobin-bound oxygen is available.[49] This still allows an adequate amount of oxygen to supply the low requirements of the profoundly hypothermic myocardium.

The laboratory comparisons of crystalloid and blood cardioplegia vary considerably in the duration of aortic cross-clamp time, the temperature of the solutions and myocardium, and the degree to which variables other than the presence or absence of blood are controlled.[7,9,16,32,61,180,192] Catinella and co-workers[32] compared the two solutions in dogs undergoing 180 minutes of arrest, with myocardial temperature maintained near 15°C during arrest. They found that ventricular function and compliance were statistically unchanged in both groups, but high-energy phosphates were better preserved in the blood cardioplegia group.

A number of randomized clinical studies comparing cold crystalloid to cold blood cardioplegia have been performed.[31,41,70,99,143] These have been performed in patients undergoing coronary artery bypass with average cross-clamp times varying from 47[31] to 70[45] minutes and with hematocrits of the cardioplegic solutions varying from 6[31] to 21.[46] These studies have shown either no difference[31,143] or a slight superiority[41,70,99] with cold blood cardioplegia.

There are a number of other characteristics of cold blood cardioplegia, in addition to its oxygen delivery, that make it attractive.[7,23,25,26] The red cell is a powerful buffer. Blood is an effective scavenger of oxygen free radicals.[189] Blood provides onconicity, lessening the likelihood of myocardial edema, and it has favorable rheologic properties. There are experimental data to suggest that blood cardioplegia is superior to crystalloid cardioplegia in the neonatal heart.[46]

With the growing proportion of patients coming to surgery with poor ventricular function or with chronic or acute ischemia, and with the increasing complexity of operations and the consequent longer aortic cross-clamp times, cold blood cardioplegia is likely to give superior results to those achieved with cold crystalloid cardioplegia.

Operative Techniques

Operative techniques of cold cardioplegia are based on the following principles: (1) rapid induction and continuous maintenance of cardiac arrest and profound myocardial hypothermia; (2) avoidance of injury to the coronary arteries, coronary sinus, or myocardium as a result of solution infusion; (3) avoidance of injury from reperfusion of blood after release of the aortic cross-clamp; and (4) maintenance of optimal cardiac physiology during the period of recovery from cold cardioplegic arrest.

Monitoring
The effect of cold blood cardioplegia is closely related to the level of myocardial hypothermia. For this reason, monitoring myocardial temperature can be helpful in assuring adequate delivery of solution and attainment of the desired level of hypothermia. We usually monitor the septal temperature and seek a temperature below 20°C, preferably near 15°C. If other areas of the myocardium have poorer blood supply than the interventricular septum, temperature in these areas can be measured.

Antegrade Infusion
A number of commercially available cardioplegic solution infusion systems are now available that precisely control and monitor infusion solution temperature, infusion flow rate, infusion pressure, and myocardial temperature. These systems make the administration of cold cardioplegia simple and safe.

In patients undergoing coronary artery bypass or mitral valve procedures, we usually use antegrade and retrograde infusion.[24] Antegrade infusion is performed through a cannula in the ascending aorta that also serves as a left ventricular vent.[82] Infusion flow rates are usually around 200 ml/min and the aortic root pressure is kept below 100 mm Hg. Excessive infusion pressure can cause myocardial edema.[103] For aortic valve replacement we usually infuse the solution directly into the coronary ostia through hand-held cannulas, as well as retrogradely through a coronary sinus catheter.

Retrograde Coronary Sinus Infusion
Lillehei[123] and Gott[76] described continuous perfusion of the coronary sinus with normothermic blood in the 1950s in patients undergoing procedures on the aortic valve. The use of the coronary sinus fell into disuse until the reports of retrograde coronary sinus cardioplegia by Menasche[136-139] and Fabiani[60] in the 1980s. Menasche described direct cannulation of the coronary sinus through a small incision in the right atrium. Fabiani described infusion into the right atrium with tapes snared around the caval cannulae and the aorta and pulmonary artery occluded. There was subsequent development of special catheters that could be placed "blindly" through the right atrium and directed into the coronary sinus.[28,51,79] These catheters also have inflatable or self-inflating balloons and the ability to measure pressure in the coronary sinus during infusion. The ability to place these catheters without bicaval cannulation or isolation of the right atrium, and their safety and reliability, have made their use widespread.[35]

Studies in dog hearts have questioned the adequacy of perfusion of the right ventricle and interventricular septum via the coronary sinus.[170,179] Studies in humans, however, have shown good preservation of right ventricular function following retrograde coronary sinus cardioplegia.[50,62,138,139]

Experimental studies have shown that retrograde coronary sinus cardioplegia is superior to antegrade cardioplegia in the presence of coronary artery obstruction[79,150] and that antegrade and retrograde cardioplegia provides better myocardial protection than either technique alone.[149] These studies have been confirmed in humans.[139]

Retrograde cardioplegia is particularly useful in reoperative coronary artery surgery, where the technique not only provides superior delivery of solution, but can flush out atheromatous material that may have embolized down the coronary arteries.[80,125] Retrograde coronary sinus infusion is also effective in patients undergoing coronary artery bypass who have mild aortic regurgitation, for reinfusion of solution during mitral valve repair, and for patients undergoing complex procedures on the aortic root.

Reinfusion

Reinfusion of cold cardioplegic solution is necessary for maintenance of arrest and hypothermia.[57,116,146] If proper reinfusion is performed, topical hypothermia is unnecessary[3,26] and the potential for pulmonary morbidity that is associated with iced slush-induced injury to the phrenic nerve[14,130,161] is avoided. Reinfusion also washes out metabolic end products[73,124] and may replenish glucose for anaerobic metabolism. The heart rewarms with the passage of time because of the warmer temperatures that surround it, the blood coming back to the left ventricle from bronchial flow, and the blood perfusing the myocardium via noncoronary collaterals.[20] Noncoronary collateral flow can also wash out the cardioplegic solution, resulting in return of electromechanical activity and its undesired consequence of higher energy consumption. The rate of myocardial temperature rise can be slowed by systemic hypothermia, total bypass, and topical hypothermia.[147] Reinfusion also maintains the electromechanical arrest that may be affected by noncoronary collateral flow.[146]

We usually reinfuse every 20–30 minutes, whenever the myocardial temperature rises above 20°C, or whenever there is return of electromechanical activity. If the aortic clamp is to be removed shortly, reinfusion is not performed, so that prolonged rewarming and recovery of the heart is avoided following release of the clamp.

Reperfusion and Recovery

Both reperfusion of blood following release of the cross-clamp and recovery of the heart prior to weaning from cardiopulmonary bypass are critical periods. Engelman[58] demonstrated that myocardial injury can occur secondary to high arterial pressure following release of the aortic cross-clamp. It seems likely that the cold, flaccid heart of cardioplegia would be particularly susceptible to this type of injury. Therefore we maintain the pressure around 50 mm Hg during and following the release of the aortic clamp for a minute or two until the heart attains tone. The heart is usually in a stable rhythm with excellent mechanical function 15–20 minutes following aortic unclamping and is ready for weaning from bypass.

Warm Blood Cardioplegia

Warm Blood Cardioplegia Induction and Reperfusion

Buckberg and colleagues[23] have proposed the concepts of warm blood cardioplegia reperfusion and induction and have studied them extensively. Follette and colleagues[66] studied dog hearts undergoing 1 hour of ischemic arrest with topical hypothermia followed by reperfusion with unmodified warm blood or with warm blood that was hypocalcemic, hyperkalemic, alkalotic, and hyperosmolar. Reperfusion with the modified warm blood resulted in superior recovery of myocardial performance, improved restoration of compliance, and less postischemic edema. Teoh and colleagues[181] studied this method clinically in a prospective randomized trial in patients undergoing elective coronary artery bypass. They found that terminal warm blood accelerated myocardial metabolic recovery, preserved high-energy phosphates, improved the metabolic response to postoperative hemodynamic stresses, and reduced left atrial pressures. However, there was no significant difference in systolic function (the relation between systolic blood pressure and end-systolic volume index) or myocardial performance (the relation between stroke work index and end-diastolic volume index).

Rosenkranz and co-workers[157-159] performed several studies in dog hearts that had been injured by normothermic ischemia, investigating the use of a period of warm blood cardioplegia infusion followed by cold blood cardioplegia. They found that modified warm blood induction, with glutamate and aspartate, allowed complete recovery of myocardial metabolism and function compared to cold blood cardioplegia alone and may be used as a form of "active resuscitation" of energy-depleted hearts. They applied these principles in a group of patients requiring intraaortic balloon and inotropic drug support for cardiogenic shock, comparing the group to another concurrent but nonrandomized group of similar patients.[156] They concluded that improved results in this high-risk group of patients came from warm blood cardioplegic induction, glutamate enrichment, meticulous attention to cardioplegic distribution, warm cardioplegic reperfusion before unclamping, and graft perfusion during construction of proximal anastomoses.

More studies will be needed, particularly prospective randomized studies, before the clinical indications for the use of modified warm blood induction and reperfusion are defined.

Continuous Retrograde Warm Blood Cardioplegia

Lichtenstein, Salerno, and colleagues[122,162] at the University of Toronto began using continuous warm antegrade cardioplegia in 1987. They reasoned that the low oxygen requirements of the normothermic potassium-arrested heart (1.1 ml/100 g/min)[27,134] could be easily supplied by infusing warm blood cardioplegia at 150–250 ml/min, thereby completely avoiding any period of ischemia during aortic cross-clamping. They subsequently evolved a technique involving initial antegrade infusion of high-potassium warm blood cardioplegia followed by continuous retrograde infusion of a lower-potassium solution.[163] They have described their initial clinical results,[120,121,164] suggesting that the warm blood cardioplegia technique may be superior to their previous technique of cold blood cardioplegia.

Engelman[56] found no difference in results comparing the techniques of warm blood cardioplegia and cold blood cardioplegia in a prospective randomized study of patients undergoing coronary artery bypass. Kay[110] found no difference in the methods in "low-risk" patients but suggested that retrograde continuous warm blood cardioplegia appears to provide superior protection for "high-risk" patients.

Retrograde warm blood cardioplegia has potential disadvantages.[164] The retrograde cannula can become displaced, leaving the heart ischemic at normothermia. The blood coming out of the coronary artery during coronary surgery can obscure the surgical field, affecting the precision of the anastomosis. A catheter-directed constant stream of oxygen has been used to address this problem.[182] Normothermic cardiopulmonary bypass results in lower systemic vascular resistance, often requiring large volume infusion and the use of phenylephrine.[39] The safety of normothermic cardiopulmonary bypass has not been established in patients with severe cerebrovascular disease and renal impairment.

Further studies will be necessary, particularly prospective randomized studies, to determine whether continuous retrograde warm blood cardioplegia is superior to intermittent cold blood cardioplegia, and if so, in which patient groups.

References

1. Adams PX, Cunningham JN, Trehan NK, Brazier JR, Reed GE, Spencer FC: Clinical experience using potassium-induced cardioplegia with hypothermia in aortic valve replacement. J Thorac Cardiovasc Surg 75:564,1978.
2. Allard JR, Shizgal HM, Dobell ARC: Distribution of myocardial blood flow during cardiopulmonary bypass in normal and hypertrophied left ventricles. Surg Forum 24:178,1973.
3. Allen BS, Buckberg GD, Rosenkranz ER, Plested W, Skow J, Mazzei E, Scanlan R: Topical cardiac hypothermia in patients with coronary disease: an unnecessary adjunct to cardioplegic protection and cause of pulmonary morbidity. J Thorac Cardiovasc Surg 104:626,1992.
4. Appelbaum A, Kouchoukos NT, Blackstone EH, Kirklin JW: Early risks of open heart surgery for mitral valve disease. Am J Cardiol 37:201,1976.
5. Apstein CS, Deckelbaum L, Mueller M, Hagopian L, Hood WB Jr: Graded global ischemia and reperfusion: cardiac function and lactate metabolism. Circulation 55:864,1977.
6. Ashmore PG, Svitek V, Ambrose P: The incidence and effects of particulate aggregation and microembolism in pump-oxygenator systems. J Thorac Cardiovasc Surg 55:691,1968.
7. Barner HB: Blood cardioplegia: a review and comparison with crystalloid cardioplegia. Ann Thorac Surg 52:1354,1991.
8. Barner HB, Jellinek M, Sandeven JW, Menz LJ, Hahn JW: Cold blood-diltiazem cardioplegia. Ann Thorac Surg 33:55,1982.
9. Barner HB, Laks H, Codd JE, Standeven JW, Jellinek M, Kaiser GC, Menz LJ, Tyras DH, Pennington GC, Hahn JW, Willman VL: Cold blood as the vehicle for potassium cardioplegia. Ann Thorac Surg 28:509,1979.
10. Barner HB, Standeven JW, Jellinek M, Menz LJ, Hahn JW: Topical cardiac hypothermia for myocardial preservation. J Thorac Cardiovasc Surg 73:856,1977.
11. Barner HB, Swartz MT, Devine JE, Williams GA, Janosik D: Diltiazem as an adjunct to cold blood potassium cardioplegia: a clinical assessment of dose and prospective randomization. Ann Thorac Surg 43:191,1987.
12. Baroldi G, Milam JD, Wukasch DC, Sandiford FM, Romagnoli A, Cooley DA: Myocardial damage in "stone hearts." J Mol Cell Cardiol 6:395,1974.
13. Behrendt DM, Jochim KE: Effect of temperature of cardioplegic solution. J Thorac Cardiovasc Surg 76:353,1978.
14. Benjamin JJ, Cascade PN, Rubenfire M, Wajszczuk W, Kerin N: Left lower lobe atelectasis and consolidation following cardiac surgery: the effect of topical cooling on the phrenic nerve. Radiology 142:11,1982.
15. Bernard WF, Schwartz HF, Mallick NP: Elective hypothermic cardiac arrest in normothermic animals. Ann Surg 153:43,1961.
16. Bing OHL, LaRaia PJ, Gaasch WH, Spadard J, Franklin A, Weintraub RM: Independent protection provided by red blood cells during cardioplegia. Circulation 66(Suppl 1):81,1982.
17. Bixler TJ, Gardner TJ, Flaherty JT, Goldman RA, Gott VL: Effects of procaine-induced cardioplegia on myocardial ischemia, myocardial edema and post-arrest ventricular function: a comparison with potassium-induced cardioplegia and hypothermia. J Thorac Cardiovasc Surg 75:886,1978.
18. Bloodwell RD, Kidd JN, Hallman GL, Burdette WJ, McMurtrey MJ, Cooley DA: Cardiac valve replacement without coronary perfusion: clinical and laboratory observation. *In* Brewer, LA (ed): Prosthetic Heart Valves. Springfield, Ill, Charles C Thomas, 1969, p 397.
19. Bodenhamer RM, DeBoer LWV, Geffin GA, O'Keefe DD, Fallon JT, Aretz TH, Haas GS, Daggett WM: Enhanced myocardial protection during ischemic arrest.

Oxygenation of a crystalloid cardioplegic solution. J Thorac Cardiovasc Surg 85: 769,1983.

20. Brazier J, Hottenrott C, Buckberg GD: Noncoronary collateral myocardial blood flow. Ann Thorac Surg 19:426,1975.

21. Bretschneider HJ, Hubner G, Knoll D, Lohr B, Nordbeck H, Spieckermann PG: Myocardial resistance and tolerance to ischemia: physiological and biochemical basis. J Thorac Cardiovasc Surg 16:241,1975.

22. Brody WR, Reitz BA, Andrews MJ, Roberts WC, Michaelis LL: Long-term morphologic and hemodynamic evaluation of the left ventricle after cardiopulmonary bypass: a comparison of normothermic anoxic arrest, coronary artery perfusion and profound topical hypothermia. J Thorac Cardiovasc Surg 70:1073,1975.

23. Buckberg GD: Strategies and logic of cardioplegic delivery to prevent, avoid, and reverse ischemic and reperfusion damage. J Thorac Cardiovasc Surg 93:127,1987.

24. Buckberg GD: Antegrade/retrograde blood cardioplegia to ensure cardioplegic distribution: operative techniques and objectives. J Card Surg 4:216,1989.

25. Buckberg GD: Oxygenated cardioplegia: blood is a many splendored thing. Ann Thorac Surg 50:175,1990.

26. Buckberg GD: Myocardial temperature management during aortic clamping for cardiac surgery: protection, preoccupation, and perspective. J Thorac Cardiovasc Surg 102:895,1991.

27. Buckberg GD, Brazier JR, Nelson RL, Goldstein SM, McConnell DH, Cooper N: Studies of the effects of hypothermia on regional myocardial blood flow and metabolism during cardiopulmonary bypass. I. The adequately perfused beating, fibrillating, and arrested heart. J Thorac Cardiovasc Surg 73:87,1977.

28. Buckberg GD, Drinkwater DC, Laks H: A new technique for delivering antegrade/retrograde blood cardioplegia without right heart isolation. Eur J Cardiothorac Surg 4:163,1990.

29. Buckberg GD, Towers B, Paglia D, Mulder DG, Maloney JV: Subendocardial ischemia after cardiopulmonary bypass. J Thorac Cardiovasc Surg 64:699,1972.

30. Buja LM, Levitsky S, Ferrans VJ, Souther SG, Roberts WC, Morrow AG: Acute and chronic effects of normothermic anoxia on canine hearts. Light and electron microscopic evaluation. Circulation 43 (Suppl I):I-44,1971.

31. Buttner EE, Karp RB, Reves JG, Oparil S, Brummet C, McDaniel HG, Smith LR, Kreusch G: A randomized comparison of crystalloid and blood-containing cardioplegic solutions in 60 patients. Circulation 69:973,1984.

32. Catinella FP, Cunningham JN, Spencer FC: Myocardial protection during prolonged aortic crossclamping: comparison of blood and crystalloid cardioplegia. J Thorac Cardiovasc Surg 88:411,1984.

33. Cerra FB, Lajos TZ, Montes M, Siegel JH: Structural-functional correlates of reversible myocardial anoxia. J Surg Res 16:140,1974.

34. Chitwood WR (ed): Myocardial Preservation: Clinical Applications. Philadelphia, Hanley & Belfus, 1988.

35. Chitwood WR: Retrograde cardioplegia: current methods. Ann Thorac Surg 53: 352,1992.

36. Chitwood WR, Sink JD, Hill RC, Wechsler AS, Sabiston DC: The effects of hypothemia on myocardial oxygen consumption and transmural coronary blood flow in the potassium-arrested heart. Ann Surg 190:106,1979.

37. Chrislieb IY, Clark RE, Sobel BE: Three-hour preservation of the hypothermic globally ischemic heart with nifedipine. Surgery 90:947,1981.

38. Christakis FT, Fremes SE, Weisel RD, Tittley JG, Mickle DAG, Ivanov J, Madonik MM, Benak AM, McLaughlin PR, Baird RJ: Diltiazem cardioplegia: a balance of risk and benefit. J Thorac Cardiovasc Surg 91:647,1986.

39. Christakis GT, Koch JP, Deemar KA, Fremes SE, Sinclair L, Chen E, Salerno TA, Goldman BS, Lichtenstein SV: A randomized study of the systemic effects of warm heart surgery. Ann Thorac Surg 54:449,1992.

40. Clark RE, Christlieb IY, Ferguson TB, Weldon CS, Marbarger JP, Sobel BE, Roberts R, Henry PD, Ludbrook PA, Biello D, Clark BK: Laboratory and initial clinical studies of nifedipine, a calcium antagonist for improved myocardial preservation. Ann Surg 193:719,1981.

41. Codd JE, Barner HB, Pennington DG, Merjavy JP, Kaiser GC, Devine JE, Willman VL: Intraoperative myocardial protection: a comparison of blood and asanguineous cardioplegia. Ann Thorac Surg 39:125,1985.

42. Cohn LH, Collins JJ Jr: Local cardiac hypothermia for myocardial protection. Ann Thorac Surg 17:135,1974.
43. Cohn LH, Fujiwara Y, Kirk E, Collins JJ Jr: Effects of local cardiac hypothermia on the magnitude and distribution of coronary blood flow and on myocardial function and metabolism. Ann Thorac Surg 19:10,1975.
44. Conti VR, Bertranou EG, Blackstone EH, Kirklin JW, Digerness SB: Cold cardioplegia versus hypothermia for myocardial protection: randomized clinical study. J Thorac Cardiovasc Surg 76:577,1978.
45. Cooley DA, Reul GJ, Wukasch DC: Ischemic contracture of the heart: "stone heart." Am J Cardiol 29:575,1972.
46. Corno AF, Bethencourt DM, Laks H, Haas GS, Bhuta S, Davtyan HG, Flynn WM, Drinkwater DC, Laidig C, Chang P: Myocardial protection in the neonatal heart: a comparison of topical hypothermia and crystalloid and blood cardioplegic solutions. J Thorac Cardiovasc Surg 93:163,1987.
47. Cunkingnan RA, Carey JS: Normothermic coronary perfusion during aortic valve replacement. Ann Throrac Surg 25:215,1978.
48. Daggett WM, Randolph JD, Jacobs M, O'Keefe DD, Geffin GA, Swinski LA, Boggs BR, Austen WG: The superiority of cold oxygenated dilute blood cardioplegia. Ann Thorac Surg 43:397,1987.
49. Digerness SB, Vanini V, Wideman FE: In vitro comparison of oxygen availability from asanguinous and sanguinous cardioplegia. Circulation 64(Suppl II):II-80,1981.
50. Douville EC, Kratz JM, Spinale FG, Crawford FA, Alpert CC, Pearce A: Retrograde versus antegrade cardioplegia: impact on right ventricular function. Ann Thorac Surg 54:56,1992.
51. Drinkwater DC, Laks H, Buckberg GD: A new simplified method of optimizing cardioplegic delivery without right heart isolation: antegrade/retrograde blood cardioplegia. J Thorac Cardiovasc Surg 100:56,1990.
52. Ebert PA, Greenfield LJ, Austen WG, Morrow AG: Experimental comparison of methods for protecting the heart during aortic occlusion. Ann Surg 155:25,1962.
53. Effler DB, Knight HF, Groves LK, Kolff WJ: Elective cardiac arrest for open heart surgery. Surg Gynecol Obstet 105:407,1957.
54. Ellis RJ, Pryor W, Ebert PA: Advantages of potassium cardioplegia and perfusion hypothermia in left ventricular hypertrophy. Ann Thorac Surg 24:299,1977.
55. Engedahl H, Skagseth E, Saetersdal TS, Myklebus R: Cardiac hypothermia evaluated by ultrastructural studies in man. J Thorac Cardiovasc Surg 75:548,1978.
56. Engelman RM, Levitsky S (eds): A Textbook of Cardioplegia for Difficult Clinical Problems. Mount Kisco, New York, Futura Publishing Co, 1992.
57. Engelman RM, Levitsky S, O'Donoghue MJ, Auvil J: Cardioplegia and myocardial preservation during cardiopulmonary bypass. Circulation 58(Suppl I):I-107,1978.
58. Engelman RM, Levitsky S, Wyndam CRC: Optimal conditions for reperfusion during cardiopulmonary bypass. Circulation 56(Suppl II):II-148,1977.
59. Engelman RJ, Rousou J, Lemeshow S, Dobbs WA: The metabolic consequences of blood and crystalloid cardioplegia. Circulation 64(Suppl 2):75,1981.
60. Fabiani JN, Deloche A, Swanson J, Carpentier A: Retrograde cardioplegia through the right atrium. Ann Thorac Surg 41:101,1986.
61. Feindel CM, Tait GA, Wilson GJ, Klement P, MacGregor DC: Multidose blood versus crystalloid cardioplegia: comparison by quantitative assessment of irreversible myocardial injury. J Thorac Cardiovasc Surg 87:585,1984.
62. Fiore AC, Naunheim KS, Kaiser GC, Willman VL, McBride LR, Pennington C, Barner HB: Coronary sinus versus aortic root perfusion with blood cardioplegia in elective myocardial revascularization. Ann Thorac Surg 47:684,1989.
63. Fiore AC, Naunheim KS, Taub J, Braun P, McBride LR, Pennington G, Kaiser GC, Willman VL, Barner HB: Myocardial preservation using lidocaine blood cardioplegia. Ann Thorac Surg 50:771,1990.
64. Fishman NH, Youker JE, Roe BB: Mechanical injury to the coronary arteries during operative cannulation. Am Heart J 75:26,1968.
65. Foglia RP, Steed DL, Follette DM, DeLand EC, Buckberg GD: Creation and avoidance of myocardial edema by potassium cardioplegia. Surg Forum 28:226,1977.
66. Follette DM, Fey K, Buckberg GD, Helly JJ: Reducing post-ischemic damage by

temporary modification of reperfusate calcium, potassium, pH, and osmolarity. J Thorac Cardiovasc Surg 82:221,1981.

67. Follette DM, Fey K, Mulder DG, Maloney JV, Buckberg G: Prolonged safe aortic cross clamping by combining membrane stabilization, multi-dose cardioplegia, and appropriate pH reperfusion. J Thorac Cardiovasc Surg 74:682,1977.

68. Follette DM, Mulder DG, Maloney JV, Buckberg GD: Advantages of blood cardioplegia over continuous coronary perfusion or intermittent ischemia: experimental and clinical study. J Thorac Cardiovasc Surg 76:604,1978.

69. Follette DM, Steed DL, Foglia R, Fey K, Buckberg GD: Advantages of intermittent blood cardioplegia over intermittent ischemia during prolonged hypothermic aortic clamping. Circulation 58(Suppl I):I-200,1978.

70. Fremes SE, Christakis GT, Weisel RD, Mickle DAG, Madonik MM, Ivanov J, Hardings R, Seawright SJ, Houle S, McLaughlin PR, Baird RJ: A clinical trial of blood and crystalloid cardioplegia. J Thorac Cardiovasc Surg 88:726,1984.

71. Fuhrman GJ, Fuhrman FA, Field J: Metabolism of rat heart slices, with special reference to effects of temperature and anoxia. Am J Physiol 163:642,1950.

72. Gay WA, Ebert PA: Functional, metabolic, and morphologic effects of potassium-induced cardioplegia. Surgery 74:284,1973.

73. Gehl H: Experimentelle Untersuchungen zur bestimming der Dauer eines gut reversiblen Herzstillstandes bei selektiver tiefer Hypothermie durch intermitteirende Coronarperfusion. Z Gesamte Exp Med 139:663,1965.

74. Gott VL, Bartlett M, Long DH, Lillihei CW, Johnson JA: Myocardial energy substances in the dog heart during potassium and hypothermic arrest. J Appl Physiol 17:815,1962.

75. Gott VL, Dutton RC, Young WP: Myocardial rigor mortis as an indication of cardiac metabolic function. Surg Forum 13:172,1962.

76. Gott VL, Gonzalez JI, Zuhdi MN, Varco RL, Lillihei CW: Retrograde perfusion of the coronary sinus for direct-vision aortic surgery. Surg Gynecol Obstet 104:319,1957.

77. Greenberg JJ, Edmunds LH, Brown RB: Myocardial metabolism and post-arrest function in the cold and chemically arrested heart. Surgery 48:31,1960.

78. Griepp RB, Stinson EB, Shumway NE: Profound local hypothermia for myocardial protection during open heart surgery. J Thorac Cardiovasc Surg 66:731,1973.

79. Gundry SR, Kirsh MM: A comparison of retrograde cardioplegia versus antegrade cardioplegia in the presence of coronary artery obstruction. Ann Thorac Surg 38:124,1984.

80. Gundry SR, Razzouk AJ, Vigesaa RE, Wang N, Bailey LL: Optimal delivery of cardioplegic solution for "redo" operations. J Thorac Cardiovasc Surg 103:896,1992.

81. Guyton RA, Dorsey LMA, Craver JM, Bone DK, Jones EL, Murphy DA, Hatcher CR: Improved myocardial recovery after cardioplegic arrest with an oxygenated crystalloid solution. J Thorac Cardiovasc Surg 89:877,1985.

82. Harlan BJ, Kyger ER, Reul GJ, Cooley DA: Needle suction of the aorta for left heart decompression during aortic cross-clamping. Ann Thorac Surg 23:259,1977.

83. Harlan BJ, Ross D, Macmanus Q, Knight R, Luber J, Starr A: Cardioplegic solutions for myocardial preservation: analysis of hypothermic arrest, potassium arrest, and procaine arrest. Circulation 58(Suppl I):I-114,1978.

84. Hearse DJ, Braimbridge MV, Jynge P: Protection of the Ischemic Myocardium: Cardioplegia. New York, Raven Press, 1981.

85. Hearse DJ, Chain EB: The role of glucose in the survival and "recovery" of the anoxic isolated perfused rat heart. Biochem J 128:1125,1972.

86. Hearse DJ, Garlick PB, Humphrey SM: Ischemic contracture of the myocardium: mechanisms and prevention. Am J Cardiol 39:986,1977.

87. Hearse DJ, Humphrey SM, Boink ABTJ, Ruigrok TJC: The calcium paradox: metabolic, electrophysiological, contractile and ultrastructural characteristics in four species. Eur J Cardiol 7:241,1978.

88. Hearse DJ, Stewart DA, Braimbridge MV: Cellular protection during myocardial ischemia: the development and characterization of a procedure for the induction of reversible ischemic arrest. Circulation 54:193,1976.

89. Hearse DJ, Stewart DA, Braimbridge MV: Myocardial protection during bypass and arrest: a possible hazard with lactate-containing infusates. J Thorac Cardiovasc Surg 72:880,1976.

90. Heitmiller RF, DeBoer LWV, Geffin GA, Toal KW, Fallon JT, Drop LJ, Teplick RS, O'Keefe DD, Daggett WM: Myocardial recovery after hypothermic arrest: a comparison of oxygenated crystalloid to blood cardioplegia. The role of calcium. Circulation 72(Suppl 2):241,1985.

91. Hoffman JIE: Determinants and prediction of transmural myocardial perfusion. Circulation 58:381,1978.

92. Holland CE, Olson RE: Prevention by hypothermia of paradoxical calcium necrosis in cardiac muscle. J Mol Cell Cardiol 7:917,1975.

93. Holman WL, Spruell RD, Digerness SB, Dudelston J, Pacifico AD: Oxyhemoglobin dissociation during hypothermic blood cardioplegia arrest. Circulation 86(Suppl II):II-339,1992.

94. Hooker DR: On the recovery of the heart in electric shock. Am J Physiol 91: 305,1929.

95. Hottenrott CE, Towers B, Kurkji HJ, Maloney JV, Buckberg GD: The hazard of ventricular fibrillation in hypertrophied ventricles during cardiopulmonary bypass. J Thorac Cardiovasc Surg 66:742,1973.

96. Hufnagel CA, Conrad PW, Schanno J, Pifarre R: Profound cardiac hypothermia. Ann Surg 153:790,1961.

97. Hurley EJ, Lower RR, Dong E, Pillsbury RC, Shumway NE: Clinical experience with local hypothermia in elective cardiac arrest. J Thorac Cardiovasc Surg 47: 50,1964.

98. Isom OW, Kutin ND, Falk EA, Spencer FC: Patterns of myocardial metabolism during cardiopulmonary bypass and coronary perfusion. J Thorac Cardiovasc Surg 66:705,1973.

99. Iverson LIG, Young JN, Ennix CL Jr, Ecker RR, Moretti RL, Lee J, Hayes RL, Farrar MP, May RD, Masterson R, May I: Myocardial protection: a comparison of cold blood and cold crystalloid cardioplegia. J Thorac Cardiovasc Surg 87: 509,1984.

100. Iyengar SRK, Ramchand S, Charrette EJP, Iyengar CKS, Lynn RB: Anoxic cardiac arrest: an experimental and clinical study of its effects. J Thorac Cardiovasc Surg 66:722,1973.

101. Jennings RB, Ganote CE: Structural changes in myocardium during acute ischemia. Circ Res 34,35(Suppl III):III-156,1974.

102. Jennings RB, Ganote CE, Reimer KA: Ischemic tissue injury. Am J Pathol 81: 179,1975.

103. Johnson RE, Dorsey LM, Moye SJ, Hatcher CR, Guyton RA: Cardioplegic infusion: the safe limits of pressure and temperature. J Thorac Cardiovasc Surg 83: 813,1982.

104. Johnson RG, Jacocks MA, Aretz TH, Geffin GA, O'Keefe DD, DeBoer LWV, Guyton RA, Fallon JT, Daggett WM: Comparison of myocardial preservation with hypothermic potassium and nifedipine arrest. Circulation 66(Suppl 1): 73,1982.

105. Jynge P, Hearse DJ, Braimbridge MV: Myocardial protection during ischemic cardiac arrest: a possible hazard with calcium-free cardioplegic infusates. J Thorac Cardiovasc Surg 73:848,1977.

106. Jynge P, Hearse DJ, Braimbridge MV: Protection of the ischemic myocardium: volume-duration relationships and the efficacy of myocardial infusates. J Thorac Cardiovasc Surg 76:698,1978.

107. Jynge P, Hearse DJ, de Leiris J, Feuvray D, Braimbridge MV: Protection of the ischemic myocardium: ultrastructural, enzymatic, and functional assessment of the efficacy of various cardioplegic infusates. J Thorac Cardiovasc Surg 76:2,1978.

108. Karp RB, Lell W: Evaluating techniques of myocardial preservation for aortic valve replacement: operative risk. J Thorac Cardiovasc Surg 72:206,1976.

109. Kay EB, Nogueria C, Suzuki A, Postigo J, Mendelsohn D: Myocardial protection during aortic valvular surgery. Ann Surg 154:159,1961.

110. Kay GL, Aoki A, Zubiate P, Prejean C, Ruggio J, Kay JH: Superior myocardial protection by normothermic aerobic arrest over ischemic arrest for high-risk patients. Ann Thorac Surg: In Press.

111. Kay HR, Levine FH, Fallon JT, Grotte GJ, Butchart EG, Rao S, McEnany MT, Austen WG, Buckley MJ: Effect of cross-clamp time, temperature, and cardioplegic agents on myocardial function after induced arrest. J Thorac Cardiovasc Surg 76:590,1978.

112. Kirsch U, Rodewald G, Kalmar P: Induced ischemic arrest: clinical experience with cardioplegia in open-heart surgery. J Thorac Cardiovasc Surg 63:121,1972.

113. Kubler W, Spieckermann PG: Regulation of glycolysis in the ischemic and anoxic myocardium. J Mol Cell Cardiol 1:351,1970.

114. Kyo S, Laraia PJ, Magrassi P, Levine FH, Tsai C, Austen G, Buckley MJ: Myocardial protection by lidocaine during cardioplegia. J Surg Res 34:533,1983.

115. Laks H, Barner HB, Kaiser G: Cold blood cardioplegia. J Thorac Cardiovasc Surg 77:319,1979.

116. Laks H, Barner HB, Standeven JW, Hahn JW, Jellinek M, Menz LJ: Myocardial protection by intermittent perfusion with cardioplegic solution versus intermittent coronary perfusion with cold blood. J Thorac Cardiovasc Surg 76:158,1978.

117. Lee WH, Krumhaar D, Fonkalsrud EW, Schjeide EW, Maloney JV: Denaturation of plasma proteins as a cause of morbidity and death after intracardiac operations. Surgery 50:29,1961.

118. Levitsky S, Sloane RE, Mullin EM, McIntosh CL, Morrow AG: Normothermic myocardial anoxia: effects on the canine heart with left ventricular outflow obstruction. Ann Thorac Surg 11:229,1971.

119. Levitsky S, Wright RN, Rao KS, Holland C, Roper K, Engelman R, Feinberg H: Does intermittent coronary perfusion offer greater myocardial protection than continuous aortic cross-clamping? Surgery 82:51,1977.

120. Lichtenstein SV, Abel JG, Salerno TA: Warm heart surgery and results of operation for recent myocardial infarction. Ann Thorac Surg 52:455,1991.

121. Lichtenstein SV, Ashe KA, El Dalati H, Cusimano RJ, Panos A, Slutsky AS: Warm heart surgery. J Thorac Cardiovasc Surg 101:269,1991.

122. Lichtenstein SV, El Dalati H, Panos A, Slutsky AS: Long cross-clamp time with warm heart surgery (letter). Lancet 1:1443,1989.

123. Lillehei CW, DeWall RA, Gott VL, Varco RL: The direct vision correction of calcific aortic stenosis by means of a pump oxygenator and retrograde coronary sinus perfusion. Dis Chest 30:123,1956.

124. Lolley DM, Ray JF, Myers WO, Sheldon G, Sautter RD: Reduction of intraoperative myocardial infarction by means of exogenous anaerobic substrate enhancement: prospective randomized study. Ann Thorac Surg 26:515,1978.

125. Loop FD, Lytle BW, Cosgrove DM, Woods EL, Stewart RW, Golding LAR, Goormastic M, Taylor PC: Reoperation for coronary atherosclerosis: changing practice in 2059 consecutive patients. Ann Surg 212:378,1990.

126. MacGregor DC, Wilson GJ, Tanaka S, Holness DE, Lixfield W, Silver MD, Rubis LJ, Goldstein W, Guntensen J: Ischemic contracture of the left ventricle: production and prevention. J Thorac Cardiovasc Surg 70:945,1975.

127. Macmanus Q, Grunkemeier G, Lambert L, Dietl C, Starr A: Aortic valve replacement and aorta-coronary bypass surgery: results with perfusion of proximal and distal coronary arteries. J Thorac Cardiovasc Surg 75:865,1978.

128. Magee PG, Flaherty JT, Bixler TJ, Gardner TJ, Bulkley BH, Gott VL: Comparison of myocardial protection with nifedipine and potassium. Circulation 60(Suppl 1): 151,1979.

129. Magovern GJ, Dixon CM, Burkholder JA: Improved myocardial protection with nifedipine and potassium-based cardioplegia. J Thorac Cardiovasc Surg 82: 239,1981.

130. Marco JD, Hahn JW, Barner HB: Topical cardiac hypothermia and phrenic nerve injury. Ann Thorac Surg 23:235,1977.

131. McFarland JA, Thomas LB, Gilbert JW, Morrow AG: Myocardial necrosis following elective cardiac arrest induced with potassium citrate. J Thorac Cardiovasc Surg 40:200,1960.

132. McGoon DC: The ongoing quest for ideal myocardial protection: a catalog of the recent English literature. J Thorac Cardiovasc Surg 89:639,1985.

133. McGoon DC, Pestana C, Moffitt EA: Decreased risk of aortic valve surgery. Arch Surg 91:779,1965.

134. McKeever WP, Gregg DE, Canney PC: Oxygen uptake of the nonworking left ventricle. Circ Res 6:612,1958.

135. Melrose DG, Dreyer B, Bentall HH, Baker JBE: Elective cardiac arrest. Lancet 2: 21,1955.

136. Menasche P, Kucharski K, Mundler O, Veyssie L, Subayi J, Le Pimpec F, Fauchet

M, Piwnica A: Adequate preservation of right ventricular function after coronary sinus cardioplegia: a clinical study. Circulation(Suppl III):III-19,1989.

137. Menasche P, Kural S, Fauchet M, Lavergne A, Commin P, Bercot M, Touchot B, Georgiopoulos G, Piwnica A: Retrograde coronary sinus perfusion: a safe alternative for ensuring cardioplegic delivery in aortic valve surgery. Ann Thorac Surg 34:647,1982.

138. Menasche P, Subayi J, Piwnica A: Retrograde coronary sinus cardioplegia for aortic valve operations: a clinical report on 500 patients. Ann Thorac Surg 49: 556,1990.

139. Menasche P, Subayi JB, Veyssie L, LeDref O, Chevret S, Piwnica A: Efficacy of coronary sinus cardioplegia in patients with complete coronary artery occlusions. Ann Thorac Surg 51:418,1991.

140. Merchant FJ, Feinberg H, Levitsky S: Sequential analysis of altered myocardial metabolism and contractility induced by normothermic arrest and reperfusion. J Surg Res 16:153,1974.

141. Midell AI, DeBoer A, Bermudez G: Postperfusion coronary ostial stenosis. J Thorac Cardiovasc Surg 72:80,1976.

142. Mulder DG, Olinger LN, McConnell DH, Maloney JV, Buckberg GD: Myocardial protection during aortic valve replacement. Ann Thorac Surg 21:123,1976.

143. Mullen JC, Christakis GT, Weisel RD, Fremes SE, Ivanov J, Madonik M, Houle S, McLaughlin PR: Late postoperative ventricular function after blood and crystalloid cardioplegia. Circulation 74(Suppl 3):89,1986.

144. Murphy ES, Rosch J, Rahimtoola SH: Frequency and significance of coronary arterial dominance in isolated aortic stenosis. Am J Cardiol 39:505,1977.

145. Najafi H, Henson D, Dye WS, Javid H, Hunter JA, Callaghan R, Eisenstein R, Julian OC: Left ventricular hemorrhagic necrosis. Ann Thorac Surg 7:550,1969.

146. Nelson RL, Fey KH, Follette DM, Livesay JJ, DeLand EC, Maloney JV, Buckberg GD: Intermittent infusion of cardioplegic solution during aortic cross-clamping. Surg Forum 27:241,1976.

147. Nelson RL, Goldstein SM, McConnell DH, Maloney JV Jr, Buckberg GD: Improved myocardial performance after aortic cross clamping by combining pharmacologic arrest with topical hypothermia. Circulation 54(Suppl III):III-11,1976.

148. Nelson RL, Goldstein SM, McConnell DH, Maloney JV Jr, Buckberg GD: Studies of the effects of hypothermia on regional myocardial blood flow and metabolism during cardiopulmonary bypass. V. Profound topical hypothermia during ischemia in arrested hearts. J Thorac Cardiovasc Surg 73:201,1977.

149. Partington MT, Acar C, Buckberg GD, Julia PL: Studies of retrograde cardioplegia: II. Advantages of antegrade/retrograde cardioplegia to optimize distribution in jeopardized myocardium. J Thorac Cardiovasc Surg 97:613,1989.

150. Partington MT, Acar C, Buckberg GD, Julia P, Kofsky ER, Bugyi HI: Studies of retrograde cardioplegia: I. Capillary flow distribution to myocardium supplied by open and occluded arteries. J Thorac Cardiovasc Surg 97:605,1989.

151. Puppello DE, Blank RH, Bessone LN, Connar RG, Carlton LM Jr: Local deep hypothermia for combined valvular and coronary heart disease. Ann Thorac Surg 21:508,1976.

152. Richardson JV, Kouchoukos NT, Wright JO, Karp RB: Combined aortic valve replacement and myocardial revascularization: results in 220 patients. Circulation 59:75,1979.

153. Ringer S: A further contribution regarding the influence of the different constituents of the blood on the contraction of the heart. J Physiol 4:29,1883.

154. Roberts AJ (ed): Myocardial Protection in Cardiac Surgery. New York, Marcel Dekker, 1987.

155. Roe BB, Hutchinson JC, Fishman NH, Ullyot DJ, Smith DL: Myocardial protection with cold, ischemic, potassium-induced cardioplegia. J Thorac Cardiovasc Surg 73:366,1977.

156. Rosenkranz ER, Buckberg GD, Laks H, Mulder DG: Warm induction of cardioplegia with glutamate-enriched blood in coronary patients with cardiogenic shock who are dependent on inotropic drugs and intraaortic balloon support. J Thorac Cardiovasc Surg 86:507,1983.

157. Rosenkranz ER, Okamoto F, Buckberg GD, Robertson JM, Vinten-Johansen J, Bugyi H: Safety of prolonged aortic clamping with blood cardioplegia: III. Aspar-

tate enrichment of glutamate blood cardioplegia in energy-depleted hearts after ischemic and reperfusion injury. J Thorac Cardiovasc Surg 91:428,1986.

158. Rosenkranz ER, Okamoto F, Buckberg GD, Vinten-Johansen J, Robertson JM, Bugyi H: Safety of prolonged aortic clamping with blood cardioplegia: II. Glutamate enrichment in energy-depleted hearts. J Thorac Cardiovasc Surg 88: 402,1984.

159. Rosenkranz ER, Vinten-Johansen J, Buckberg GD, Okamoto F, Edwards H, Bugyi H: Benefits of normothermic induction of blood cardioplegia in energy-depleted hearts, with maintenance of arrest by multidose cold blood cardioplegic infusion. J Thorac Cardiovasc Surg 84:667,1982.

160. Rossiter SJ, Hultgren HN, Kosek JC, Wuerflein RD, Angell WW: Ischemic myocardial injury with aortic valve replacement and coronary bypass. Arch Surg 109: 652,1974.

161. Rousou JA, Parker T, Engelman RM, Breyer RH: Phrenic nerve paresis associated with the use of iced slush and the cooling jacket for topical hypothermia. J Thorac Cardiovasc Surg 89:921,1985.

162. Salerno TA: Invited letter concerning: Myocardial temperature management during aortic clamping for cardiac surgery—protection, preoccupation, and perspective. J Thorac Cardiovasc Surg 103:1019,1992.

163. Salerno TA, Christakis GT, Abel J, Houck J, Barrozo CAM, Fremes SE, Cusimano RJ, Lichtenstein SV: Technique and pitfalls of retrograde continuous warm blood cardioplegia. Ann Thorac Surg 51:1023,1991.

164. Salerno TA, Houck JP, Barrozo CAM, Panos A, Christakis GT, Abel JG, Lichtenstein SV: Retrograde continuous warm blood cardioplegia: a new concept in myocardial protection. Ann Thorac Surg 51:245,1991.

165. Sapsford RN, Blackstone EH, Kirklin JW, Karp RB, Kouchoukos NT, Pacifico AD, Roe CR, Bradley EL: Coronary perfusion versus cold ischemic arrest during aortic valve surgery: a randomized study. Circulation 49:1190,1974.

166. Schaff HV, Dombroff R, Faherty JT, Bulkley BH, Hutchins GM, Goldman RA, Gott VL: Effect of potassium cardioplegia on myocardial ischemia and post arrest ventricular function. Circulation 58:240,1978.

167. Schraut W, Lamberti JJ, Kampman K, Anagnostopoulos C, Replogle R, Glagov S: Does local cardiac hypothermia during cardiopulmonary bypass protect the myocardium from long-term morphological and functonal injury? Ann Thorac Surg 24:31,1977.

168. Sealy WC, Young WG, Brown IW, Harris JS, Merritt DH: Potassium, magnesium and neostigmine for controlled cardioplegia. J Thorac Surg 37:655,1959.

169. Severinghaus JW: Oxyhemoglobin dissociation curve correction for temperature and pH variation in human blood. J Appl Physiol 12:485,1958.

170. Shiki K, Masuda M, Yonenaga K, Asou T, Tokunaga K: Myocardial distribution of retrograde flow through the coronary sinus of the excised normal canine heart. Ann Thorac Surg 41:265,1986.

171. Shragge BW, Digerness SB, Blackstone EH: Complete recovery of myocardial function following cold exposure. Circulation 57,58(Suppl II):II-97,1978.

172. Shragge BW, Digerness SB, Blackstone EH: Complete recovery of the heart following exposure to profound hypothermia. J Thorac Cardiovasc Surg 81:455, 1981.

173. Shumway NE, Lower RR: Topical cardiac hypothermia for extended periods of anoxic arrest. Surg Forum 10:563,1959.

174. Standeven JW, Jellinek M, Menz LJ, Kolata RJ, Barner HB: Cold blood potassium diltiazem cardioplegia. J Thorac Cardiovasc Surg 87:201,1984.

175. Starr A, Edwards ML: Mitral replacement: clinical experience with a ball valve prosthesis. Ann Surg 154:726,1961.

176. Starr A, Edwards ML, McCord C, Griswold HE: Aortic replacement: experience with a semirigid ball valve prosthesis. Circulation 27:779,1963.

177. Stemmer EA, Joy I, Aronow WS, Thibault W, McCart P, Connolly JE: Preservation of myocardial ultrastructure. J Thorac Cardiovasc Surg 70:666,1975.

178. Stiles QR, Hughes RK, Lindesmith GG: The effectiveness of topical cardiac hypothermia. J Thorac Cardiovasc Surg 73:176,1977.

179. Stirling MC, McClanahan TB, Schott RJ, Lynch MJ, Bolling SF, Kirsh MM, Gallagher KP: Distribution of cardioplegic solution infused antegradely and retrogradely in normal canine hearts. J Thorac Cardiovasc Surg 98:1066,1989.

180. Takamoto S, Levine FH, LaRaia PJ, Adzick NS, Fallon JT, Austen WG, Buckley MJ: Comparison of single-dose and multiple-dose crystalloid and blood potassium cardioplegia during prolonged hypothermic aortic occlusion. J Thorac Cardiovasc Surg 79:19,1980.
181. Teoh KH, Christakis GT, Weisel RD, Fremes SE, Mickle DAG, Romaschin AD, Harding RS, Ivanov J, Madonik MM, Ross IM, McLaughlin PR, Baird RJ: Accelerated myocardial metabolic recovery with terminal warm blood cardioplegia. J Thorac Cardiovasc Surg 91:888,1986.
182. Teoh KHT, Panos AL, Harmantas AA, Lichtenstein SV, Salerno TA: Optimal visualization of coronary artery anastomoses by gas jet. Ann Thorac Surg 52:564,1991.
183. Trump BF, Mergner WJ, Kahng MW, Saldino AJ: Studies on the subcellular pathophysiology of ischemia. Circulation 53(Suppl I):I-17,1976.
184. Tyers GFO, Manley NJ, Williams EH, Shaffer CW, Williams DR, Kurusz M: Preliminary clinical experience with isotonic hypothermic potassium-induced arrest. J Thorac Cardiovasc Surg 74:674,1977.
185. Tyers GFO, Todd GJ, Neely JR, Waldhausen JA: The mechanism of myocardial protection from ischemic arrest by intracoronary tetrodotoxin administration. J Thorac Cardiovasc Surg 69:190,1975.
186. Tyers GFO, Todd GJ, Neibauer IM, Manley NJ, Waldhausen JA: The mechanism of myocardial damage following potassium citrate (Melrose) cardioplegia. Surgery 78:45,1975.
187. Tyers GFO, Williams EH, Hughes HC, Todd GJ: Effect of perfusate temperature on myocardial protection from ischemia. J Thorac Cardiovasc Surg 73:766,1977.
188. Urschel HC, Greenberg JJ: Differential cardiac hypothermia for elective cardioplegia. Ann Surg 152:845,1960.
189. Van Asbeck B, Hoidal J, Vercellotti GM, Schwartz BA, Moldow CF, Jacob HS: Protection against lethal hyperoxia by tracheal insufflation of erythrocytes: role of red cell glutathione. Science 227:756,1985.
190. Vouhe PR, Helias J, Grondin CM: Myocardial protection through cold blood cardioplegia using a calcium antagonist (diltiazem). Ann Thorac Surg 30:342,1980.
191. Waldhausen JA, Braunwald NS, Bloodwell RD, Cornell WP, Morrow AG: Left ventricular function following elective cardiac arrest. J Thorac Cardiovas Surg 39:799,1960.
192. Warner KG, Josa M, Marston W, Butler MD, Gherardi PC, Assousa SN, Cavanaugh AC, Hunt H, Khuri SF: Reduction in myocardial acidosis using blood cardioplegia. J Surg Res 42:247,1987.
193. Wheeldon DR, Bethune DW, Gill RD, English TAH: A simple cooling circuit for topical cardiac hypothermia. Thorax 31:565,1976.
194. Wukasch DC, Reul GJ, Milam JD, Hallman GL, Cooley DA: The "stone heart" syndrome. Surgery 72:1071,1972.
195. Zimmerman ANE, Daems W, Hulsmann WC, Snijder J, Wisse E, Durrer D: Morphological changes of heart muscle caused by successive perfusion with calcium-free and calcium-containing solutions (calcium-paradox). Cardiovasc Res 1:201,1967.

7

Postoperative Care

Postoperative care has evolved over the years into a scientific method of maintaining desirable physiologic states or changing abnormal states. This chapter discusses our routine postoperative monitoring and therapy and reviews common problems occurring in the postoperative period, with an outline of our therapies.

Routine Monitoring

There are routine postoperative order sheets for children and adults. A 24-hour flow sheet is used in the recovery room and intensive care unit for recording vital signs and other data.

Blood pressure, electrocardiogram, pulmonary artery pressure,[42] and central venous pressure are displayed on a four-channel scope. With a constant infusion device, heparinized saline is infused into the arterial line. Infusions as low as 2 ml/h can be achieved in infants, maintaining patency of small indwelling monitoring lines without excessive fluid administration. Oxygen saturation and end tidal CO_2 are also monitored on most patients.

Urine output is collected and recorded at hourly intervals. Chest output is collected in an autotransfusion device and recorded at 15-minute intervals until bleeding has slowed, and then at hourly intervals.

Blood studies, including hematocrit, platelet count, prothrombin time, partial thromboplastin time, electrolytes, renal panel, and arterial blood gases, are performed when the patient arrives in the cardiac recovery room. A portable chest x-ray is obtained and checked to assure proper expansion of the lungs and proper position of the endotracheal tube, nasogastric tube, and venous monitoring lines. The immediate postoperative chest x-ray also serves as a baseline from which to gauge changes in the mediastinal shadow. A 12-lead electrocardiogram is obtained.

Routine Therapy

Blood

In adults, the shed mediastinal blood is infused every 4 hours or more often if necessary[21] for the first 12 hours postoperatively. Autologous or homologous whole blood or packed cells are usually administered in order to keep hematocrit over 25 in adults and over 30 in infants and children.

Fluids

The usual maintenance fluid is 5% dextrose in water, and the rate for the first 24 hours is usually 50 ml/h for adults. For infants, 50% of the calculated maintenance dose is administered during the first 24 hours.

Electrolytes

Potassium is the most important electrolyte in the postoperative period. Changes in serum potassium following cardiopulmonary bypass are common. Body losses and internal shifts during the postoperative period usually result in some hypokalemia, which should be corrected since it can cause ventricular irritability. We administer potassium to adults in doses up to 10 mEq over a 30-minute period if renal function and urine output are normal. Repeat serum potassiums are obtained in order to determine requirements. In infants calcium is replaced as serum levels indicate.

Medications

A cephalosporin is continued in the postoperative period at a dose of 1–2 g every 8 hours in adults. Antibiotics are usually continued until all indwelling lines and catheters are removed. A similar postoperative antibiotic regimen is given to infants and children, with dosage adjusted appropriately.

For pain, morphine is usually administered intravenously in the early postoperative period in an adult dosage of 2–4 mg every 1–2 hours as needed. Later, when oral medication is tolerated, a codeine compound or aspirin is given.

Respiratory Management

Ventilatory Support

Patients undergoing open heart surgery are routinely returned to the recovery room intubated and are placed on mechanically supported ventilation. The majority of our adult patients receive morphine for anesthesia and therefore require supported ventilation during the initial postoperative period. Mechanical ventilation is preferred in infants and children because it decreases the amount of cardiac work and stabilizes the respiratory status in the early postoperative period. Changes in hemodynamics can then be managed without being influenced by the respiratory status.

Adult patients are maintained on a volume ventilator with an initial tidal volume of 15 ml/kg and a rate of 12 respirations/min. Infants weighing less than 10 kg are placed on a pressure-cycled ventilator, which is more sensitive to the weak inspiratory efforts in infants. Patients on pressure-cycled ventilators require particularly close monitoring, since the inspiratory volume may change substantially and suddenly owing to changes in lung or chest wall compliance and endotracheal tube or airway resistance.

Management of the endotracheal tube in infants is of utmost importance. The short trachea of an infant makes accidental extubation more likely. The endotracheal tube's small internal luminal diameter makes passing a suction catheter more difficult, and stenosis or occlusion by a mucous plug is a potential complication. Constant attention to the position and patency of the endotracheal tube by the nurses and physicians is necessary.

Most patients are started on an inspired oxygen concentration of 100% and a positive end-expiratory pressure (PEEP) of 5 cm. Respiratory adjustment is made as indicated by the arterial blood gas analyses, pulse oximetry, and end tidal CO_2. If the patient is being hyperventilated, as indicated by a pCO_2 of less than 36 mm Hg, the rate is decreased or the patient is placed on intermittent mandatory ventilation. The tidal volume can also be decreased, but this may predispose to development of atelectasis.

Hypoventilation, as indicated by a pCO_2 over 44, can be treated by increasing the tidal volume 10%–15%; this is the preferred initial step if it can be accomplished without a rise in inspiratory pressure. Increasing the respiratory rate can improve ventilation but may impair pulmonary blood flow.

Inspired oxygen concentration is adjusted to keep the arterial pO_2 in the range of 80–100 mm Hg. This allows some margin over the pO_2 at which hemoglobin is 90% saturated (60 mm Hg) and thereby allows for some drop in arterial pO_2 without rapidly reaching a dangerous level of hypoxemia. Management of respiratory failure is covered later in this chapter.

Weaning from Assisted Ventilation
As the patient awakens from anesthesia, ventilatory support can be progressively diminished by changing to intermittent mandatory ventilation (IMV), which allows a gradual transition from mechanical ventilation to spontaneous breathing. This is accomplished by providing a continuous source of fresh gas from which the patient can breathe as ventilator rates are decreased.[23] This method of weaning is psychologically and physiologically beneficial to the patient and is easily managed by the professional staff.[9] Patients with no respiratory or circulatory problems are placed on IMV soon after surgery. Monitoring is by oximetry and end tidal CO_2, with arterial blood gases being checked if a smooth progression is not occurring. Progression to spontaneous ventilation usually occurs by the morning following surgery. With modification of anesthesia, same-day extubation is possible in good-risk patients.

Extubation
Our guidelines for extubation of the uncomplicated cardiac patient are shown in Table 7–1. These simple guidelines are suitable for most patients. Ventilation management and decision regarding extubation should always be individualized. Patients with preoperative respiratory impairment may not be able to acheive the levels of pCO_2 or pO_2 required of normal patients. A patient with chronic obstructive pulmonary disease may have persistent hypercarbia. Knowledge of the patient's preoperative respiratory state, particularly room-air arterial blood gases, can be used to make rational decisions regarding postoperative management.

Respiratory Care After Extubation
Good respiratory care following extubation is necessary for smooth postoperative recovery. Pulmonary secretions must be coughed up and development of atelectasis prevented. The educated cooperation of the patient is essential, as are the cooperative efforts of nurses, respiratory therapists, and physi-

Table 7–1. Respiratory Guidelines for Initiation of Spontaneous Ventilation and Subsequent Extubation

1. Patients placed on spontaneous ventilation should be:
   a. Awake and responsive
   b. Hemodynamically stable
   c. Not having any premature ventricular contractions

2. Ventilatory support should resume if any of the following occur:
   a. Respiratory rate increases over 25
   b. Heart rate increases or decreases by more than 15
   c. Blood pressure drops below 100 systolic or rises more than 20 mm systolic
   d. Ventricular irritability occurs
   e. pCO_2 is less than 30 or more than 46
   f. pO_2 is less than 70

3. The following should be present in order to extubate:
   a. pCO_2 less than 46
   b. pO_2 more than 70 on FIO_2 of 40%

cians. We encourage ambulation and coughing and deep breathing. Our use of intermittent positive-pressure breathing (IPPB) treatments is infrequent. Studies[19,29] have shown that verbal encouragement of deep breathing is just as effective as IPPB. Incentive spirometers or blow bottles are more effective than IPPB in reducing pulmonary complications, are less expensive, and are associated with fewer side effects.

Problems

Shivering

Shivering can occur in the recovery room as the patient rewarms, resulting in an increase in CO_2 production. We usually treat shivering with vecuronium, 5–10 mg every hour, for the first 5 hours as needed, with the patient fully supported on the ventilator and well sedated.

Fever

Fever is a common occurrence in the early period following open heart surgery. This may be related to a compensatory response to the hypothermia during cardiopulmonary bypass. Fever increases the metabolic rate of the body and thereby increases cardiac output and the work of the heart. For this reason, therapy must be effective and timely. We routinely give acetaminophen if the temperature goes over 100°F in the postoperative period. Fever after the first 48 postoperative hours requires investigation for an infectious cause.

Supraventricular Arrhythmias

Supraventricular arrhythmias following open heart surgery are frequent.[1] Their physiological effect is related to the ventricular rate and the hemodynamic effect of the loss of sinus rhythm, and therapy is indicated by the rate of ventricular response and the degree of hemodynamic impairment. Our initial management of atrial flutter or fibrillation is intravenous administration of digoxin in a dose of 0.125 mg for adults. This dose is repeated every 30–60 minutes until the rhythm reverts to sinus or the ventricular rate falls below 100. If a ventricular rate cannot be controlled by digoxin and the rate results in an impaired hemodynamic state, verapamil can be administered intravenously in 5- to 10-mg doses to control the ventricular response and improve the hemodynamic state.[33]

Supraventricular arrhythmias that cause hemodynamic impairment and that do not respond to medical therapy require electroconversion. A synchronized defibrillator that prevents discharge of the defibrillating current on the T wave should be readily available and can be used in emergency or elective situations to reverse supraventricular arrhythmias. Some supraventricular arrhythmias, particularly atrial flutter, may be treated by atrial overdrive pacing.[45]

Ventricular Arrhythmias

Ventricular arrhythmias are potentially fatal. Careful monitoring should diagnose their occurrence rapidly, and appropriate therapy should be instituted immediately. Frequent premature ventricular contractions (PVCs), multifocal PVCs, and runs of PVCs or short bursts of ventricular tachycardia all require rapid institution of therapy in order to prevent progression to persistent ventricular tachycardia or ventricular fibrillation. We treat unifocal PVCs that occur more than five times per minute and treat any multifocal PVCs or runs of two or more PVCs. Initial treatment of unifocal PVCs is to increase the heart rate with atrial pacing,[17] up to 110. If the more rapid atrial pacing does not override the ventricular irritability, treatment in the adult consists of an intravenous bolus of lidocaine (50 or 100 mg) followed by a lidocaine infusion of 0.5–4.0 mg/min. Electrolytes are rechecked. Determination of magnesium levels and replenishment of magnesium stores may be effective.

Persistent ventricular tachycardia or ventricular fibrillation requires immediate electrical defibrillation and administration of lidocaine. External cardiac massage is required if immediate hemodynamic stability is not reinstated. Other resuscitative measures, such as administration of sodium bicarbonate and other drugs, should be performed if satisfactory cardiac output does not return.

All episodes of ventricular arrhythmias require careful search for the cause, which may be hypoxia, hypercarbia, acidosis, hypokalemia, hypotension, myocardial ischemia or infarction, or other factors. Reanalysis of arterial blood gases, serum electrolytes, the electrocardiogram, chest x-ray, and a hemodynamic evaluation of the patient are required. Persistence of a ventricular arrhythmia in spite of high doses of intravenous lidocaine (4 mg/min) may require treatment with drugs such as propranolol,[27] procaineamide,[24] bretylium tosylate,[3] or other antiarrhythmics.

Excessive Bleeding

Management of postoperative bleeding can be quite simple or can require educated and refined clinical judgment. Some bleeding is normal, of course, in every postoperative cardiac patient. Bleeding that causes either tamponade or hypotension requires urgent reoperation. The amount of bleeding that is acceptable is determined by its hemodynamic effect, the size of the patient, the clotting status of the patient, the extensiveness of the operation, and other factors. We have no hard rules for the timing of reoperation. This clinical judgment is arrived at by consideration of all the previously mentioned factors.

Patients who have had reoperations, preoperative hepatic impairment, or complicated procedures with prolonged cardiopulmonary bypass present the most difficult decisions concerning reoperation. Absence of any hemodynamic impairment from the bleeding, such as tamponade or hypovolemia, is required for any delay in reoperation.

Clotting studies should be performed in the presence of persistent postoperative bleeding. Appropriate replacement of deficient clotting factors is often successful in stopping bleeding.[47] Desmopressin acetate (DDAVP), a synthetic vasopressin analogue that lacks vasoconstrictor activity, can reduce postoperative bleeding. Although DDAVP does not reduce postoperative bleeding when administered prophylactically following routine coronary artery bypass,[16] it does appear to reduce bleeding when administered to those patients having excessive postoperative bleeding.[2,7,37] The usual dose is 0.3 μg/kg.

Epsilon-aminocaproic acid, a fibrinolytic agent, may decrease postoperative bleeding, particularly in those patients with excessive fibrinolysis.[44]

Judicious use of mild hypotension can be effective in the treatment of postoperative bleeding. Hypotension is safe if properly used. Systolic blood pressure may be lowered to below 100 mm Hg but usually not below 90 mm Hg using nitroprusside. Careful monitoring of cardiac output is necessary to make sure that a serious decrease in cardiac output is not occurring.

Sudden and life-threatening bleeding occasionally occurs in the recovery room or intensive care unit. This requires bold and speedy therapy. We keep equipment available in the recovery room and intensive care unit for emergency opening of the chest and do not hesitate to open the chest if massive bleeding or serious tamponade abruptly occurs. Often a bleeding point can be controlled by digital pressure while blood volume is replaced and the patient resuscitated. If definitive surgical control of the bleeding cannot be obtained in the recovery room, the patient is returned to the operating room. Open resuscitation in the recovery room or intensive care unit is effective and associated with a low incidence of wound infection.[30]

Hypotension and Low Cardiac Output

Hypotension and low cardiac output are major problems and are the subjects of Chapter 8.

Tamponade

Tamponade is often easily diagnosed by rising atrial pressures, decreasing arterial pressure, and widening mediastinal shadow on x-ray. Pulsus paradoxus may also be present. However, tamponade can occur without any change in mediastinal shadow. Transthoracic or transesophageal echocardiography can be helpful in the diagnosis of tamponade. Decreased myocardial performance is the most difficult syndrome to differentiate from tamponade, and definite diagnosis sometimes requires reexploration to rule out tamponade.

Pericardial fluid or blood can collect slowly weeks or months following surgery, resulting in late tamponade requiring surgical relief.[12,38] Diagnosis of this condition is also aided by echocardiography.

Hypertension

Hypertension occurs in 30%–50% of patients following cardiopulmonary bypass.[15] Hypertension is undesirable in the postoperative period because it predisposes to bleeding, can cause suture line disruption and aortic dissection, results in an increased oxygen requirement by the myocardium, and can depress myocardial performance. Hypertension is more common postoperatively among those patients with a history of hypertension. We usually treat systolic pressure of over 130 mm Hg. Nitroprusside, a vasodilator that acts directly on the smooth muscle of the arterioles and veins, is our drug of choice.[36] The usual dose is from 0.5–2 μg/kg/min. The effect of nitroprusside, with its rapid onset and short duration, is more easily controlled than that of other vasodilators.[40] Nitroglycerin is also effective in treating postoperative hypertension and may be the preferred drug for patients with suspected perioperative ischemia.[13]

Respiratory Failure

Respiratory failure in the postoperative cardiac surgical patient is usually manifested by intrapulmonary shunting that results in poor oxygenation, requiring high levels of inspired oxygen to maintain an adequate arterial oxygen level. Such respiratory failure may be due to preexisting pulmonary impairment, pulmonary impairment secondary to cardiopulmonary bypass, blood transfusion, atelectasis, or infection, pulmonary impairment caused by poor cardiac function, or a combination of these factors. Treatment of respiratory failure requires diagnosis of its cause or causes and initiation of appropriate therapy.

Preexisting pulmonary disease should be diagnosed and defined during the preoperative evaluation (see Chapter 1). Evaluation of postoperative cardiac function, especially left-sided filling pressures, can determine whether there is a cardiogenic factor involved in the respiratory failure. Any fluid overload should be treated with diuresis. Depressed cardiac performance should be treated pharmacologically or mechanically as outlined in Chapter 8.

Most respiratory failure is transient and responds readily to vigorous adjustment of respiratory management, particularly the use of PEEP. PEEP can favorably affect the pulmonary shunt fraction and resulting hypoxia by opening collapsed alveolar units.[35] Increasing levels of PEEP can cause decreases in cardiac output and blood pressure.[20]

If PEEP is not already being used, we usually initiate it if an inspired oxygen concentration (FIO_2) of 70% does not result in an arterial pO_2 over 70 mm Hg. Increments of 2–5 cm of PEEP are instituted and the cardiovascular effects are carefully noted. Mild hypotension, which may occur if atrial pressures are low, can usually be reversed by volume expansion. Arterial blood gases and cardiac output are checked to assess the effect of PEEP.

Adjustment of PEEP requires assessment of its effect on both respiratory and cardiac function. The optimum end-expiratory airway pressure varies widely from patient to patient and ranges up to 15 cm H_2O in most patients.[41] Continuous assessment of arterial blood gases and cardiac output is required for determination of the optimum level of PEEP.

As pulmonary function improves, inspired oxygen concentration is decreased until an FIO_2 of 60%–70% is reached, and then PEEP is decreased, usually in increments of 2–5 cm H_2O.

Treatment of respiratory failure may require prolonged intubation and a decision as to whether a tracheostomy should be performed. The use of low-pressure soft-cuff endotracheal tubes has essentially eliminated tracheal-esophageal fistula and tracheal stenosis.[25] These tubes are well tolerated through the vocal cords for weeks, and although hoarseness is common after prolonged intubation, it usually resolves and permanent complications are rare. For these reasons, some consider endotracheal intubation for periods of up to 4 weeks preferable to tracheostomy.[25] We generally support this view and do not consider tracheostomy until after at least 2 weeks of endotracheal intubation. We avoid tracheostomy even more vigorously in infants and children and rarely perform tracheostomy in this group.

Sternal Infection, Mediastinitis

Sternal wound infection with mediastinitis is one of the most serious infectious complications following cardiac surgery. Prompt recognition and appropriate treatment can minimize morbidity and mortality. Presentation of sternal wound infection and mediastinitis can range from sepsis with few localizing symptoms or signs to obvious wound infection with dehiscence and purulent drainage. A chest computerized tomographic (CT) scan or white blood cell scan can help to establish the diagnosis. Diagnosis of sternal infection requires prompt surgical treatment. Surgical exploration is occasionally required to confirm or disprove the diagnosis of sternal infection and mediastinitis.

Surgical therapy consists of mediastinal drainage, debridement of the sternal edges, provision for mediastinal irrigation, and tight and stable reapproximation of the sternum. The infected sternal edges are cleaned back to healthy, bleeding tissue with a bone curet. Large drainage tubes and an irrigation tube are placed in the mediastinum. Wires are used to reapproximate the sternum, and many may be required. Figure-of-eight wires and parallel wires through the sternum or around adjacent ribs may be necessary for sternal stability. The presternal fascia and subcutaneous tissue are closed. The skin may be left open or loosely approximated.

Antibiotic therapy is continued for 2 to 4 weeks. The mediastinum is irrigated with either antibiotic solution[6] or povidone-iodine solution[43] for 1 or 2 weeks. After irrigation has been stopped for several days and there is no evidence of persisting infection, the mediastinal tubes are removed.

Postpericardiotomy Syndrome

The postpericardiotomy syndrome can occur days to months following cardiac surgery. It is characterized by fever and the symptoms and signs of a pleuropericardial process that may include chest pain, a pericardial rub, electrocardiographic ST-segment and T-wave abnormalities, enlarged cardiac silhouette on chest x-ray, pleural effusions, and leukocytosis.[10] Heart-reactive antibody has been detected in a high proportion of patients with this syndrome.[11] Pericardial rubs or unexplained postoperative fever can occur without chest pain or any other finding characteristic of the syndrome.[26]

The postpericardiotomy syndrome usually responds promptly to aspirin. If that is not effective, indomethacin or steroids should be tried.

Prosthetic Valve Endocarditis

Infection of a prosthetic heart valve is one of the most catastrophic complications following cardiac surgery. Early diagnosis, prompt initiation of antibiotic treatment, and timely reoperation, if necessary, are required for satisfactory outcome. Any persistent fever in the postoperative period should raise the suspicion of prosthetic endocarditis. Multiple blood cultures should be obtained. Positive blood cultures in the absence of any other source indicate prosthetic valve endocarditis.

Prompt and appropriate antibiotic therapy should be instituted. Reoperation has been advocated as soon as the diagnosis of prosthetic endocarditis is made. This may prove to be the proper approach, since reoperation is required in a large proportion of patients with endocarditis, particulary those with endocarditis in the early postoperative period. Our present policy is to reoperate if there is uncontrolled infection, development of a perivalvular leak, multiple or large systemic emboli, valve obstruction, or development of congestive heart failure.[39] Antibiotic therapy is almost never successful if a perivalvular leak develops, and reoperation should be performed regardless of the hemodynamic effect of the leak.

Neurologic Impairment

With the increasing average age of patients undergoing cardiac surgery and the increasing proportion of complex procedures, there has been an increase in the incidence of neurologic complications.[4] This has stimulated a number of novel approaches to the diagnosis and management of atherosclerosis of the ascending aorta, the most common cause of neurologic injury.[22,32,46] Some postoperative neurologic deficits are minor, transient, and of short duration, requiring little more than ordinary care; they resolve within 2 or 3 days. More severe or persistent deficits require a more exhaustive neurologic evaluation.

Renal Failure

Renal failure following cardiopulmonary bypass was a substantial problem during the early years of cardiac surgery[34] but has decreased to around 2% in recent years.[14,31] The mortality of acute oliguric renal failure is 25%–35%.[5,14] Preoperatively elevated serum creatinine, advanced age, and more complicated procedures increase the risk of postoperative renal failure.[5] Low-dose dopamine can improve renal function after cardiopulmonary bypass,[8] and we frequently use this treatment in patients in the high risk group. Treatment for acute renal failure after cardiac surgery is basically no different from that for renal failure in other contexts, although the patient's hemodynamic status may make hemodialysis difficult, requiring the use of alternate methods of dialysis.[28] Early and aggressive dialysis probably decreases the mortality of acute oliguric renal failure after cardiopulmonary bypass.[14]

Gastrointestinal Complications

Although the incidence of gastrointestinal complications is low following cardiopulmonary bypass, occurring in approximately 1% of patients, the mortality of gastrointestinal complications is high.[18] Gastrointestinal bleeding is the most frequent complication, followed by intestinal infarction and acute pancreatitis.[18] An aggressive approach to diagnosis and treatment of these complications is necessary to decrease morbidity and mortality.

References

1. Angelini P, Feldman MI, Lufschanowski R, Leachman RD: Cardiac arrhythmias during and after heart surgery: diagnosis and management. Prog Cardiovasc Dis 16:469,1974.
2. Ansell J, Klassen V, Lew R, Ball S, Weinstein M, VanderSalm T, Okike N, Gratz I, Leslie J, Roberts A, Fleming N, Salzman P: Does desmopressin acetate prophylaxis reduce blood loss after valvular heart operations? J Thorac Cardiovasc Surg 104:117,1992.
3. Bernstein JG, Koch-Weser J: Effectiveness of bretylium tosylate against refractory ventricular arrhythmias. Circulation 45:1024,1972.
4. Blauth CI, Cosgrove DM, Webb BW, Ratliff NB, Boylan M, Piemonte MR, Lytle BW, Loop FD: Atheroembolism from the ascending aorta: an emerging problem in cardiac surgery. J Thorac Cardiovasc Surg 103:1104,1992.
5. Corwin HL, Sprague SM, DeLaria GA, Norusis MJ: Acute renal failure associated with cardiac operations. J Thorac Cardiovasc Surg 98:1107,1989.
6. Culliford AT, Cunningham JN Jr, Zeff RH, Isom OW, Teiko P, Spencer FC: Sternal and costochondral infections following open-heart surgery: a review of 2,594 cases. J Thorac Cardiovasc Surg 72:714,1976.
7. Czer LSC, Bateman TM, Gray RJ, Raymond M, Stewart ME, Lee S, Goldfinger D, Chaux A, Matloff JM: Treatment of severe platelet dysfunction and hemorrhage after cardiopulmonary bypass: Reduction in blood product usage with desmopressin. J Am Coll Cardiol 9:1139,1987.
8. Davis RF, Lappas DG, Kirklin JK, Buckley MJ, Lowenstein E: Acute oliguria after cardiopulmonary bypass: renal functional improvement with low-dose dopamine infusion. Crit Care Med 10:852,1982.
9. Downs JB, Klein EF Jr, Desautels D, Modell JH, Kirby RR: Intermittent mandatory ventilation: a new approach to weaning patients from mechanical ventilators. Chest 64:331,1973.
10. Engle MA, Ito T: The postpericardiotomy syndrome. Am J Cardiol 7:73,1961.
11. Engle MA, McCabe JC, Ebert PA, Zabriskie J: The postpericardiotomy syndrome and antiheart antibodies. Circulation 49:401,1974.
12. Fraser DG, Ullyot DJ: Mediastinal tamponade after open-heart surgery. J Thorac Cardiovasc Surg 66:629,1973.
13. Fremes SE, Weisel RD, Mickle DAG, Teasdale SJ, Aylmer AP, Christakis GT, Madonik MM, Ivanov J, Houle S, McLaughlin PR, Baird RJ: A comparison of nitroglycerin and nitroprusside: I. Treatment of postoperative hypertension. Ann Thorac Surg 39:53,1985.
14. Gailiunas P Jr, Chawla R, Lazarus JM, Cohn L, Sanders J, Merrill JP: Acute renal failure following cardiac operations. J Thorac Cardiovasc Surg 79:241,1980.
15. Gray RJ: Postcardiac surgical hypertension. J Cardiothorac Anesth 2:678,1988.
16. Hackmann T, Gascoyne RD, Naiman SC, Growe GH, Burchill LD, Jamieson WRE, Sheps SB, Schechter MT, Townsend GE: A trial of desmopressin (l-desamino-8-d-arginine vasopressin) to reduce blood loss in uncomplicated cardiac surgery. N Engl J Med 321:1437,1989.
17. Hodam RP, Starr A: Temporary postoperative epicardial pacing electrodes, their value and management after open-heart surgery. Ann Thorac Surg 8:506,1969.
18. Huddy SPJ, Joyce WP, Pepper JR: Gastrointestinal complications in 4473 patients who underwent cardiopulmonary bypass surgery. Br J Surg 78:293,1991.
19. Iverson LIG, Ecker RR, Fox HE, May IA: A comparative study of IPPB, the incentive spirometer, and blow bottles: the prevention of atelectasis following cardiac surgery. Ann Thorac Surg 25:197,1978.

20. Jardin F, Farcot J, Boisante L, Curien N, Margairaz A, Bourdarias J: Influence of positive end-expiratory pressure on left ventricular performance. N Engl J Med 304:387,1981.

21. Johnson RG, Rosenkrantz KR, Preston RA, Hopkins C, Daggett WM: The efficacy of postoperative autotransfusion in patients undergoing cardiac operations. Ann Thorac Surg 36:173,1983.

22. Katz ES, Tunick PA, Rusinek H, Ribakove G, Spencer FC, Kronzon I: Protruding aortic atheromas predict stroke in elderly patients undergoing cardiopulmonary bypass: experience with intraoperative transesophageal echocardiography. J Am Coll Cardiol 20:70,1992.

23. Klein EF Jr: Weaning from mechanical breathing with intermittent mandatory ventilation. Arch Surg 110:345,1975.

24. Koch-Weser J, Klein SW: Procaineamide dosage schedules, plasma concentrations, and clinical effects. JAMA 215:1454,1971.

25. Lewis FR, Blaisdell W, Schlobohm RM: Incidence and outcome of posttraumatic respiratory failure. Arch Surg 112:436,1977.

26. Livelli FD Jr, Johnson RA, McEnany MT, Sherman E, Newell J, Block PC, DeSanctis RW: Unexplained in-hospital fever following cardiac surgery. Natural history, relationship to postpericardiotomy syndrome, and prospective study of therapy with indomethacin versus placebo. Circulation 57:968,1978.

27. Matloff JM, Wolfson S, Gorlin R, Harken DE: Control of postcardiac surgical tachycardias with propranolol. Circulation 37(Suppl II):II-133,1968.

28. Mazze RI: Critical care of the patient with acute renal failure. Anesthesiology 47: 138,1977.

29. McConnell DH, Maloney JV, Buckberg GD: Postoperative intermittent positive-pressure breathing treatments. J Thorac Cardiovasc Surg 68:944,1974.

30. McKowen RL, Magovern GJ, Liebler GA, Park SB, Bukholder JA, Maher TD: Infectious complications and cost-effectiveness of open resuscitation in the surgical intensive care unit after cardiac surgery. Ann Thorac Surg 40:388,1985.

31. McLeish KR, Luft FC, Kleit SA: Factors affecting prognosis in acute renal failure following cardiac operations. Surg Gynecol Obstet 145:28,1977.

32. Mills NL, Everson CT: Atherosclerosis of the ascending aorta and coronary artery bypass: pathology, clinical correlates, and operative management. J Thorac Cardiovasc Surg 102:546,1991.

33. Plumb V, Karp RB, Kouchoukos NT, Zorn GL, James TN, Waldo AL: Verapamil therapy of atrial fibrillation and atrial flutter following cardiac operation. J Thorac Cardiovasc Surg 83:590,1982.

34. Porter GA, Starr A: Management of postoperative renal failure following cardiovascular surgery. Surgery 65:390,1969.

35. Powers SR Jr, Mannal R, Neclerio M, English M, Marr C, Leather R, Ueda H, Williams G, Custead W, Dutton R: Physiologic consequences of positive end-expiratory pressure (PEEP) ventilation. Ann Surg 178:265,1973.

36. Roberts AJ, Niarchos AP, Subramanian VA, Abel RM, Hoover EL, McCabe JC, Case DB, Laragh JH, Gay WA Jr: Hypertension following coronary artery bypass graft surgery. Comparison of hemodynamic responses to nitroprusside, phentolamine, and converting enzyme inhibitor. Circulation 58(Suppl I):I-43,1977.

37. Salzman EW, Weinstein MJ, Weintraub RM, Ware JA, Thurer RL, Robertson L, Donovan A, Gaffney T, Bertele V, Troll J, Smith M, Chute, LE: Treatment with desmopressin acetate to reduce blood loss after cardiac surgery: a double-blind randomized trial. N Engl J Med 314:1402,1986.

38. Simpkin P, Brown AH, Ersoz A, Braimbridge MV: Chronic left heart tamponade. J Thorac Cardiovasc Surg 65:531,1973.

39. Slaughter L, Morris JE, Starr A: Prosthetic valvular endocarditis, a 12 year review. Circulation 47:1319,1973.

40. Stinson EB, Holloway EL, Derby G, Oyer PE, Hollingsworth J, Griepp RB, Harrison DC: Comparative hemodynamic responses to chlorpromazine, nitroprusside, nitroglycerin, and trimethaphan immediately after open-heart operations. Circulation 51(Suppl I):I-26,1975.

41. Suter PM, Fairley HB, Isenberg MD: Optimum end expiratory airway pressure in patients with acute pulmonary failure. N Engl J Med 292:284,1975.

42. Swan HJC, Ganz W, Forrester J, Marcus H, Diamond G, Chonette D: Catheteriza-

tion of the heart in man with use of a flow-directed balloon-tipped catheter. N Engl J Med 283:447,1970.

43. Thurer RJ, Bognolo D, Vargas A, Isch JH, Kaiser GA: The management of mediastinal infection following cardiac surgery: an experience utilizing continuous irrigation with povidone-iodine. J Thorac Cardiovasc Surg 68:962,1974.

44. Vander Salm TJ, Ansell JE, Okike ON, Marsicano TH, Lew R, Stephenson WP, Rooney K: The role of epsilon-aminocaproic acid in reducing bleeding after cardiac operation: a double-blind randomized study. J Thorac Cardiovasc Surg 95: 538,1988.

45. Waldo AL, MacLean WAH, Cooper TB, Kouchoukos NT, Karp RB: Use of temporarily placed epicardial atrial wire electrodes for the diagnosis and treatment of cardiac arrhythmias following open-heart surgery. J Thorac Cardiovasc Surg 76: 500,1978.

46. Wareing TH, Davila-Roman VG, Barzilai B, Murphy SF, Kouchoukos NT: Management of the severely atherosclerotic ascending aorta during cardiac operations. J Thorac Cardiovasc Surg 103:453,1992.

47. Woodman RC, Harker LA: Bleeding complications associated with cardiopulmonary bypass. Blood 76:1680,1990.

8

Low Cardiac Output: Pathophysiology and Treatment

Low cardiac output is often the most critical physiologic abnormality in the cardiac surgery patient. The basic thrust of the surgeon should be to prevent low cardiac output by proper preoperative preparation, excellent anesthesia, precise surgery, meticulous myocardial preservation, and proper postoperative care. However, low cardiac output may exist in spite of proper perioperative care. The determinants of low cardiac output must be understood and the syndrome properly treated to achieve a successful outcome of surgery.

Recent advances have occurred in the understanding of the mechanisms of low cardiac output and in the pharmacologic and mechanical means of improving cardiac output. This chapter reviews the determinants of cardiac output and myocardial performance and the means by which they can be therapeutically manipulated, discusses the indications for institution of mechanical circulatory support using the intraaortic balloon, and presents the techniques of intraaortic balloon insertion.

Determinants of Cardiac Output

Cardiac output is the product of the stroke volume of the heart and the heart rate. Some improvement in cardiac output can be achieved by increasing heart rate alone.[2] However, in the presence of heart rates in the physiologic range, substantial improvement in cardiac output is achieved by increasing stroke volume.

The stroke volume, or volume of blood ejected each beat, is determined by three factors: (1) preload of the ventricle, (2) afterload of the ventricle, and (3) myocardial contractility. The preload of the ventricle is the diastolic volume, which is a function of the end-diastolic pressure and the compliance of the myocardium. It is difficult to measure diastolic volume or compliance in clinical situations, so the filling pressure of the ventricle, or atrial pressure, is used as the indicator of preload.

Afterload is impedance to left ventricular emptying. The major determinants of impedance are arterial compliance and arteriolar resistance. Systemic vascular resistance is an accurate indicator of afterload. Mean arterial blood pressure can be an accurate reflection of afterload.

Myocardial contractility is the velocity, force, and extent of myocardial fiber shortening. Both preload and afterload affect myocardial contractility, making it difficult to determine accurately the contractile state of the intact human heart, even with the sophisticated equipment of the cardiac catheterization laboratory.

The most accurate methods of assessing myocardial contractility involve intraventricular pressure measurements in association with ventriculography.[21,30,33] Such methods are obviously impractical in the clinical setting, requiring that the diagnosis of depressed myocardial contractility be made by exclusion of other factors that may cause low cardiac output. Such factors include hypovolemia, cardiac tamponade, excessive afterload, and possible valve prosthesis malfunction.

Preload, afterload, and myocardial contractility can all be manipulated to attain the maximum stroke volume and best level of cardiac output. Such manipulations must be performed with knowledge of their effect on myocardial oxygen supply/demand balance.

Manipulation of Preload

Preload can be increased by volume infusion or venoconstriction and decreased by diuresis, venodilatation, or increased stroke volume. The proper left ventricular filling pressure postoperatively is determined by the preoperative state of the ventricle, the operation, and other factors. Some ventricles are stiff or noncompliant and require high filling pressures in order to attain a satisfactory diastolic volume, such as the markedly hypertrophied ventricle associated with aortic stenosis. The preoperative atrial and ventricular end-diastolic pressures can indicate what pressure might be required in the postoperative period in such a ventricle. In most hearts, however, filling pressures should not exceed 15 mm Hg in either the right or left ventricle unless preoperative evidence of decreased myocardial compliance is present. Filling pressures over 15 mm Hg in hearts with normal compliance do not result in improved cardiac output.[18]

Hypovolemia is deficient preload and is a frequent cause of decreased cardiac output following cardiac surgery. Hypovolemia is diagnosed by abnormally low atrial pressures and may by corroborated by absence of pulmonary venous engorgement on chest x-ray. It is treated by volume replacement and is usually the most easily treated cause of low cardiac output.

Manipulation of Afterload

Afterload reduction can improve cardiac output and myocardial performance in the postoperative period.[1,6,19,22,42] Systemic vascular resistance is often elevated following cardiopulmonary bypass.[28,34] Vasodilators reduce systemic vascular resistance and improve cardiac output. Benzing and co-workers[5] studied the effects of nitroprusside immediately after open heart surgery in 11 children who had a cardiac index below 2.0 L/min/m². Left atrial pressure was maintained around 15 cm H_2O. During infusion of nitroprusside, systemic vascular resistance decreased 54%, mean arterial pressure decreased 19%, and cardiac index increased 77%. Bixler and colleagues[6] found improved cardiac output following nitroprusside infusion in adult patients with postoperative left ventricular failure.

Drugs that improve myocardial contractility, such as dopamine, may be combined with nitroprusside for further improvement in myocardial performance.[27] When nitroprusside and dopamine are administered together for treatment of severe chronic congestive heart failure, the increase in cardiac output can be significantly greater than with either agent alone.[40]

Manipulation of Myocardial Contractility

Choice of Inotropic Drug

The administration of inotropic drugs increases the force and extent of myocardial fiber shortening, resulting in improved emptying of the ventricle with each beat, thereby improving cardiac output. The ideal inotropic drug would increase myocardial contractility and would not affect heart rate, cause cardiac rhythm disturbances, or increase peripheral resistance. Such an ideal inotropic agent does not presently exist. As a result, there are several drugs from which to choose, each with a somewhat different spectrum of action.

Dopamine, a naturally occurring catecholamine that is a precursor of norepinephrine, and dobutamine, a synthetic sympathomimetic amine,[44] are the two most appropriate inotropic agents at present in most clinical situations. Dopamine does not possess the disturbing chronotropic and arrhythmogenic effects of isoproterenol,[39] although dopamine may produce tachycardia and elevations in peripheral vascular resistances, especially at higher dosages.[37] Dopamine and epinephrine have similar hemodynamic effects, except on the kidneys. Dopamine increases renal blood flow, glomerular filtration rate, and sodium excretion.[36] It increases urine flow, whereas epinephrine causes a decrease in urine flow.[41]

Dobutamine increases cardiac output, usually with a decrease in left ventricular pressure and systemic vascular resistance.[11,15,38] Dobutamine maintains a satisfactory myocardial oxygen supply/demand ratio (as discussed in the following section), probably through improved myocardial energetics and an increase in myocardial blood flow.[9,14,45]

The choice of dopamine or dobutamine should be based on the hemodynamics and clinical condition of the individual patient. A patient with a low systemic vascular resistance and renal impairment would be better treated with dopamine, whereas a patient with elevated pulmonary or systemic vascular resistance would be better treated with dobutamine. Dopamine and dobutamine can also be used in combination.

Amrinone, a phosphodiesterase-III inhibitor, is a newer drug that increases cardiac output.[4,10] Amrinone increases cardiac output by increasing myocardial contractility and lowering systemic vascular resistance and does not cause an increase in heart rate.[3,13] Amrinone can also lower pulmonary vascular resistance and may be especially useful in patients with elevated pulmonary vascular resistance.[35]

Metabolic Effects of Inotropic Drugs

Inotropic agents cause an increase in myocardial oxygen demand, and this increased demand must be met by increased myocardial blood flow, or myocardial ischemia and necrosis can occur. Myocardial oxygen demand must be weighed against myocardial blood flow to determine whether a proper balance exists. If an imbalance of myocardial oxygen supply/demand exists in spite of the use of inotropic agents and afterload-reducing agents, mechanical circulatory support should be instituted.

Inotropic drugs usually increase myocardial oxygen demand by increasing heart rate, increasing ventricular wall tension, and increasing myocardial contractility. This increase in oxygen demand should be met by an increase in oxygen supply. Clinical assessment of coronary blood flow is necessary in order to assure adequate oxygen supply.

The main determinants of myocardial blood flow are the diastolic pressure gradient across the myocardium (arterial diastolic pressure minus ventricular diastolic pressure) and the time of diastole. These determinants have been described as the diastolic pressure-time index (DPTI).[8] Myocardial blood flow is therefore decreased by decreased diastolic arterial pressure, increased ventricular diastolic pressure, and increased heart rate. As myocardial blood flow decreases, the subendocardial area is affected first, with subsequent involvement of the midmyocardial and subepicardial layers. Ventricular hypertrophy and coronary artery disease can be additional factors impairing coronary blood flow.

Indications for Intraaortic Balloon Counterpulsation

Institution of mechanical circulatory support is required if an abnormal myocardial oxygen supply/demand balance exists either in spite of or because of the use of inotropic drugs. The most definitive method of determining the myocardial oxygen supply/demand balance is evaluation of myocardial lactate metabolism by arterial blood and coronary sinus lactate analysis. Lack of myocardial lactate production indicates a satisfactory myocardial oxygen supply/demand balance. Coronary sinus lactate sampling, however, is not possible in the usual clinical setting. Other more indirect methods of determining myocardial oxygen supply/demand balance are therefore required.

A ratio of myocardial oxygen supply as indicated by the DPTI and oxygen demand as indicated by the systolic pressure-time index has been recommended as a measurement of the adequacy of subendocardial perfusion.[31,32] This ratio has been termed the endocardial viability ratio (EVR) and can be calculated using a computer. An EVR over 0.8 is reported as indicating a satisfactory myocardial oxygen supply/demand balance.

It is likely that simpler methods of assessing myocardial metabolism can be used in the absence of coronary artery disease in order to determine the need for intraaortic balloon pumping (IABP). The following physiologic parameters are indicative of an adequate left ventricular myocardial blood flow: (1) diastolic arterial pressure over 75 mm Hg, (2) left atrial pressure below 20 mm Hg, and (3) heart rate below 110. Attaining these levels of blood pressure, atrial pressure, and heart rate by utilizing an inotropic drug, possibly in combination with a vasodilator agent, is not likely to cause subendocardial ischemia. On the other hand, if normal arterial pressures are achieved with pharmacologic support but atrial pressure or heart rate remains high, a myocardial oxygen supply/demand disparity is likely to exist and IABP should be instituted.

IABP frequently improves systemic perfusion, coronary blood flow, and myocardial metabolism.[12,23] Decreased afterload lowers myocardial oxygen demand. Increased arterial diastolic pressure improves myocardial blood flow and oxygen supply. IABP may also decrease ventricular diastolic pressure, further improving myocardial oxygen supply.

IABP is a valuable advance in the management of poor cardiac output secondary to depressed myocardial performance.[24] It has a particularly important role in the management of low cardiac output in patients with associated coronary artery disease. Beyond intraaortic balloon pumping is another plane of therapy using ventricular assist devices.

Technique of Intraaortic Balloon Insertion

The intraaortic balloon is usually inserted into the common femoral artery and advanced into the descending aorta (Fig. 8–1). Percutaneous placement has largely replaced the earlier method of surgical insertion.[7] Aortoiliac or femoral artery atherosclerosis may preclude use of the femoral artery. Alternative sites of insertion have been described, including the ascending aorta[16,17,20] and the subclavian artery.[26]

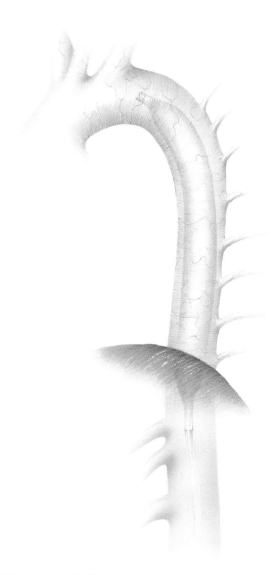

Figure 8–1 Balloon in ascending aorta.

Placement of the intraaortic balloon in the femoral artery can result in major vascular complications, requiring removal of the balloon as well as thrombectomy, repair of the artery, or repair of false aneurysm.[25,29,43]

References

1. Appelbaum A, Blackstone EH, Kouchoukos NT, Kirklin JW: Afterload reduction and cardiac output in infants early after intracardiac surgery. Am J Cardiol 39: 445,1977.
2. Armstrong PW, Gold HK, Buckley JM, Willerson JT, Sanders CA: Hemodynamic evaluation of rate augmentation produced by atrial pacing and isoproterenol in the early postoperative phase of cardiac valve surgery. Circulation 44:649,1971.
3. Benotti JR, Grossman W, Braunwald E, Carabello BA: Effects of amrinone on myocardial energy metabolism and hemodynamics in patients with severe congestive heart failure due to coronary artery disease. Circulation 62:28,1980.
4. Benotti JR, Grossman W, Braunwald E, Davolos DD, Alousi AA: Hemodynamic assessment of amrinone: a new inotropic agent. N Engl J Med 299:1373,1978.
5. Benzing G, Helmsworth JA, Schrieber JT, Loggie J, Kaplan S: Nitroprusside after open-heart surgery. Circulation 54:467,1976.

6. Bixler TJ, Gardner TJ, Donahoo JS, Brawley RK, Potter A, Gott VL: Improved myocardial performance in postoperative cardiac surgical patients with sodium nitroprusside. Ann Thorac Surg 25:444,1978.

7. Bregman D, Casarella WJ: Percutaneous intraaortic balloon pumping: initial clinical experience. Ann Thorac Surg 29:153,1980.

8. Buckberg GD, Fixler DE, Archie JP: Experimental subendocardial ischemia in dogs with normal coronary arteries. Circ Res 30:67,1972.

9. Chatterjee K: Effects of dobutamine on coronary hemodynamics and myocardial energetics. *In* Chatterjee K (ed): Dobutamine: A Ten-Year Review. New York, NCM Publishers Inc, 1989, pp 49–67.

10. Colucci WS, Wright RF, Braunwald E: New positive inotropic agents in the treatment of congestive heart failure: mechanisms of action and recent clinical developments. N Engl J Med 314:349,1986.

11. DiSesa VJ, Gold JP, Shemin RJ, Collins JJ Jr, Cohn LH: Comparison of dopamine and dobutamine in patients requiring postoperative circulatory support. Clin Cardiol 9:253,1986.

12. Dunkman WB, Leinbach RC, Buckley MJ, Mundth ED, Kantrowitz AR, Austen WG, Sanders CA: Clinical and hemodynamic results of intra-aortic balloon pumping and surgery for cardiogenic shock. Circulation 46:465,1972.

13. Dupuis J-Y, Bondy R, Cattran C, Nathan HJ, Wynands JE: Amrinone and dobutamine as primary treatment of low cardiac output syndrome following coronary artery surgery: a comparison of their effects on hemodynamics and outcome. J Cardiothorac Vasc Anesth 6:542,1992.

14. Fowler MB, Alderman EL, Oesterle SN, Derby G, Daughters GT, Stinson EB, Ingels NB, Mitchell RS, Miller DC: Dobutamine and dopamine after cardiac surgery: greater augmentation of myocardial blood flow with dobutamine. Circulation 70(Suppl I):I-103,1984.

15. Goldstein RA, Passamani ER, Roberts R: A comparison of digoxin and dobutamine in patients with acute infarction and cardiac failure. N Engl J Med 303:846, 1980.

16. Gueldner TL, Lawrence GH: Intra-aortic balloon assist through cannulation of the ascending aorta. Ann Thorac Surg 19:88,1975.

17. Hazelrigg SR, Auer JE, Seifert PE: Experience in 100 transthoracic balloon pumps. Ann Thorac Surg 54:528,1992.

18. Kouchoukos NT, Kirklin JW, Sheppard LC, Roe P: Effect of elevation of left atrial pressure by blood infusion on stroke volume early after cardiac operations. Surg Forum 22:126,1971.

19. Kouchoukos NT, Sheppard LC, Kirklin JW: Effect of alterations in arterial pressure on cardiac performance early after open intracardiac operations. J Thorac Cardiovasc Surg 64:563,1972.

20. Krause AH, Bigelow JC Jr, Page S: Transthoracic intra-aortic balloon cannulation to avoid repeat sternotomy for removal. Ann Thorac Surg 21:562,1976.

21. Kreulen TH, Bove AA, McDonough MT, Sands MJ, Spann JF: The evaluation of left ventricular function in man: a comparison of methods. Circulation 51: 677,1975.

22. Lappas DG, Ohtaka M, Fahmy NR, Buckley MJ: Systemic and pulmonary effects of nitroprusside during mitral valve replacement in patients with mitral regurgitation. Circulation 58(Suppl I):I-18,1978.

23. Leinbach RC, Buckley MJ, Austen WG, Petschek HE, Kantrowitz AR, Sanders CA: Effects of intra-aortic balloon pumping on coronary flow and metabolism in man. Circulation 43,44(Suppl I):I-77,1971.

24. Maccioli GA, Lucas WJ, Norfleet EA: The intra-aortic balloon pump: a review. J Cardiothorac Anesth 2:365,1988.

25. Martin RS, Moncure AC, Buckley MJ, Austen WG, Akins C, Leinback RC: Complications of percutaneous intra-aortic balloon insertion. J Thorac Cardiovasc Surg 85:186,1983.

26. Mayer JH: Subclavian artery approach for insertion of intra-aortic balloon. J Thorac Surg 76:61,1978.

27. Miller RR, Awan NA, Joye JA, Maxwell KS, DeMaria AN, Amsterdam EA, Mason DT: Combined dopamine and nitroprusside therapy in congestive heart failure: greater augmentation of cardiac performance by addition of inotropic stimulation to afterload reduction. Circulation 55:881,1977.

28. Parr FVS, Blackstone EH, Kirklin JW: Cardiac performance and mortality early after intra-cardiac surgery in infants and young children. Circulation 51:867,1975.

29. Perler BA, McCabe CJ, Abbott WM, Buckley MJ: Vascular complications of intra-aortic balloon counterpulsation. Arch Surg 118:957,1983.

30. Peterson KL, Uther JB, Shabetai R, Braunwald E: Assessment of left ventricular performance in man. Circulation 47:924,1973.

31. Phillips PA, Bregman D: Intraoperative application of intra-aortic balloon counterpulsation determined by clinical monitoring of the endocardial viability ratio. Ann Thorac Surg 23:45,1977.

32. Phillips PA, Marty AT, Miyamoto AM: A clinical method for detecting subendocardial ischemia after cardiopulmonary bypass. J Thorac Cardiovasc Surg 69: 30,1975.

33. Rackley CE: Quantitative evaluation of left ventricular function by radiographic techniques. Circulation 54:862,1976.

34. Roberts AJ, Niarchos AP, Subramanian VA, Abel RM, Hoover EL, McCabe JC, Case DB, Laragh JH, Gay WA Jr: Hypertension following coronary artery bypass graft surgery. Comparison of hemodynamic responses to nitroprusside, phentolamine, and converting enzyme inhibitor. Circulation 58(Suppl I):I-43,1977.

35. Robinson BW, Gelband H, Mas MS: Selective pulmonary and systemic vasodilator effects of amrinone in children: new therapeutic implications. J Am Coll Cardiol 21:1461,1993.

36. Rosenblum R, Tai AR, Lawson D: Dopamine in man: cardiorenal hemodynamics in normotensive patients with heart disease. J Pharmacol Exp Ther 183:256,1972.

37. Salomon NW, Plachetka JR, Copeland JG: Comparison of dopamine and dobutamine following coronary artery bypass grafting. Ann Thorac Surg 33:48,1982.

38. Sethna DH, Gray RJ, Moffitt EA, Bussell JA, Raymond MJ, Conklin CM, Matloff JM: Dobutamine and cardiac oxygen balance in patients following myocardial revascularization. Anesth Analg 61:917,1982.

39. Steen PA, Tinker JH, Pluth JR, Barnhorst DA, Tarhan S: Efficacy of dopamine, dobutamine, and epinephrine during emergence from cardiopulmonary bypass in man. Circulation 57:378,1978.

40. Stemple DR, Kleiman JH, Harrison DC: Combined nitroprusside-dopamine therapy in severe chronic congestive heart failure. Dose-related hemodynamic advantages over single drug infusions. Am J Cardiol 42:267,1978.

41. Stephenson LW, Blackstone EH, Kouchoukos NT: Dopamine vs epinephrine in patients following cardiac surgery: randomized study. Surg Forum 27:727,1976.

42. Stinson EB, Holloway EL, Derby GC, Copeland JG, Oyer PE, Beuhler DL, Griepp RB: Control of myocardial performance early after open-heart operations by vasodilator treatment. J Thorac Cardiovasc Surg 73:523,1977.

43. Todd GJ, Bregman D, Voorhees AB, Reemtsma K: Vascular complications associated with percutaneous intra-aortic balloon pumping. Arch Surg 118:963,1983.

44. Tuttle RR, Mills HL: Dobutamine. Development of a new catecholamine to selectively increase cardiac contractility. Circ Res 36:185,1975.

45. Van Trigt P, Spray TL, Pasque MK, Peyton RB, Pellom GL, Wechsler AS: The comparative effects of dopamine and dobutamine on ventricular mechanics after coronary artery bypass grafting: a pressure-dimension analysis. Circulation 70(Suppl I):I-112,1984.

9

Coronary Artery Surgery

The development of direct coronary artery surgery by Favaloro[47] and Johnson[73] is one of the outstanding achievements in the history of cardiac surgery. Properly performed coronary artery bypass results in immediate and predictable improvement in myocardial blood flow in the majority of patients.[93,103,121] This increase in myocardial blood flow results in alleviation of anginal symptoms, increased exercise tolerance, freedom from medications, and overall improvement in the quality of life. In many patients coronary bypass clearly improves survival.

The 1970s saw a great expansion in coronary artery surgery, accompanied by improvements in anesthesia, myocardial preservation, and surgical technique. The 1980s saw the advent of percutaneous transluminal coronary angioplasty (PTCA),[63] which has greatly affected the patient mix coming to surgery, with patients who have less severe disease undergoing PTCA instead of surgery. Other factors, such as the aging population and the growing number of patients who have had coronary bypass surgery, have caused a continuing trend toward patients coming to surgery who are older, have more extensive coronary disease, worse ventricular function, more severe coexistent medical problems, and a higher likelihood of having had a previous coronary operation.[34,74,82,116] Coronary artery surgeons in the 1990s will find increasing numbers of these more complex and challenging patients.

In this chapter we review coronary anatomy, present our indications for surgery in the various anatomic and clinical subsets of coronary disease, discuss our operative strategy and techniques in detail, and review the results that can be achieved with the proper performance of coronary surgery.

Coronary Artery Anatomy

The most frequently occurring anatomy is described in this section. Many variations in coronary anatomy exist; these have been exhaustively described by McAlpine.[107]

Right Coronary Artery

The right coronary artery arises from the anterior aorta and courses in the atrioventricular groove around the margin of the right ventricle (Fig. 9–1). It usually bifurcates at the junction of the right and left atria and the interventricular septum (the crux) into the posterior descending branch and a distal posterolateral branch. The posterior descending artery courses down the pos-

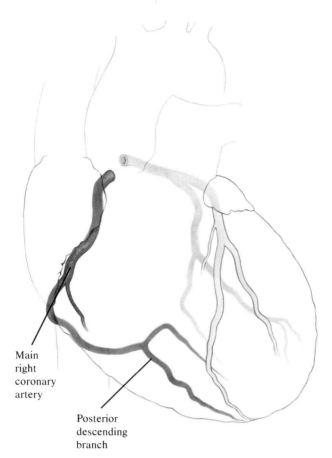

Main
right
coronary
artery

Posterior
descending
branch

Figure 9–1 Right coronary artery.

terior interventricular septum, supplying blood to the inferior portion of the ventricular septum.

The posterior descending artery comes from the right coronary artery in approximately 90% of cases, an anatomic pattern referred to as *right dominant*. The posterior descending can arise from the circumflex coronary artery, a pattern referred to as *left dominant*, or there can be two posterior descending arteries, one from the right coronary artery and one from the circumflex coronary artery, a pattern referred to as *balanced*. These terms are somewhat misleading, since the right coronary artery almost never supplies the majority of left ventricular blood flow.

The most common site of obstructive atherosclerosis in the right coronary artery is in the proximal portion, before it passes around the margin of the right ventricle. A common site of distal anastomosis is just before the bifurcation at the crux. Disease also frequently occurs at the bifurcation. In the presence of disease at the bifurcation, we perform bypass to the posterior descending artery, avoiding endarterectomy whenever possible.

Occasionally the right coronary artery has large posterior lateral branches supplying the posterior wall of the left ventricle. If large posterior lateral branches of the right coronary artery require bypass, they are approached like either posterior descending arteries or obtuse marginal arteries, with the vein being brought around the right side of the heart or the left side, as anatomy dictates. If both the posterior descending and posterolateral branches need to be bypassed, a sequential graft can be used.

Left Main Coronary Artery

The left main coronary artery arises from the posterior portion of the aortic root. The left main coronary artery is usually about 2 cm in length, bifurcating

Figure 9–2 Left anterior descending coronary artery.

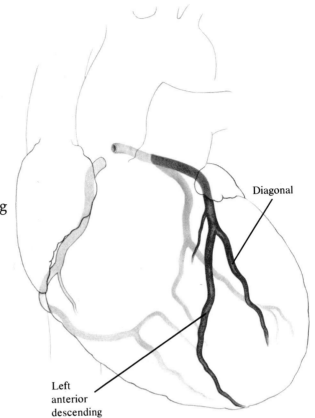

Diagonal

Left
anterior
descending

into the left anterior descending and circumflex coronary arteries. The left main coronary artery can be the site of significant stenosis—this anatomic subset of coronary disease carries the worst prognosis in terms of survival without surgery.[35,144] The left main coronary artery is not directly grafted because it is inaccessible without dividing the aorta or pulmonary artery. Grafts are placed to the left anterior descending and obtuse marginal coronary arteries for treatment of left main stenosis.

Left Anterior Descending Coronary Artery

The left anterior descending coronary artery courses around the pulmonary artery and follows the anterior interventricular groove to the apex, giving off numerous branches to the ventricular septum, as well as a variable number of diagonal branches, which pass laterally over the anterior wall of the left ventricle (Fig. 9–2). The left anterior descending coronary artery and its branches supply blood to the interventricular septum and anterior wall, constituting approximately 50% of total left ventricular blood flow.

The left anterior descending is the most frequently diseased coronary artery. The distal anastomosis on the left anterior descending coronary artery is usually placed from the midpoint on. Diagonal branches that are 1–1.5 mm in diameter or larger, have proximal stenoses, or are compromised by left anterior descending artery stenoses before and after their origin are also bypassed.

Circumflex Coronary Artery

The circumflex coronary artery courses in the atrioventricular groove beneath the left atrial appendage, around the lateral aspect of the left ventricle, to

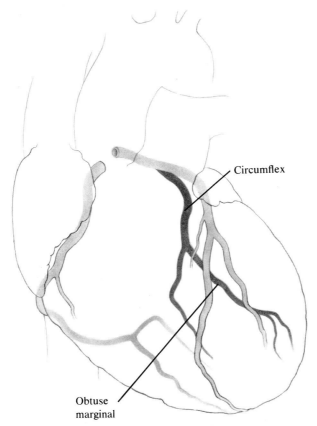

Circumflex

Figure 9–3 Circumflex coronary artery.

Obtuse
marginal

the posterior atrioventricular groove, giving off a variable number of obtuse marginal branches which supply the lateral and inferior walls of the left ventricle (Fig. 9–3). The circumflex artery is usually located below the great cardiac vein and a layer of fat and is difficult or dangerous to approach directly in the atrioventricular groove. For this reason the circumflex artery system is bypassed by placing grafts to obtuse marginal branches. Obtuse marginals frequently have proximal stenoses.

Tertiary Left Main Coronary Artery Branch

In a small number of cases the left main coronary artery trifurcates. The artery between the left anterior descending and circumflex has been called the ramus medianus, ramus marginalis, and ramus medialis. Knowledge of the anatomy of this vessel is important, since it can be a large vessel supplying a large area of lateral left ventricle. The ramus passes anterior to the left atrial appendage, is usually subepicardial for its first few centimeters, then is often covered by a thin layer of myocardium. It is frequently 2 mm or more in diameter. The unusual submyocardial location can make the ramus difficult to locate, but it should be sought and bypassed whenever it is stenotic and of sufficient size.

Coronary Arteriography

Selective coronary arteriography, as developed by Sones[139] and modified by Judkins,[75] provides the means of accurately diagnosing the presence and extent of coronary artery disease. Selective coronary arteriography has made possible the modern era of coronary artery surgery and can be performed at extremely low risk.[37] It can demonstrate the extent, severity, and location of coronary artery stenoses and the quality and size of the distal coronary arteries.[132] Ventriculography demonstrates the global and segmental function of the left ventricle. Proper assessment of the location and severity of arterial stenosis, the size and quality of the distal vessel, and the ventricular function is necessary to determine operability, operative risk, and probability of operative result.[92]

Coronary arteriography has limitations, as does any radiographic study. There is considerable observer variability in the interpretation of arteriograms,[42,157] and misinterpretation may occur, particularly underestimation of the severity of stenosis.[70,150] Recognition of the limitations and pitfalls of coronary arteriography is important in making clinical and operative decisions.

Indications for Coronary Arteriography

We believe the indications for coronary arteriography should be broad, since information gained about coronary anatomy is vital to the proper management of patients. The clinical manifestation of angina may correlate poorly with the severity of the disease and the patient's prognosis. Noninvasive techniques are useful, but not as accurate as arteriography, in determining the severity of disease.

Angina pectoris is the main indication for coronary arteriography and it is also often indicated in acute myocardial infarction. Postinfarction angina, recurrent infarction, resistant ventricular arrhythmias, and moderate hemodynamic instability may all be benefited by surgery. Coronary arteriography should be performed in patients over 40 years of age with valvular disease. It

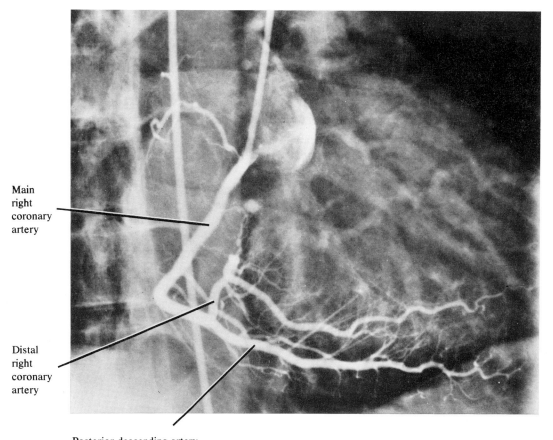

Main
right
coronary
artery

Distal
right
coronary
artery

Posterior descending artery

Figure 9-4 Right coronary artery, right anterior oblique projection.

may also be indicated in the asymptomatic patient with a positive stress test or strong family history for coronary artery disease and sudden death, in the postoperative evaluation of coronary artery surgery, and in the evaluation of atypical chest pain.

Ventriculogram

A ventriculogram is performed before selective injection of the coronary arteries. The ventriculogram is performed first because selective arteriography can reduce ventricular function.[37] We use the right anterior oblique projection to compute the ejection fraction. The ventriculogram is also analyzed to determine areas of segmental wall motion abnormalities. Nitroglycerin may be given and a repeat ventriculogram performed to detect changes in wall motion. Improvement of wall motion following nitroglycerin administration has been correlated with improvement following bypass surgery.[33]

Right Coronary Arteriogram

The right anterior oblique (RAO) projection (Fig. 9–4) and the left anterior oblique (LAO) projection (Fig. 9–5) are both good for visualizing the proximal portion of the right coronary artery. The LAO view provides a better view of the distal artery and the bifurcation. In the presence of an occluded proximal right coronary artery, the distal artery and branches may be visualized via collaterals. The right coronary artery may be filled by collaterals from the distal circumflex or from the left anterior descending via septal perforators or

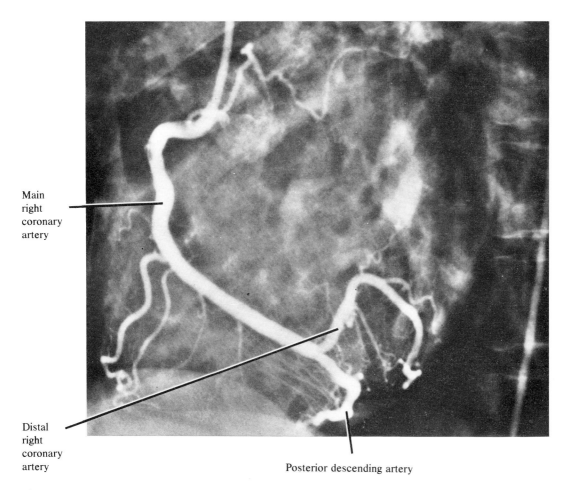

Main right coronary artery

Distal right coronary artery

Posterior descending artery

Figure 9–5 Right coronary artery, left anterior oblique projection.

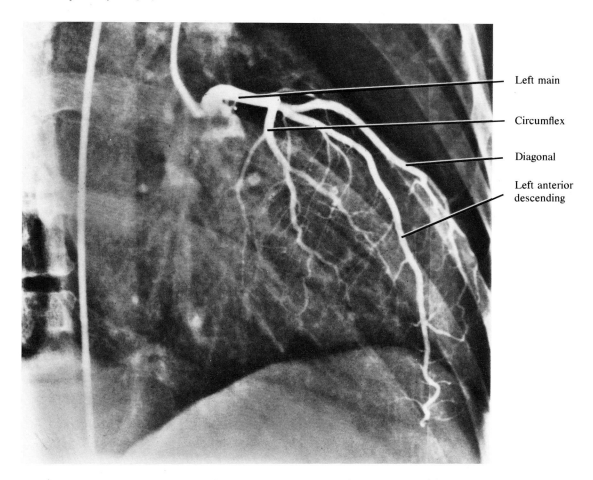

Left main

Circumflex

Diagonal

Left anterior
descending

Figure 9–6 Left coronary artery, right anterior oblique projection.

by connection around the apex. Visualization of an occluded right coronary artery via collaterals often gives good indication that a vessel suitable for operation will be found at the time of surgery.

Left Coronary Arteriogram

The left main coronary artery is usually seen best in the RAO projection (Fig. 9–6). The left anterior descending (LAD) is seen best in the RAO projection, and most stenoses can be accurately determined from this view (Fig. 9–7). Stenoses in the most proximal portion of the LAD can be obscured by overlying diagonal branches or the proximal circumflex. The LAO projection may clarify the extent of disease in the proximal LAD. Other views have been recommended for assessment of the proximal LAD.[140]

Determination of the status of the distal vessel beyond an occluded LAD is an important matter. There are several strong indicators of distal vessel operability: (1) the distal vessel fills via collaterals, (2) there is good anterior wall motion on ventriculogram, and (3) there is no evidence of an anteroseptal infarction on the electrocardiogram.

The portion of the circumflex system most frequently diseased is seen best in the RAO projection (Fig. 9–8). The RAO view also shows the obtuse marginal branches well. The relative positions of multiple obtuse marginal branches should be carefully noted so that the proper branches are bypassed at the time of surgery.

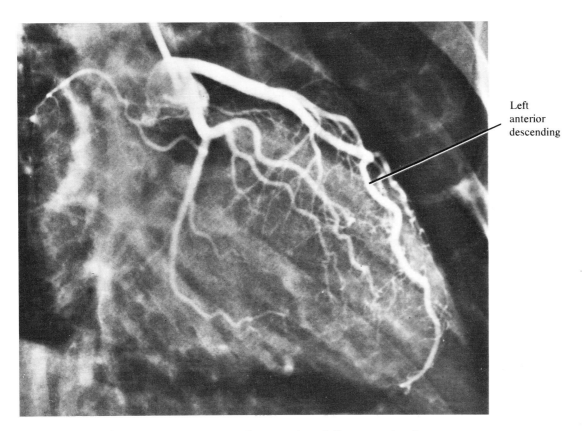

Left
anterior
descending

Figure 9–7 Left coronary artery, right anterior oblique projection.

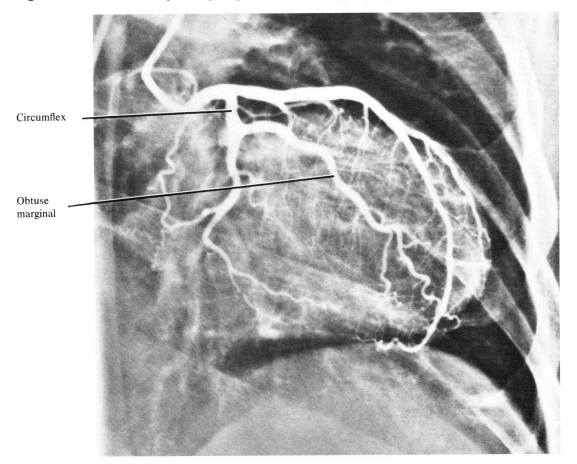

Circumflex

Obtuse
marginal

Figure 9–8 Left coronary artery, right anterior oblique projection.

Noninvasive Methods of Diagnosis of Coronary Artery Disease

Exercise Stress Test

Electrocardiographic monitoring during progressive exercise is a valuable technique for assessing myocardial ischemia. A positive test (ST-segment depression more than 1 mm) can indicate severe coronary artery disease.[44] Marked ST-segment depression[57] or hypotension[71,147] during exercise indicates the presence of very severe coronary artery disease, such as left main stenosis or triple-vessel disease. Markedly positive tests are associated with poor prognosis with medical treatment only. The exercise test must be kept in proper perspective in the overall diagnosis of ischemic heart disease. A positive test does not always indicate coronary artery disease, and a negative test does not always exclude its presence.[153]

Nuclear Cardiology

There is widespread use of radionuclides for diagnosis of cardiac disease and assessment of ventricular function. Myocardial blood flow can be assessed using thallium perfusion scans.[10,130] The presence of an acute myocardial infarction can be determined with radioactive pyrophosphate. Regional and global ventricular function can be studied.[23]

Echocardiography

Echocardiography is valuable for the evaluation of ventricular function and wall motion. Stress echocardiography can detect regional wall motion abnormalities brought on by exercise or the use of dopamine or dipyridamole. Stress echocardiography can be valuable in the diagnosis of coronary artery disease and to assess prognosis after myocardial infarction.[7,40]

Positron Emission Tomography

Positron emission tomography (PET) provides information on myocardial perfusion, metabolism, and cell membrane function through the use of radionuclides nitrogen-13-ammonia, rubidium-82, and fluoro-18-deoxyglucose.[58] PET is valuable in the diagnosis of coronary artery disease and especially valuable in identifying injured but viable myocardium potentially salvageable by revascularization.[19,43,58,135]

Indications for Surgery

Consideration of indications for surgical treatment of ischemic heart disease requires definition of what can and should be achieved with contemporary coronary bypass surgery in relation to what can be achieved with medical therapy or PTCA or other interventional techniques. All therapies must be examined in terms of their effectiveness and durability in (1) relieving angina pectoris, (2) preventing myocardial damage and serious ventricular arrhythmias, and (3) preventing cardiac death.

It should be emphasized that surgical treatment, interventional procedures, and medical treatment of myocardial ischemia are not competitive; they are often complementary. Coronary atherosclerosis is a relentless disease, and the myocardial ischemia produced can require medical treatment throughout its course, or intermittently during its course, in spite of properly timed and properly performed coronary surgery. Proper application and timing of PTCA is also of great value in the management of coronary artery disease.[81]

It is important to define properly performed coronary bypass surgery. Elective or urgent coronary artery surgery in patients with suitable distal vessels (1.5 mm or more in diameter and mild or no atherosclerotic involvement distally), suitable ventricular function (ejection fraction over 25%), and no major associated disease, should result in operative mortality below 2%, perioperative infarction rate below 5%, and a late graft patency rate of 80% or better.[55,76,99,122] If these results are achieved, we believe careful analysis of the available data supports surgery as the initial treatment of choice in a number of subsets of ischemic heart disease.

Chronic Stable Angina

A common indication for coronary artery bypass is chronic angina. Surgery provides effective, predictable relief of angina in the vast majority of patients.[55]

Unstable Angina

There are a number of anginal syndromes that lie between stable angina and myocardial infarction. These syndromes range from mere increase in the frequency of anginal attacks to a severe syndrome of prolonged pain occurring at rest, often unresponsive to any treatment except narcotics—a clinical pattern initially indistinguishable from acute myocardial infarction, yet without subsequent development of electrocardiographic and enzymatic changes diagnostic of myocardial necrosis. The milder syndrome has been called progressive or accelerated angina. The more severe syndrome has been called acute coronary insufficiency, intermediate syndrome, preinfarction angina, and unstable angina.

Rigid definition of unstable angina is necessary in the design of study protocols in order to avoid comparing dissimilar populations. Such a rigid definition has been given by the National Cooperative Study Group on Unstable Angina Pectoris[115]: angina of sufficient severity to warrant admission to an intensive care unit to rule out myocardial infarction and the occurrence of transient electrographic changes, with ST-T segment and/or T-wave changes, during episodes of pain.

Broader definitions of unstable angina are in general clinical use. The usual basic criterion is angina of such severity that the patient is admitted to a coronary care unit because of strong suspicion of acute myocardial infarction. Those patients who respond quickly to bed rest have been classified as having ''low-risk'' unstable angina. Those patients who continue to have pain at rest with reversible electrocardiographic changes have been classified as having ''high-risk'' unstable angina.[120]

Patients with the suspicion of acute myocardial infarction should be admitted to a coronary care unit and treated with bed rest and sedation. Approximately 50% of these patients will have no further pain during hospitalization.[120] Electrocardiographic and enzymatic studies should be performed to exclude acute myocardial infarction. Hypertension or congestive heart failure should be treated.

Aggressive medical management will result in control of angina in almost all patients. Half the patients still having angina after bed rest will have complete relief, and the other half will show marked improvement in the frequency and severity of their angina.[115,120]

Intraaortic balloon pumping has also been recommended for treatment of unstable angina and in one report[85] was used in 58% of patients who did not respond rapidly to medical treatment. Other reports[115,120] have not supported such frequent use of balloon pumping, and in our experience patients requiring balloon pumping amount to fewer than 1% of patients hospitalized with unstable angina.

Following medical stabilization of patients, elective coronary arteriography should be performed. Decision regarding surgery or PTCA can then be made on the basis of the clinical picture and the anatomic findings. Patients who have left main stenosis and those who have been on maximal medical therapy prior to hospitalization should undergo revascularization during the same hospitalization. Patients belonging to other anatomic subgroups can be discharged, with determination regarding surgery being made at a later time.

The National Cooperative study of 288 patients randomized as to medical or surgical therapy (with left main stenosis and failures of previous medical therapy excluded) showed that a large percentage of patients managed medically will require later surgery to relieve unacceptable angina.[115] Only 3% of the patients randomized to medical therapy required surgery during the initial hospitalization, but 13% resorted to surgery by 6 months, 19% by 1 year, and 31% by 2 years. The subsequent need for surgery did not correlate with the severity of the presenting angina or the type of electrocardiographic changes during pain. There was strong correlation between subsequent need for surgery and anatomic extent of disease, with 49% of patients with three-vessel disease requiring later surgery.

Surgical therapy during or following unstable angina results in better relief than medical therapy.[77,115,136] Surgical therapy also is associated with excellent survival. Survival in the surgical group in the Cooperative Study was 90% at 24 months in spite of an initial surgical mortality of 5%. Olinger and co-workers[120] reported no late deaths up to 30 months following surgery in a series of 53 patients who met the criteria of the Cooperative Study.

Aggressive medical therapy followed by properly performed elective surgery can result in a surgical mortality below 2% and a perioperative infarction rate below 2%.[77,115] We believe that contemporary medical treatment combined with surgery is an excellent method of managing unstable angina. It is likely that further improvements in anesthetic mangement, myocardial preservation, and operative technique will give even better results following surgical treatment of unstable angina.

Acute Myocardial Infarction

The treatment of acute myocardial infarction has been greatly affected by the advent of thrombolysis and coronary angioplasty.[90,131] The role of coronary artery bypass continues to evolve. Coronary artery bypass during the phase of acute myocardial infarction has been recommended for the following conditions: (1) uncomplicated infarction, (2) infarction with extension, (3) subendocardial infarction, (4) infarction with persistent angina, (5) infarction with refractory ventricular arrhythmias, and (6) infarction with hemodynamic impairment or cardiogenic shock.

Patients who have a clinically uncomplicated acute myocardial infarction—no recurrent pain, hemodynamic abnormality, nor rhythm disturbance—are at very low risk of in-hospital death,[50] about 1%. Although surgery has been recommended in this group of patients,[11] it can be justified only if it can be performed with a mortality of 1% or less. In addition, it should be shown that surgery either salvages "jeopardized" myocardium[138] which would otherwise progress to necrosis or improves survival when compared with no subsequent surgery or surgery performed following recovery from acute myocardial infarction. Although surgery can be performed during the acute phase of myocardial infarction without operative mortality, its role in uncomplicated acute myocardial infarction has not been defined and awaits further investigation. We do not recommend surgery during the acute phase of an uncomplicated myocardial infarction.

Acute myocardial infarction with extension is a potential indication for coronary bypass.[126] The medical methods available for control of infarct size[110] may not be sufficient to prevent continuing myocardial necrosis, as indicated by recurrent elevations of cardiac-specific enzymes. Institution of intraaortic balloon pumping may favorably affect the continuing myocardial oxygen supply/demand imbalance.[91] Surgery may also be valuable in salvaging threatened myocardium in this unstable form of acute myocardial infarction. At present, we would recommend coronary arteriography if infarct extension is occurring in the face of optimal medical management and if suitable coronary anatomy is found.

Surgery during subendocardial infarction has been recommended and should be performed if there is an unstable angina pattern. The presence of subendocardial infarction does not affect operative mortality.[101] Subendocardial infarction that is uncomplicated during initial hospitalization is associated with a high incidence of subsequent unstable angina and transmural infarction following hospitalization. Madigan and co-workers[102] reported 50 consecutive patients followed after subendocardial myocardial infarction, with a mean follow-up of 11 months. There was a 46% incidence of unstable angina, and 21% developed another myocardial infarction.

Postinfarction angina is associated with a poor hospital prognosis.[15,111,141] Bypass during this unstable phase of myocardial infarction can be performed with very low operative mortality and excellent late results.[6,53,78,84] We recommend arteriography and surgery or PTCA for postinfarction angina.

Acute myocardial infarction with cardiogenic shock is a lethal combination. Surgery for mechanical defects such as ventricular septal defect[16] and acute mitral insufficiency secondary to papillary muscle rupture[112] is well established. Coronary bypass surgery in association with mechanical circulatory support is advocated by some[112] but can be associated with an operative mortality in the 50% range. Allen and co-workers[4] recently reported a series of 80 patients undergoing coronary bypass for infarction with severe left ventricular power failure, managed with warm glutamate/aspartate blood cardioplegic induction, multidose cold blood cardioplegic replenishment, and warm reperfusate. The operative mortality in their series was 17.5%. Further hemodynamic, ventriculographic, and arteriographic correlations will be necessary to select patients who are likely to obtain long-range benefit from a surgical approach.

Acute Failure of Percutaneous Transluminal Coronary Angioplasty

Percutaneous transluminal coronary angioplasty is shown in Fig. 9–9 and Fig. 9–10. Surgical standby has been the practice for PTCA, and a number of different levels of availability of operating room and personnel have been utilized.[25] We provide standby based on the cardiologist's assessment of risk, with the highest risk having an open operating room available immediately and the next level of risk managed with the next open operating room available. Acute closure of the coronary artery requiring emergency operation occurs in 3%–7% of patients undergoing PTCA.[25,68] Mortality in patients undergoing emergency coronary artery bypass for failed PTCA has ranged from 1.4% to 12.1%.[14,145] Death is most likely to occur in women with a large

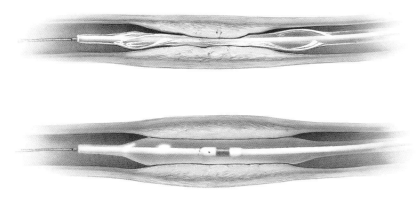

Figure 9–9 Balloon angioplasty—balloon deflated.

Figure 9–10 Balloon angioplasty—balloon inflated.

amount of potentially ischemic myocardium.[45] Patients who undergo prompt and successful surgical revascularization have excellent symptomatic relief and long-term survival.[145]

Severe Anatomic Disease

The single factor that correlates best with fatal cardiac events is the anatomic extent of coronary disease and not the degree of anginal symptoms.[20,22] The fact that sudden death makes up about 25% of initial coronary events emphasizes the treacherous nature of myocardial ischemia.[98] Because severe anatomic disease such as left main stenosis is associated with poor survival—survival that is improved by surgery—coronary bypass has been advocated for other subsets of severe anatomic disease in spite of the absence of symptoms. Patients in this asymptomatic group include those who have had angina that has been abolished by medical therapy, patients who are recovering from an acute myocardial infarction but have no angina, patients who have a positive treadmill test, and patients discovered to have severe disease upon arteriography performed because of a strong family history of coronary artery disease and sudden death.

Few would probably disagree with recommending bypass for left main disease in spite of the absence of symptoms. Recommending bypass for asymptomatic triple-vessel disease or less severe coronary disease is controversial.[36,46] It is unlikely that such controversy will ever be completely resolved. Further study of variables indicating poor prognosis in coronary artery disease is likely to clarify subsets that will have survival favorably affected by surgery. Such variables include ventricular function, response to exercise testing, results of rhythm monitoring, and radionuclide scanning at rest and during exercise.[18,56,152,156] Younis and co-workers[156] found that a reversible thallium defect most likely indicates silent myocardial ischemia in a sizable fraction of patients in this clincal subset and is associated with an unfavorable prognosis.

Combined with Valve Replacement

Valvular replacement in the presence of untreated coronary disease is associated with higher early and late mortality than valvular replacement in the absence of coronary disease.[38,94,125] Copeland and colleagues[38] found a 3-year survival of 60% in 129 patients with isolated aortic valve replacement who had untreated coronary disease. The 3-year survival following isolated aortic valve replacement in 213 patients without coronary artery disease was 85%, a statistically significant difference.

There is good evidence that performing coronary bypass for coronary artery disease at the time of valve replacement improves survival in patients with combined disease if the operative mortality is low (below 6%). Richardson and co-workers[129] reported 220 patients who underwent combined aortic valve replacement and coronary artery bypass. The cumulative survival at 3 years was 77%, a survival rate that did not differ significantly from that of their patients without coronary artery disease who had isolated aortic valve replacement during the same period.

It has been our policy since 1970 to perform coronary arteriography in all patients over 40 years of age who have valvular disease.[5,13] Coronary artery bypass is performed to vessels with 50% or more narrowing of luminal diameter and satisfactory distal vessels. Bypass is performed even if angina is not present. We also have a low threshold for replacing the aortic valve in patients whose symptoms are due to coronary artery disease but who have mild to moderate aortic stenosis.

Postoperative Recurrent Angina

Patients who have had previous coronary artery bypass and have recurrent angina are making up a larger and larger proportion of patients having coronary artery surgery.[34,74,116] Recurrent angina following coronary artery bypass can be caused by graft closure, progression of disease in the native circulation, or both.[117] Vein graft atherosclerosis has become the most common cause of reoperation.[97] Recurrence of angina should cause review of preoperative arteriograms and the operative note to determine the anatomy of the arteries bypassed, the surgeon's appraisal of the success of the operation at the time of surgery, and the state of the arteries that were not bypassed. Indications for repeating angiography should be broad. Following repeat angiography, decision regarding reoperation can be made. Reoperation has a somewhat lower level of success than an original operation. Nevertheless, reoperation should be performed if there is suitable anatomy, since it can be performed at a very low risk and will relieve or improve angina in the great majority of patients.[3,97]

Surgical Strategy

Selection of Conduit: Saphenous Vein or Internal Mammary Artery

The saphenous vein is our usual conduit for bypassing the right coronary artery and its branches and the circumflex coronary artery system. The internal mammary artery is our conduit of choice for the left anterior descending coronary artery. The patency of internal mammary artery grafts to the left anterior descending coronary artery is over 90% at 10 years whereas the patency of saphenous vein grafts is 40%–60%.[59,95] Patients who have an internal mammary artery graft to the left anterior descending have a better 10 year survival than patients with a saphenous vein graft.[96] Use of an internal mammary graft is not associated with increased surgical morbidity or mortality.[39] Use of both internal mammary arteries does increase the risk of wound infection, especially when bilateral grafts are used in insulin-dependent diabetics.[62]

Alternate Conduits

Most patients undergoing their first coronary operation will have satisfactory autogenous saphenous veins or internal mammary arteries for grafting. The growing incidence of coronary reoperations has increased the need for alternate conduits. A number of alternate conduits have been used and evaluated over the last decade. These include the lesser saphenous vein, upper extremity veins, homograft veins, gastroepiploic artery, inferior mesenteric artery, and radial artery.[51]

Lesser Saphenous Vein
The lesser saphenous vein is our autogenous vein of choice if adequate greater saphenous vein is not present.[134] The lesser saphenous vein has had acceptable patency rates when used for lower extremity revascularization, with a patency rate of 60% at 3 years.[151] Duplex scanning can be used to document the course and size of the lesser saphenous vein.

Upper Extremity Veins
The cephalic and basilic veins can also be used as conduits. The patency rate of arm veins used for coronary artery bypass is not as high as that of leg veins. Stoney and colleagues[142] reported a patency rate of 57% at 2 years. Wijnberg and colleagues[154] reported patency of 47% at 4.6 years.

Homograft Veins

Cryopreserved homograft veins are now generally available for use as alternative coronary bypass conduits.[54] The patency rates of homograft veins are quite low, however, ranging from 15% at 6–12 months,[154] to 41% at a mean of 7 months,[87] and 47% at 1–68 months.[12] These low patency rates make homograft veins the conduits of last resort. Their use is appropriate in patients in whom the primary consideration is operative risk rather than long-term result.

Gastroepiploic Artery

The gastroepiploic artery was described as an alternate arterial conduit in 1987.[127,143] A retrogastric route is preferable for the right coronary and circumflex systems and an antegastric route for the left anterior descending.[146] The gastroepiploic artery can also be used as a free graft.[100] Reports of early graft patency have been as high as 92%[72] and 100%.[100] Although there is histologic similarity between the gastroepiploic artery and the internal mammary artery, suggesting that long-term results will be favorable, studies of long-term patency are not yet available.

Inferior Epigastric Artery

The inferior epigastric artery has also been used as an alternate arterial conduit.[9,21,108,109] It is usually harvested through a paramedian incision, with the rectus muscle retracted laterally or medially. Buche and colleagues[21] have reported an early patency rate of 98%. The inferior epigastric artery is also histologically similar to the internal mammary artery. Long-term patency rates are not yet available.

Radial Artery

Carpentier and colleagues[28] reported the use of the radial artery in 1973. Very high rates of graft occlusion within the first year postoperatively were soon reported, with occlusion rates as high as 50%–60%.[41,49] This prompted abandonment of the radial artery.

Recently, Acar, Carpentier, and colleagues[1] have reported use of the radial artery with an intraoperative and postoperative regimen of diltiazem to prevent the spasm which they believe predisposed the radial artery to such high rates of occlusion. In addition, aspirin was given at discharge. With this method of management they have found a patency rate of 93.5% at a mean of 9.2 months postoperatively. Harvesting the radial artery with a broad pedicle with associated veins may also be a factor in improved long-term patency.

Polytetrafluoroethylene Grafts

The use of polytetrafluoroethylene grafts is not associated with acceptable medium-term patency rates, with Chard and co-workers[29] finding only 32% of grafts patent at 2 years.

Removal and Preparation of Vein

The removal and preparation of the saphenous vein compose a critical step in the performance of the coronary artery bypass operation. Improper handling of the vein and subsequent injury can jeopardize the successful outcome of an otherwise properly performed procedure. The saphenous vein is usually removed through a leg incision beginning at the groin or ankle, often leaving a skin bridge at the knee. Skin bridges are left in several areas if the subcutaneous layer is extremely thick or if lower extremity ischemia is present. Care is taken to keep the incision directly over the vein to prevent the creation of a skin flap and increased likelihood of wound complication.

The vein is removed with very gentle handling and careful sharp dissection of the vein and its branches. The branches are tied, clipped distally with a hemoclip, and divided. Gentle handling will prevent the avulsion of the smaller, thin-walled branches of the vein.

The vein is gently irrigated with balanced salt solution or heparinized autogenous blood and any additional branches ligated. Gentle distention of the vein with the branch clamped will demonstrate the junction of the branch and the vein, and a tie can be placed in such a manner that the branch is ligated flush with the vein. This prevents gathering of adventitia at the base of the branch, which can constrict the vein circumference. Ligation flush with the vein also avoids a stump at the takeoff of the branch: such a stump may create a nidus for thrombosis and subsequent emboli.

Myocardial Preservation

The broad subject of myocardial preservation is covered in Chapter 6. Cold blood cardioplegia with antegrade, retrograde, and graft infusion (Sutter/Sacramento) and intermittent aortic clamping for distal anastomoses under moderate hypothermia (St. Vincent/Portland) are our two methods of myocardial preservation for coronary artery bypass.

Left Ventricular Venting

Decompression of the left ventricle during coronary surgery can achieve two desirable objectives: prevention of ventricular distention and provision of a bloodless field during performance of the distal coronary anastomoses. It is possible to achieve these objectives without the use of a vent, as described by Okies and colleagues.[119] The unvented left ventricle does not usually distend during recovery following an ischemic period, even with the use of hypothermic cardioplegic arrest.[133]

Many methods of left ventricular decompression have been described, either directly through the apex or indirectly through the left atrium,[137] pulmonary artery,[66] or aorta.[64] Our usual practice during coronary surgery is either not to use a vent or to use suction on an aortic vent during aortic clamping. If the technique of cold cardioplegic arrest is used, a Y connector at the aortic needle can provide for simplified switching of solution infusion and aortic suction.

Sequence of Distal Anastomoses

The sequence of distal anastomoses should not be arbitrary. Size disparity should be avoided if possible. The internal mammary artery anastomosis is the last anastomosis performed.

Distal Anastomosis: Running Versus Interrupted Technique

The distal anastomosis was performed using an interrupted technique during the early years at the Cleveland Clinic.[47] Since then the development of fine polypropylene sutures has led to popularization of the running suture technique. The slippery quality of polypropylene allows the surgeon to open areas of the anastomosis as the suture line progresses, with subsequent easy tightening of the suture. However, the surgeon must guard against production of a purse-string effect. The purse-string effect can be avoided by infusing solution under some pressure down the graft as the suture is being tied. This easy slipping while running the suture material allows the technical advantage of the interrupted suture technique while at the same time providing the simplicity and speed of a running suture line. For these reasons we run almost all distal anastomoses, usually with 7–0 or 6–0 prolene.

In some situations, such as a difficult side-to-side anastomosis or an anastomosis to a vessel with plaque in the wall, an interrupted suture technique may be preferable. Interrupted technique with all arterial stitches taken inside-out may prevent dislodgement or cracking of a mural plaque.

Distal Anastomosis: Single Versus Sequential

Sequential anastomoses (multiple anastomoses along one vein with one proximal anastomosis) can be performed with patency rates over 90% in experienced hands.[61] Sequential grafts have the theoretical advantage of a higher flow throughout most of the vein, possibly resulting in fewer graft closures. They have the disadvantages of being more susceptible to technical error and of placing all anastomoses at risk if anything happens to the proximal portion of the graft. We use single anastomoses by choice, but do not hesitate to perform sequential grafts if the amount of vein is limited or the aorta is short.

Determination of Graft Position and Length

The length of each graft is measured by occluding the distal portion as blood or cold cardioplegic solution is injected under slight pressure. This will distend and stretch the vein in a similar fashion to what will occur with arterial pressure. The course of the vein can then be assessed and its proper length determined. An empty, shrunken heart and collapsed pulmonary artery can cause error in determination of length if the prebypass size of the heart is not noted and taken into account. The pericardial cradle is useful in determining the size the heart will regain after bypass. Retarding the venous return to the oxygenator and thereby filling the right heart can also help in assessing proper graft length.

Endarterectomy

Coronary artery endarterectomy was an early direct operation and can be a valuable procedure in carefully selected patients.[32] However, we avoid endarterectomy whenever possible. In the presence of disease at the bifurcation of the right coronary artery, grafting of the posterior descending is usually performed.

Several situations may be amenable to endarterectomy and bypass. In the face of a failed graft to an extensively diseased right coronary artery, reoperation and endarterectomy are reasonable to consider. Extensive endarterectomy of the diffusely diseased left anterior descending has been described[17,123] and may be a valuable procedure in this difficult situation.

Management of Papillary Muscle Dysfunction

The management of mitral insufficiency secondary to ischemic disease of the papillary muscle is a difficult problem.[114] Mitral valve repair or replacement is generally not indicated if the murmur is intermittent, congestive failure has never occurred, and the ventriculogram shows minimal or no mitral regurgitation. Mitral valve repair or replacement is usually indicated if the mitral insufficiency is constant and long-standing, medical management of congestive heart failure is required, and the ventriculogram shows moderate to marked mitral regurgitation. Intraoperative transesophageal echocardiography can also be particularly useful in determining whether mitral valve surgery is required.

Management of Coexistent Cerebrovascular Disease

The evolution of simultaneous carotid and coronary surgery has been in response to increased risk of cerebrovascular complications if only the coronary surgery is performed or increased risk of myocardial infarction if only the carotid surgery is performed. It is our practice to perform carotid duplex studies in patients with carotid bruits or symptoms of cerebral ischemia. If there is more than a 70% carotid stenosis, and this is confirmed by arteriography, simultaneous carotid and coronary surgery is often performed. The carotid endarterectomy is performed before the patient is placed on bypass, and the neck wound is not closed until after cardiopulmonary bypass and administration of protamine.[118] In the presence of disease at the level of the arch, bypass grafts from the ascending aorta can be performed in conjunction with coronary surgery.

Reoperation

At St. Vincent/Portland reoperations are performed using the same methods as used for first operations.

At Sutter/Sacramento reoperations are performed using the techniques described by Loop and co-workers.[97] Initial dissection exposes only the ascending aorta, the most proximal portion of the grafts, and the right atrium. After aortic clamping, antegrade cardioplegia is given. The stenotic vein grafts are then divided with a scalpel near the aorta and retrograde cardioplegia is infused, with careful attention to whether the effluent cardioplegic solution coming out the divided grafts carries any atheromatous material. The rest of the heart is then dissected.

The old grafts are then divided near their distal anastomoses and the new coronary arteriotomies are made and new grafts anastomosed. If there is concern about possible atheromatous emboli, retrograde cardioplegia can be infused after each coronary arteriotomy to flush out any material before the distal anastomosis is performed. After the distal anastomosis is performed, cardioplegic solution is infused down the new vein graft as the stump of the old graft is oversewn. Aortic anastomoses are performed with the cross-clamp on while the patient is rewarmed.

Surgical Technique

Saphenous Vein Removal and Preparation

An incision is made over the saphenous vein (Figs. 9–11, 9–12), usually with a skin bridge at the knee. Bridged incisions are made if the subcutaneous tissue is thick or chronic arterial insufficiency is present. The branches of the vein should be tied at the junction (Fig. 9–13). The adventitia should not be gathered (Fig. 9–14), nor should a stump be left.

If a branch has been torn off, fine sutures should be taken longitudinally (Figs. 9–15, 9–16) so that the vein is gathered without circumferential constric-

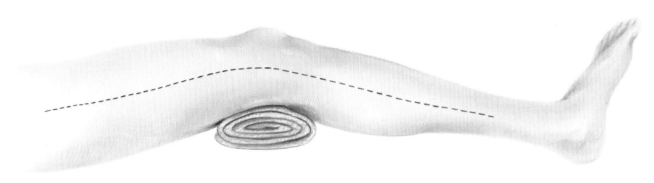

9–11

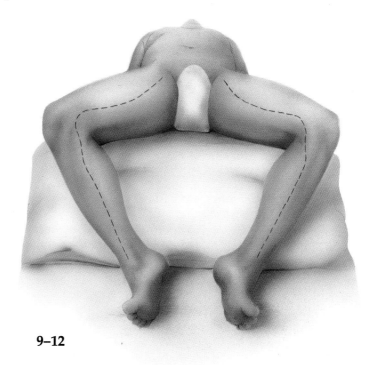

9–12

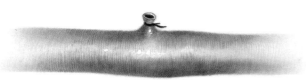

9–13

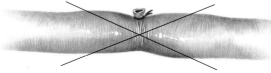

Figure 9–14 *What not to do.* The adventitia at the base of the branch should not be gathered since this can constrict the lumen.

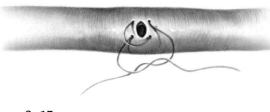

9–15

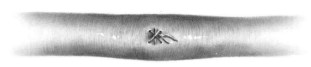

9–16

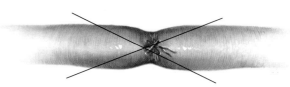

Figure 9–17 *What not to do.* Transverse sutures should not be taken since they can constrict the vein

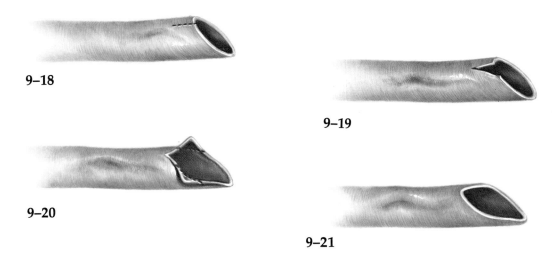

9–18

9–19

9–20

9–21

tion. Transverse sutures should not be taken, since they can constrict the vein (Fig. 9–17).

The vein end may be prepared either by simply cutting diagonally or by creation of a "cobra's head" —cutting diagonally (Fig. 9–18), extending the incision in the heel (Fig. 9–19), and trimming the edges if necessary (Fig. 9–20), resulting in a vein end (Fig. 9–21) that will lie smoothly over the arteriotomy.

Dissection of the Internal Mammary Artery

The left chest is retracted and the endothoracic fascia is cut with electrocautery 10–15 mm on each side of the internal mammary artery (IMA) (Fig. 9–22). With the electrocautery on a low current, the IMA is gently teased away from the chest wall, holding the fascia (Fig. 9–23). The IMA is not grasped with the forceps, although closed forceps can be used to push down on the IMA to better expose the branches. The branches are clipped proximally and electrocauterized distally. The IMA with its pedicle is freed from the bifurcation near the diaphragm distally to the subclavian vein proximally (Fig. 9–24).

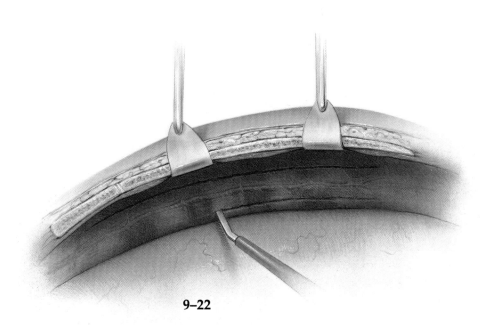

9–22

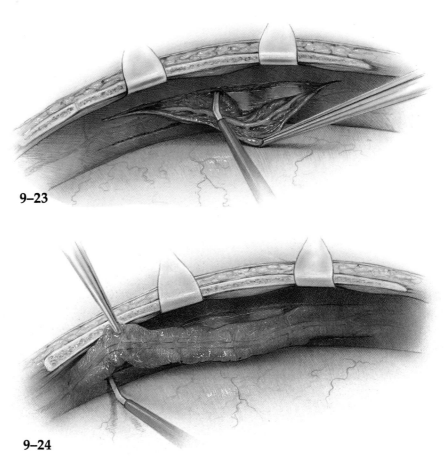

9–23

9–24

Distal Right Coronary Artery Anastomosis

Exposure of the right coronary artery at the crux can be obtained by retraction sutures (Fig. 9–25). A suture is taken in the artery and tagged. The other end of the suture is then brought through the vein, through the artery (Fig. 9–26), and through the vein, and the vein is lowered into place. The suture that had been taken first is then brought up the far side (Figs. 9–27, 9–28), around the heel (Fig. 9–29), and down the near side (Fig. 9–30). The other suture is then brought up (Fig. 9–31) to complete the suture line.

Posterior Descending Artery Anastomosis
Exposure of the posterior descending artery may be best by hand retraction of the heart, with the apex toward the patient's left shoulder. The suture line is started at the heel and brought partially up the near side, outside-inside the artery and inside-outside the vein. The other suture is then brought up the far side and around the toe, outside-inside the vein and inside-outside the artery. At St. Vincent/Portland the posterior descending artery anastomosis is performed the same as the distal right coronary artery anastomosis.

Aortic Anastomosis for Right-Sided Grafts

At St. Vincent/Portland the proximal anastomoses are performed over a partial occluding clamp after each distal anastomosis. At Sutter/Sacramento all distal anastomoses are performed and then all proximal anastomoses are performed over a partial occluding clamp.

This is the usual anastomosis for grafts to the right main coronary artery or posterior descending branch. The partial occluding clamp is placed slightly on the right side of the aorta. A circular or elliptical portion of aorta is excised.

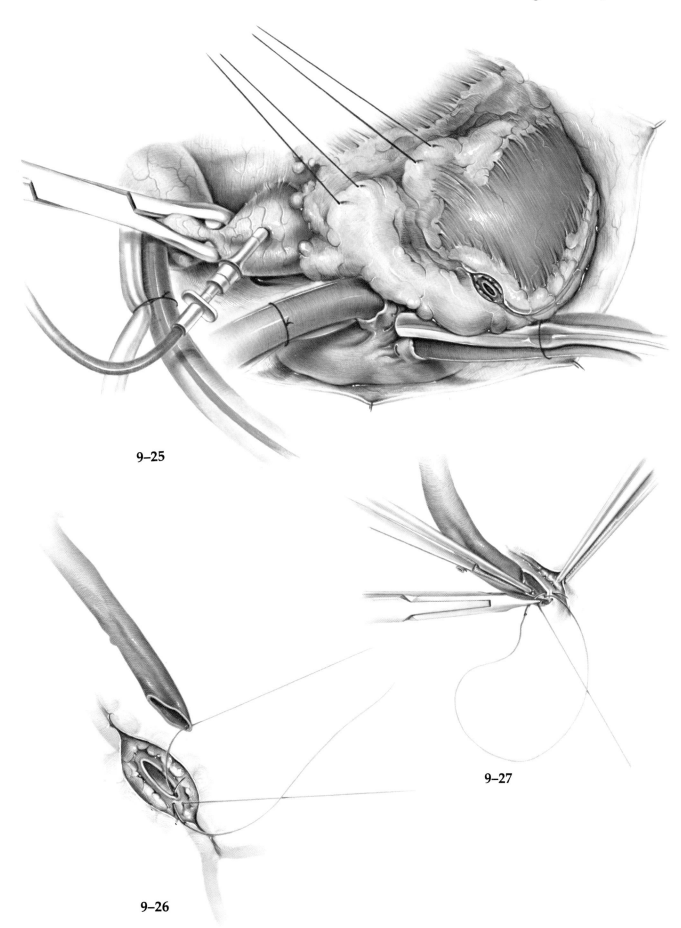

9–25

9–26

9–27

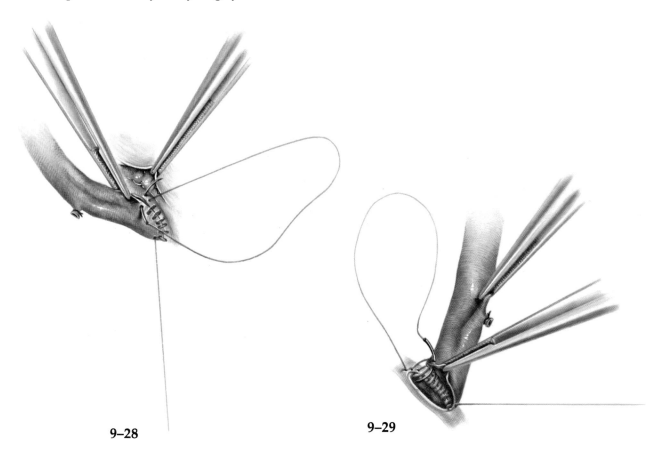

9–28

9–29

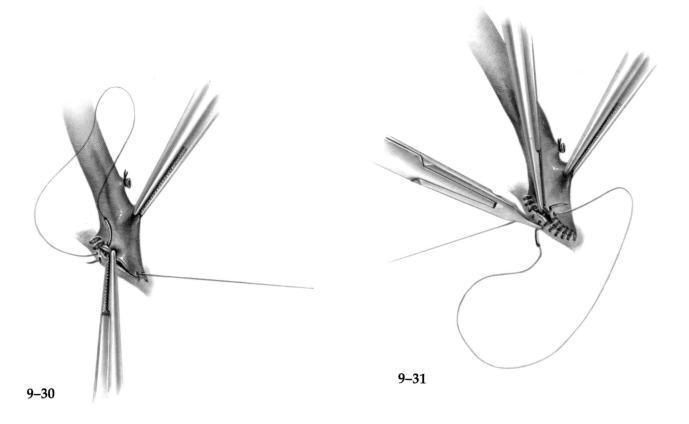

9–30

9–31

An aortic punch can facilitate this procedure. The graft is oriented longitudinally or to the right. The near suture line is brought up (Fig. 9–32), and the far suture line is brought around to meet it (Fig. 9–33).

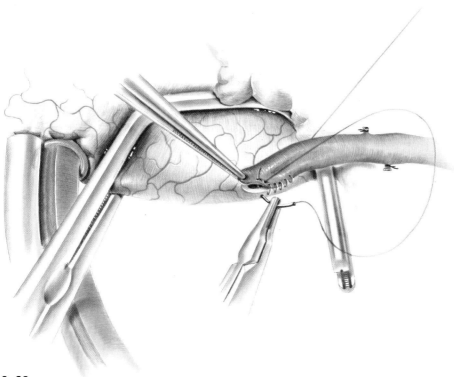

9–32

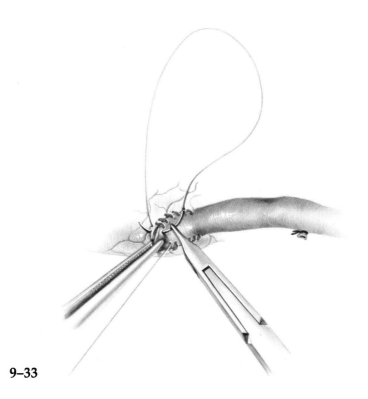

9–33

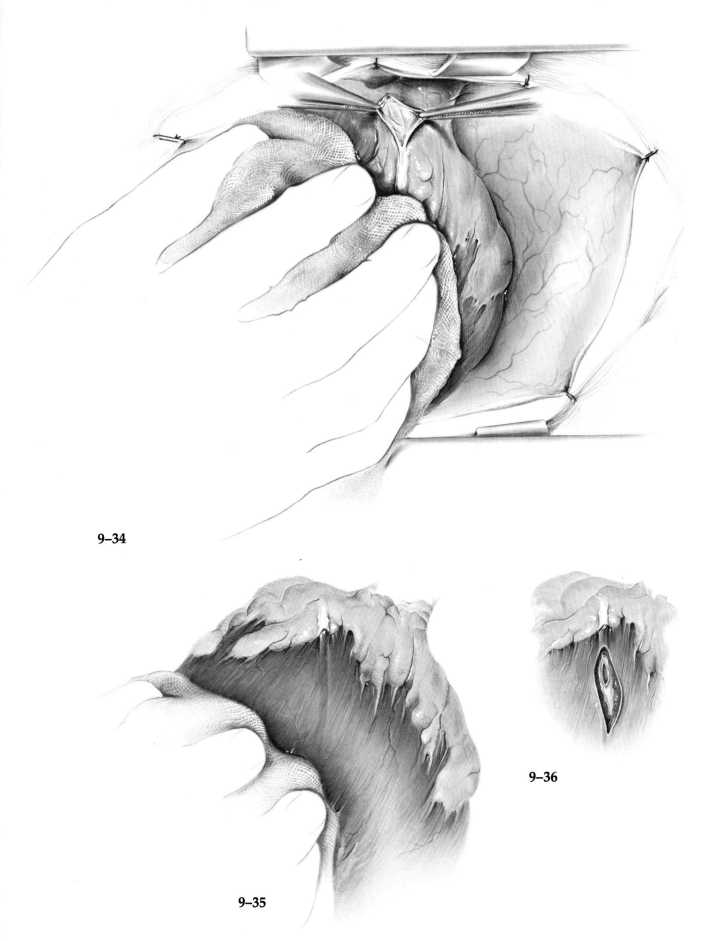

9–34

9–35

9–36

Distal Obtuse Marginal Artery Anastomosis

The heart is retracted by hand, with the apex toward the patient's right shoulder. The epicardium is incised, exposing the artery (Fig. 9–34). The obtuse marginal artery or ramus marginalis may be submyocardial. Such location is usually indicated by a groove in the myocardial surface with a light streak (Fig. 9–35). The artery can usually be seen or palpated at the atrioventricular margin before it dives below the myocardium. Identification of the artery at this point can help identify its submyocardial location. Incision through the epicardium and myocardium will then locate the artery (Fig. 9–36).

The obtuse marginal is incised with a knife (Fig. 9–37), and the incision is extended with scissors (Fig. 9–38). A suture is taken through the artery (Fig.

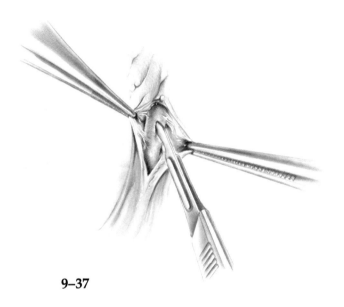

9–37

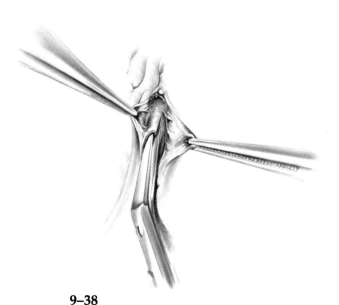

9–38

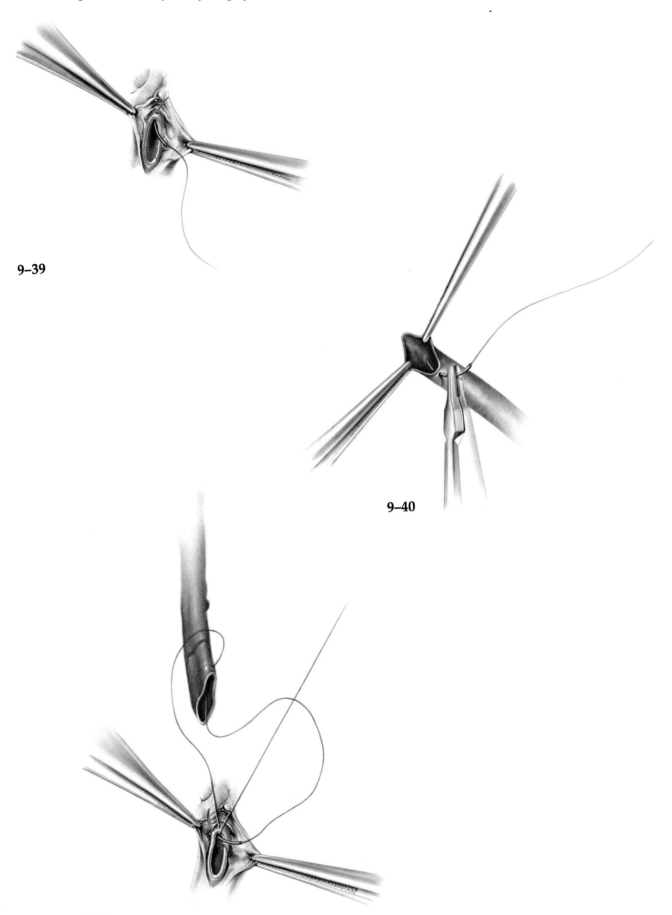

9–39

9–40

9–41

9–39), through the vein (Fig. 9–40), through the artery (Fig. 9–41), and tagged. The other end is brought through the vein (Fig. 9–42), and the vein is lowered into place. The suture line is then brought up the right side (Fig. 9–43). The other suture is brought through the heel of the vein (Fig. 9–44), through the

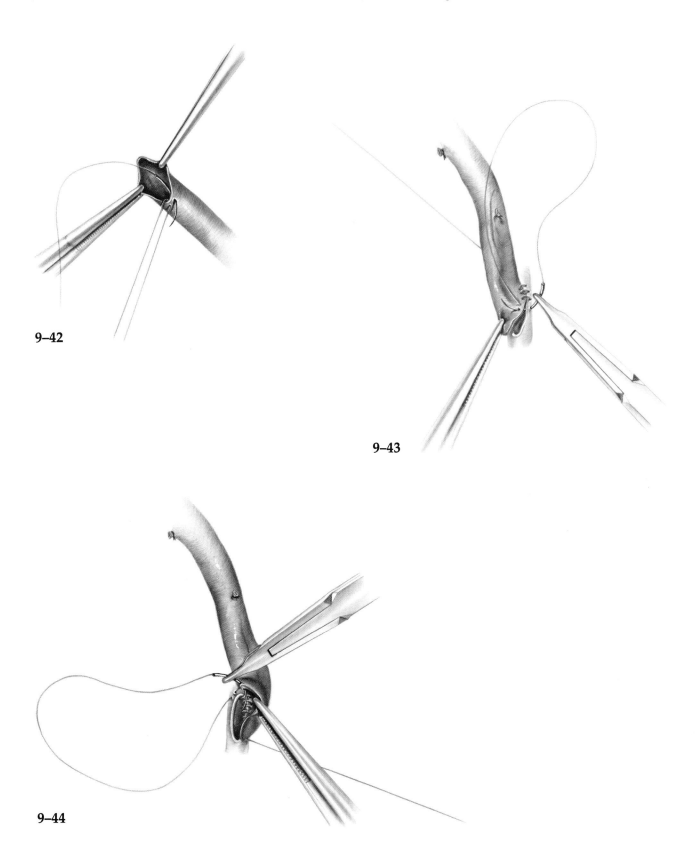

9–42

9–43

9–44

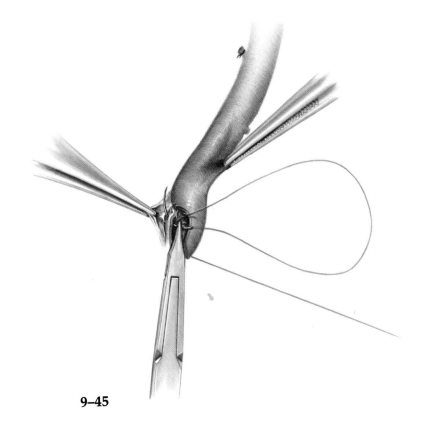

9–45

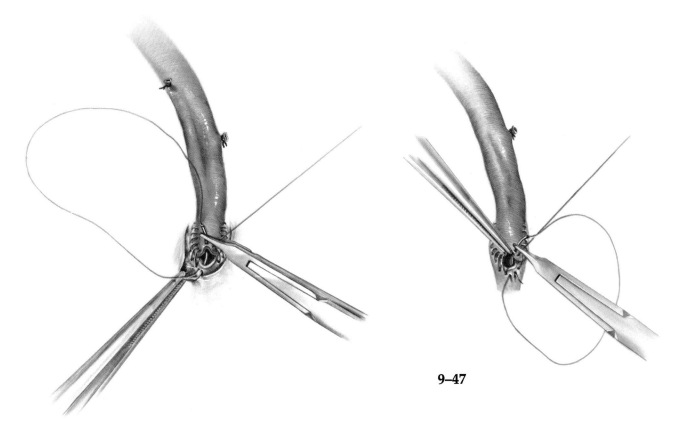

9–46

9–47

artery (Fig. 9–45), up the left side, and around the toe (Figs. 9–46, 9–47) to complete the suture line.

Obtuse Marginal Side-to-Side Anastomosis

The vein is incised longitudinally rather than transversely. This causes the least amount of constriction of the vein at the point of the anastomosis. A suture is taken inside-outside the artery and tagged. The suture line is then brought up inside-outside the vein and outside-inside the artery (Fig. 9–48). The suture line is then brought up outside-inside the vein and inside-outside the artery (Fig. 9–49) and around the end of the arteriotomy to complete the anastomosis (Fig. 9–50).

Aortic Anastomosis for Left-Sided Grafts

All left-sided grafts (left anterior descending, diagonal, and obtuse marginal) are placed on the left side of the aorta. The plane between the aorta and the pulmonary artery is opened prior to placing the clamp. A partial occluding

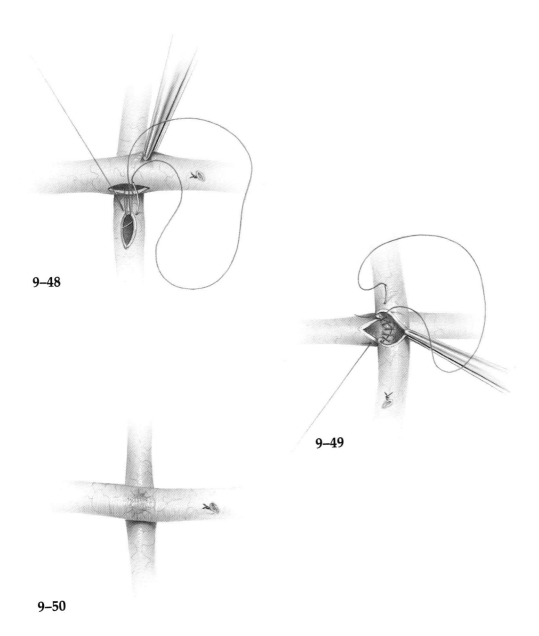

9–48

9–49

9–50

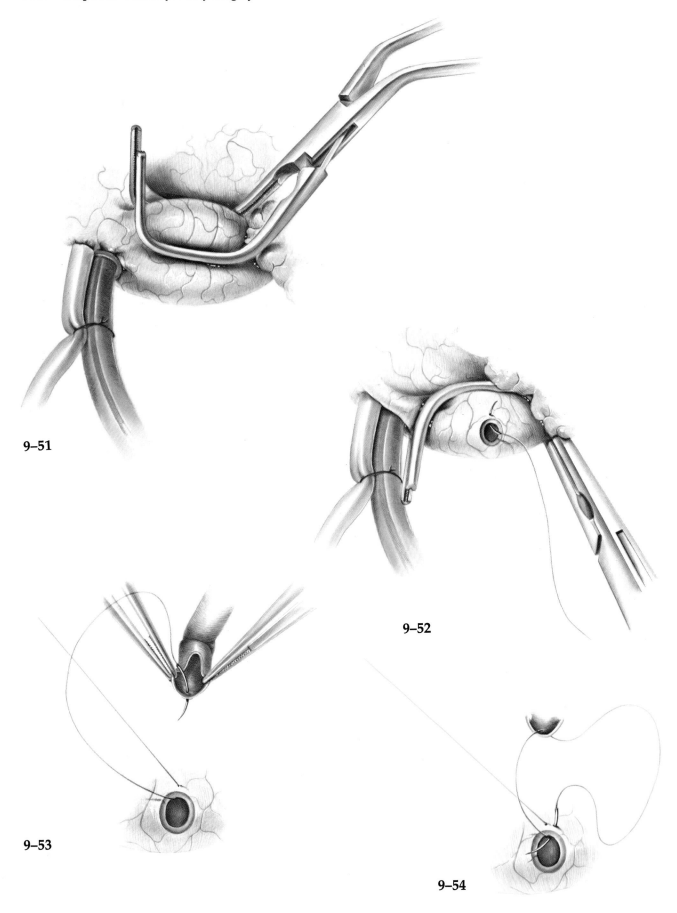

9–51

9–52

9–53

9–54

clamp is placed toward the left side (Fig. 9–51) as pump flow is temporarily decreased to lower the perfusion pressure to 50 mm Hg or lower. Lowering the pressure facilitates placement of the clamp and diminishes the likelihood of clamp injury to the aorta. A circular or elliptical piece of aorta is removed and the aortic suture taken (Fig. 9–52). This suture is passed through the vein (Fig. 9–53), the aorta (Fig. 9–54), and the vein again (Fig. 9–55). The vein is then lowered into place. The lower suture line is brought up (Fig. 9–56) and tagged. The other end of the suture is then brought through the heel of the vein (Fig. 9–57) and up (Fig. 9–58) to complete the suture line. Air is carefully

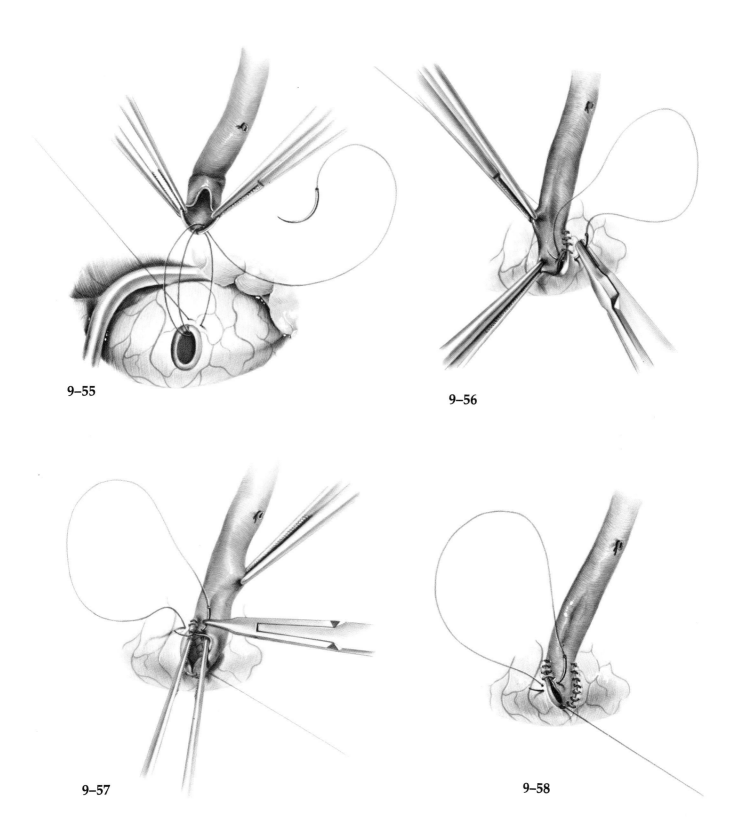

9–55

9–56

9–57

9–58

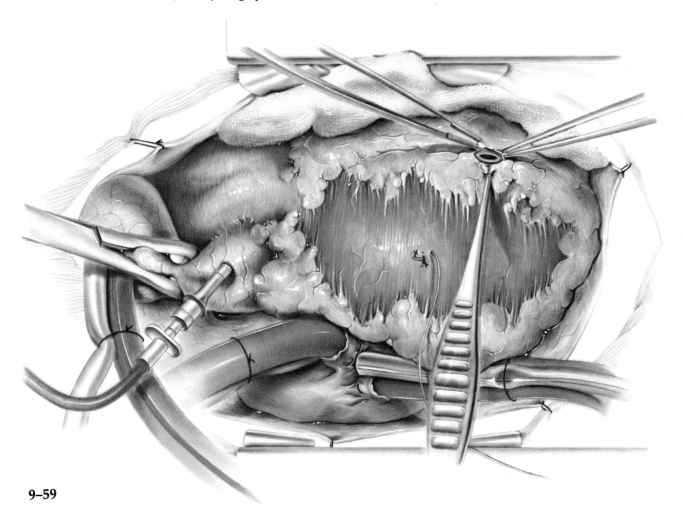

9–59

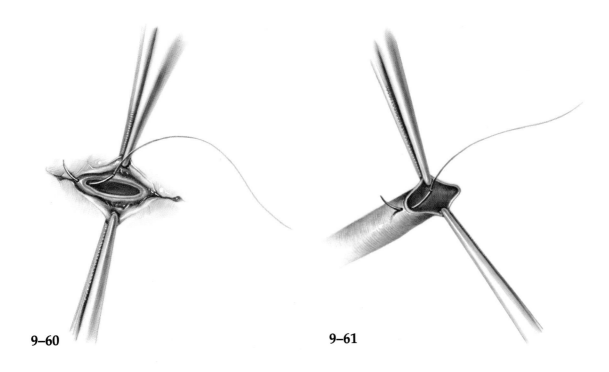

9–60   9–61

removed from the graft and excluded portion of the aorta as the clamp is released.

Distal Left Anterior Descending Artery Anastomosis

The heart is placed on pads to elevate the anterior wall and bring the left anterior descending coronary artery medially. The epicardium over the artery and the artery are incised (Fig. 9–59).

A suture is taken through the proximal end of the arteriotomy (Fig. 9–60), through the heel of the vein (Fig. 9–61), through the artery (Fig. 9–62), and through the vein (Fig. 9–63). The suture ends are then pulled and the vein is approximated to the artery.

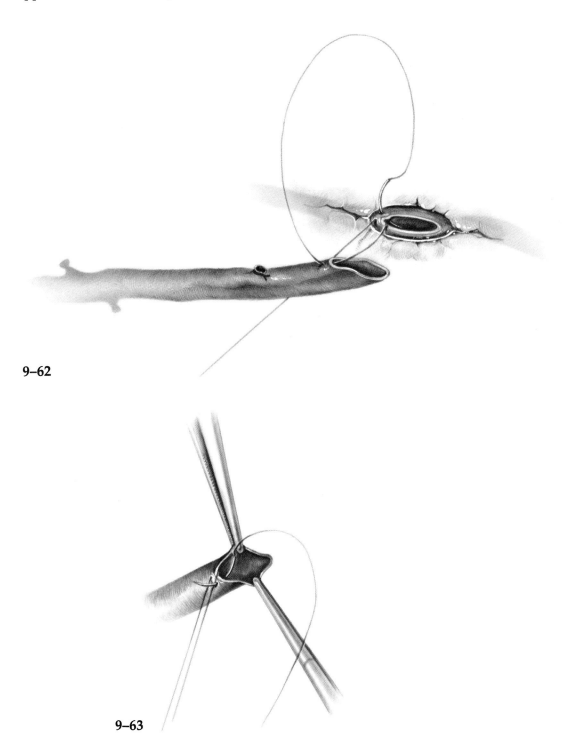

9–62

9–63

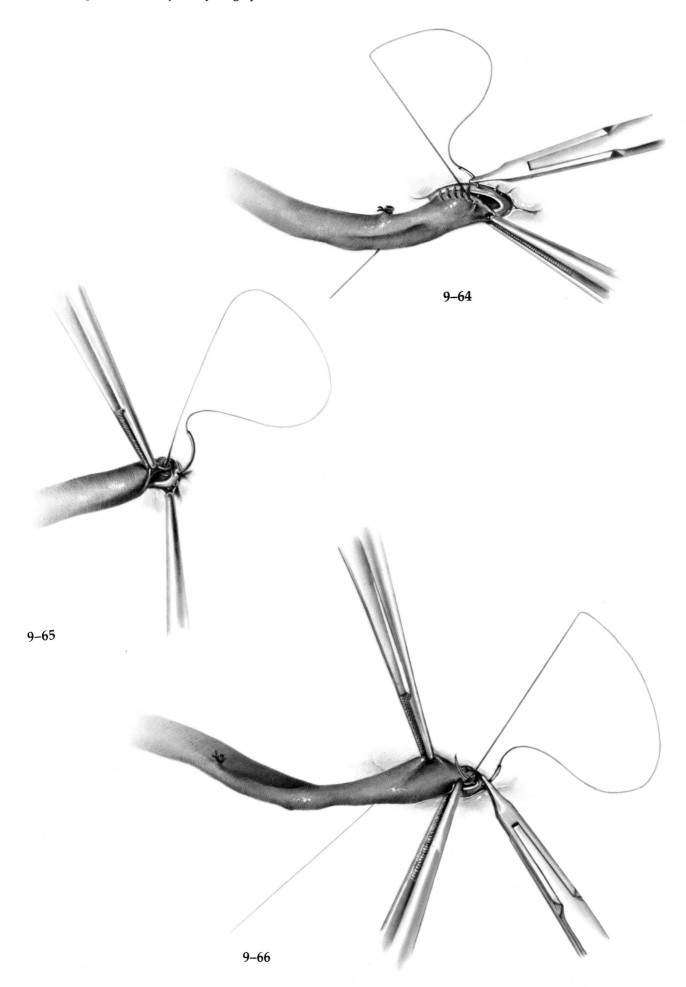

9–64

9–65

9–66

The suture line is then brought down the far side (Fig. 9–64), around the toe (Figs. 9–65, 9–66), and partially up the near side (Fig. 9–67), and tagged. The other suture is then brought through the heel of the vein and through the artery (Fig. 9–68). This suture line is then brought down to meet the other and tied, taking care to avoid any purse-string effect by injecting cardioplegic solution down the graft as the suture is tied (Fig. 9–69).

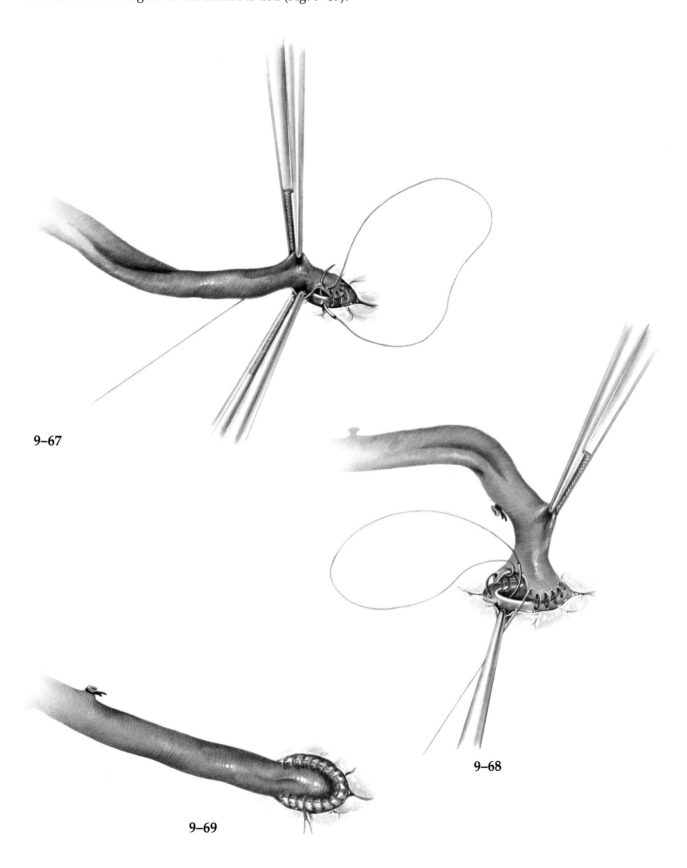

9–67

9–68

9–69

Diagonal Artery Side-to-Side Anastomosis

The far suture line is begun at the proximal end of the arteriotomy (Fig. 9–70). An alignment suture can be placed at the distal end of the arteriotomy. The suture line is then brought around (Fig. 9–71) and tagged. The other suture is brought down to complete the suture line (Fig. 9–72).

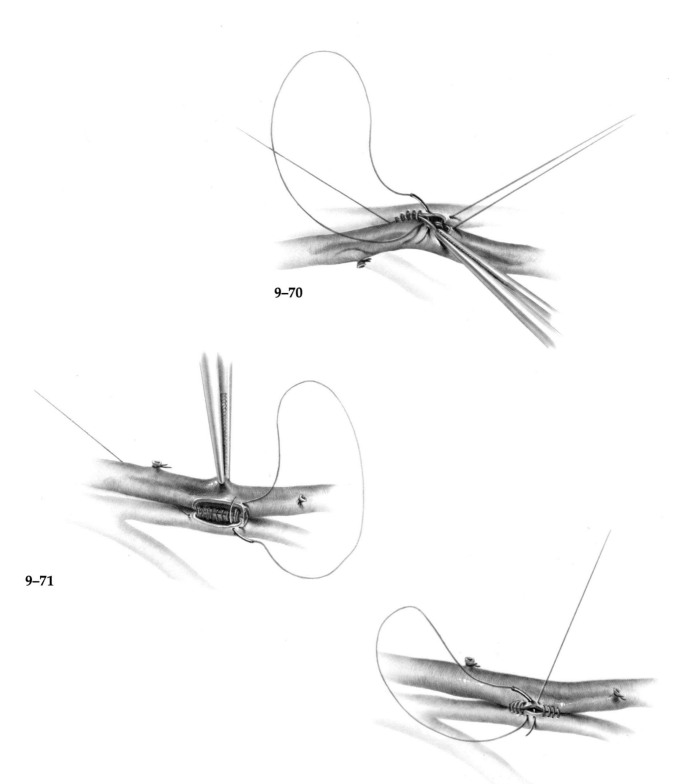

9–70

9–71

9–72

Left Internal Mammary Artery to
Left Anterior Descending Artery Anastomosis

The anastomosis is performed similar to the vein-LAD anastomosis, with the far suture line outside-inside the LAD and inside-outside the IMA. The near suture line is outside-inside the IMA and inside-outside the LAD (Fig. 9–73). The toe of the anastomosis is often sutured inside-outside the LAD to complete the anastomosis (Fig. 9–74). The pedicle is sutured to the epicardium.

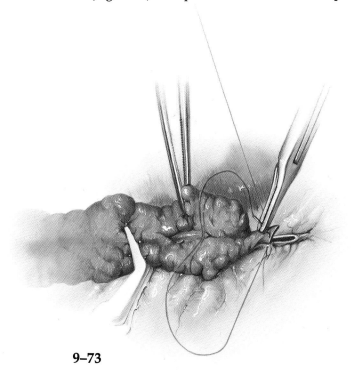

9–73

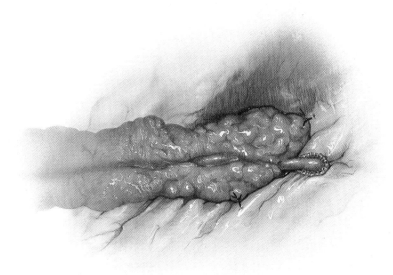

9–74

Completed Triple-Vessel Bypass

Figure 9–75 shows the right graft coursing through the atrioventricular groove to the posterior aspect of the heart. The obtuse marginal graft passes over the pulmonary artery to the posterior wall of the left ventricle. The internal mammary artery courses through a groove cut in the left side of the pleura and pericardium anterior to the phrenic nerve.

Results

Graft Patency

The occlusion rate of the saphenous vein is about 12%–20% during the first year and 2%–4% annually for the next 5 years. After this the rate doubles, so that at 10 years, approximately 50% of grafts have become occluded due to graft atherosclerosis.[60]

Patent grafts can affect the progression of disease in grafted arteries. Progression almost always occurs in that segment of coronary artery proximal to

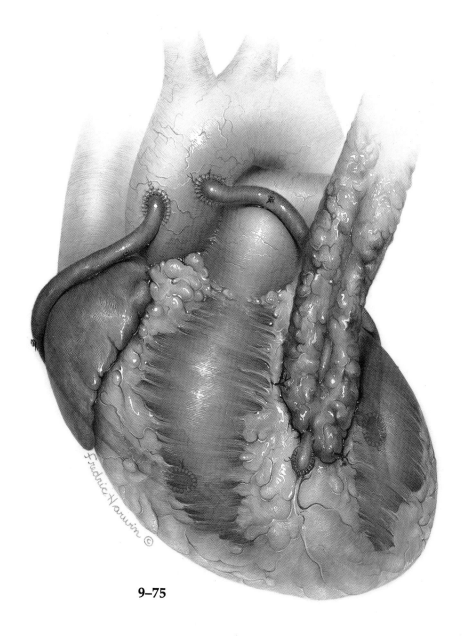

9–75

the anastomosis. At 5 years postoperatively, proximal stenoses will have progressed to occlusion in 30%–60% of arteries with patent grafts.[88,148] Development of disease in segments of coronary arteries distal to patent grafts is rare,[88] occurring in less than 2%.

Angina Relief and Quality of Life

Coronary artery bypass grafting alleviates or improves anginal symptoms in the vast majority of patients.[26,55,89] Relief of angina usually occurs in 50%–80%, with 90% being asymptomatic or improved.[69] Subjective relief of angina seems to be clearly related to improvement in regional myocardial blood flow. Symptomatic improvement correlates with graft patency,[65,106] improvement in exercise capacity,[83,86] improvement in myocardial perfusion,[130] and improvement in myocardial metabolism.[27,30,31,82]

Randomized studies of medical and surgical treatment of chronic stable angina have shown greater functional improvement in surgically treated patients.[82,104,105] Such functional improvement correlates significantly with higher exercise work loads, exercise heart rates, maximum paced heart rates, and myocardial lactate extraction.[82]

Symptomatic deterioration occurs postoperatively and is most often due to progression of atherosclerotic disease in the vein grafts and native coronary arteries. Angina recurs in approximately 20% of patients at 5 years and 40% of patients at 10 years.[2]

Left Ventricular Function

The effect of coronary artery bypass surgery on left ventricular performanc can be deterioration, no change, or improvement.[128] Deterioration in ventricular function occurring perioperatively is usually the result of an improperly performed operation. Deterioration in regional wall motion is usually associated with an occluded graft, a perioperative myocardial infarction, or both.[24,155] Normal ventricular function preoperatively should be unchanged postoperatively. A successful operation (proper intraoperative myocardial preservation and all grafts patent postoperatively) does not alter normal ventricular function.[155]

Improvement in abnormal regional or global ventricular function depends upon the reversibility of the wall motion abnormality and the success of the operation.[128,148] Areas of poor ventricular function that are associated with previous myocardial infarction do not generally show reversibility on ventriculography following nitroglycerin administration[8] and do not generally show improvement after bypass grafting.[31] Wall motion abnormality that improves after nitroglycerin administration usually improves after successful bypass grafting.[67] Abnormal wall motion seen in association with unstable angina usually improves following successful operation.[31] Abnormalities of wall motion that occur only during exercise will usually revert to normal after bypass grafting.[24,79]

Survival

The effect of coronary artery bypass on patient survival has been a controversial subject and has been a stimulus to the performance in the 1970s of several randomized trials of surgical versus medical therapy. The three main studies were the Coronary Artery Surgery Study (CASS), which enrolled patients from 1975 to 1979, the European Coronary Surgery Study Group (ECSS), which enrolled patients from 1973 to 1976, and the Veterans Administration Study, which enrolled patients from 1972 to 1974.[48] The strengths and weaknesses of these studies have been well described.[52,55] These studies were performed before the use of the internal mammary artery became widespread, before recent advances in pharmacologic management of coronary artery disease, before recent advances in myocardial preservation, and before the use of PTCA.

The survival in these heterogeneous groups of patients was 95% at 1 year, 88% at 5 years, and 75% at 10 years.[2] Survival was clearly superior in the surgical group in those patients with left main stenosis, in those patients with triple-vessel disease and an ejection fraction below 0.5, and in patients with triple-vessel disease and severe angina pectoris.[2,80,113,124,149]

References

1. Acar C, Jebara VA, Portoghese M, Beyssen B, Pagny JY, Grare P, Chachques JC, Fabiani J, Deloche A, Guermonprez JL, Carpentier AF: Revival of the radial artery for coronary artery bypass grafting. Ann Thorac Surg 54:652,1992.
2. ACC/AHA Task Force Report: Guidelines and indications for coronary artery bypass graft surgery. J Am Coll Cardiol 17:543,1991.
3. Adam M, Geisler GF, Lambert CJ, Mitchell BF Jr: Reoperation following clinical failure of aorta-to-coronary-artery bypass vein grafts. Ann Thorac Surg 14: 272,1972.
4. Allen BS, Rosenkranz E, Buckberg GD, Davtyan H, Laks H, Tillisch J, Drinkwater DC: Studies of prolonged acute regional ischemia: VI. Myocardial infarction with left ventricular power failure: a medical/surgical emergency requiring urgent revascularization with maximal protection of remote muscle. J Thorac Cardiovasc Surg 98:691,1989.
5. Anderson RP, Bonchek LI, Wood JA, Chapman RP, Starr A: The safety of combined aortic valve replacement and coronary bypass grafting. Ann Thorac Surg 15:249,1973.
6. Applebaum R, House R, Rademaker A, Garibaldi A, Davis Z, Guillory J, Chen A, Hoeksema T: Coronary artery bypass grafting within thirty days of acute myocardial infarction: early and late results in 406 patients. J Thorac Cardiovasc Surg 102:745,1991.
7. Armstrong WF: Stress echocardiography for detection of coronary artery disease. Circulation 84(Suppl I):I-43,1991.
8. Banka VS, Bodenheimer MM, Helfant RH: Determinants of reversible asynergy: the native coronary circulation. Circulation 52:810,1975.
9. Barner HB, Naunheim KS, Fiore AC, Fischer VW, Harris HH: Use of the inferior epigastric artery as a free graft for myocardial infarction. Ann Thorac Surg 52: 429,1991.
10. Beller GA: Diagnostic accuracy of thallium-201 myocardial perfusion imaging. Circulation 84(Suppl I):I-6,1991.
11. Berg R, Kendall RW, Duvoisin GE, Ganji JH, Rudy LW, Everhart FJ: Acute myocardial infarction: a surgical emergency. J Thorac Cardiovasc Surg 70: 432,1975.
12. Bical O, Bachet J, Laurian C, Camilleri JP, Goudot B, Menu P, Guilmet D: Aortocoronary bypass with homologous saphenous vein: Long-term results. Ann Thorac Surg 30:550,1980.
13. Bonchek LI, Anderson RP, Rosch J: Should coronary arteriography be performed routinely before valve replacement? Am J Cardiol 31:462,1973.
14. Borkon AM, Failing TL, Piehler JM, Killen DA, Hoskins ML, Reed WA: Risk analysis of operative intervention for failed coronary angioplasty. Ann Thorac Surg 54:884,1992.
15. Bosch X, Theroux P, Waters DD, Pelletier GB, Roy D: Early postinfarction ischemia: clinical, angiographic, and prognostic significance. Circulation 75:988,1987.
16. Brandt B III, Wright CB, Ehrenhaft JL: Ventricular septal defect following myocardial infarction. Ann Thorac Surg 27:580,1979.
17. Brenowitz JB, Kayser KL, Johnson WD: Results of coronary artery endarterectomy and reconstruction. J Thorac Cardiovasc Surg 95:1,1988.
18. Brown KA: Prognostic value of thallium-201 myocardial perfusion imaging: a diagnostic tool comes of age. Circulation 83:363,1991.
19. Brunken RC, Mody FV, Hawkins RA, Nienaber C, Phelps ME, Schelbert HR: Positron emission tomography detects metabolic viability in myocardium with

persistent 24-hour single-photon emission computed tomography Tl-201 defects. Circulation 86:1357,1992.

20. Bruschke AVG, Proudfit WL, Sones FM: Progress study of 590 consecutive non-surgical cases of coronary disease followed 5–9 years: I. Arteriographic correlations. Circulation 47:1147,1973.

21. Buche M, Schoevaerdts J, Louagie Y, Schroeder E, Marchandise B, Chenu P, Dion R, Verhelst R, Deloos M, Gonzales E, Chalant C: Use of the inferior epigastric artery for coronary bypass. J Thorac Cardiovasc Surg 103:665,1992.

22. Burggraf GW, Parker JO: Prognosis in coronary artery disease: angiographic, hemodynamic, and clinical factors. Circulation 51:146,1975.

23. Burrow RD, Strauss HW, Singleton R, Pond M, Rehn T, Bailey IK, Griffith LC, Nickoloff E, Pitt B: Analysis of left ventricular function from multiple gated acquisition cardiac blood pool imaging. Circulation 56:1024,1977.

24. Bussman WD, Mayer V, Kober G, Kaltenbach M: Ventricular function at rest, during leg raising and physical exercise before and after aortocoronary bypass surgery. Am J Cardiol 43:488,1979.

25. Cameron DE, Stinson DC, Greene PS, Gardner TJ: Surgical standby for percutaneous transluminal coronary angioplasty: a survey of patterns of practice. Ann Thorac Surg 50:35,1990.

26. Cannom DS, Miller C, Shumway NE, Fogarty TJ, Daily PO, Hu M, Brown B Jr, Harrison DC: The long-term follow-up of patients undergoing saphenous vein bypass surgery. Circulation 49:77,1974.

27. Carlson RG, Kline S, Apstein C, Scheidt S, Brachfeld N, Killip T, Lillehei CW: Lactate metabolism after aortocoronary artery vein bypass grafts. Ann Surg 176: 680,1972.

28. Carpentier A, Guermonprez JL, Deloche A, Frechette C, DuBost C: The aorta-to-coronary radial artery bypass graft. Ann Thorac Surg 16:111,1973.

29. Chard RB, Johnson DC, Nunn GR, Cartmill TB: Aorta-coronary bypass grafting with polytetrafluoroethylene conduits. J Thorac Cardiovasc Surg 94:132,1987.

30. Chatterjee K, Matloff JM, Swan HJC, Ganz W, Kaushik VS, Magnusson P, Henis MM, Forrester JS: Abnormal regional metabolism and mechanical function in patients with ischemic heart disease: improvement after successful regional revascularization by aortocoronary bypass. Circulation 52:390,1975.

31. Chatterjee K, Swan MB, Parmley WW, Sustailta H, Marcus HS, Matloff J: Influence of direct myocardial revascularization on left ventricular asynergy and function in patients with coronary heart disease: with and without previous myocardial infarction. Circulation 47:276,1973.

32. Cheanvechai C, Groves LK, Reyes EA, Shirey EK, Sones FM Jr: Manual coronary endarterectomy. J Thorac Cardiovasc Surg 70:524,1975.

33. Chesebro JH, Ritman EL, Frye RL, Smith HC, Rutherford BD, Fulton RE, Pluth JR, Barnhorst DA: Regional myocardial wall thickening response to nitroglycerin: a predictor of myocardial response to aortocoronary bypass surgery. Circulation 57:952,1978.

34. Christakis GT, Ivanov J, Weisel RD, Birnbaum PL, David TE, Salerno TA: The changing pattern of coronary artery bypass surgery. Circulation 79(Suppl I): I-151,1989.

35. Cohen MV, Gorlin R: Main left coronary artery disease: clinical experience from 1964 to 1974. Circulation 52:275,1975.

36. Cohn PF: Severe asymptomatic coronary artery disease: a diagnostic, prognostic and therapeutic puzzle. Am J Cardiol 62:565,1977.

37. Conti CR: Coronary arteriography. Circulation 55:227,1977.

38. Copeland JG, Griepp RB, Stinson EB, Shumway NE: Long-term follow-up after isolated aortic valve replacement. J Thorac Cardiovasc Surg 74:875,1977.

39. Cosgrove DM, Loop FD, Lytle BW, Goormastic M, Stewart RW, Gill CC, Golding LR: Does mammary artery grafting increase surgical risk? Circulation 72(Suppl II):II-170,1985.

40. Crawford MH: Risk stratification after myocardial infarction with exercise and doppler echocardiography. Circulation 84(Suppl I):I-163,1991.

41. Curtis JJ, Stoney WS, Alford WC Jr, Burrus GR, Thomas CS Jr: Intimal hyperplasia: a cause of radial artery aortocoronary bypass graft failure. Ann Thorac Surg 20:628,1975.

42. DeRouen TA, Murray JA, Owen W: Variability in the analysis of coronary arteriograms. Circulation 55:324,1977.

43. Dilsizian V, Bonow RO: Current diagnostic techniques of assessing myocardial viability in patients with hibernating and stunned myocardium. Circulation 87: 1,1993.

44. Ellestad MH, Wan MKC: Predictive implications of stress testing: follow-up of 2700 subjects after maximum treadmill stress testing. Circulation 51:363,1975.

45. Ellis SG, Roubin GS, King SB III, Douglas JS Jr, Shaw RE, Stertzer SH, Myler RK: In-hospital cardiac mortality after acute closure after coronary angioplasty: analysis of risk factors from 8,207 procedures. J Am Coll Cardiol 11:211,1988.

46. Epstein SE, Kent KM, Goldstein RE, Borer JS, Rosing DR: Strategy for evaluation and surgical treatment of the asymptomatic or mildly symptomatic patient with coronary artery disease. Am J Cardiol 43:1015,1979.

47. Favoloro RG: Surgical Treatment of Coronary Arteriosclerosis. Baltimore, Williams & Wilkins, 1970.

48. Fisher LD, Davis KB: Design and study similarities and contrasts: the Veterans Administration, European, and CASS randomized trials of coronary artery bypass graft surgery. Circulation 72(Suppl V):V-110,1985.

49. Fisk RL, Brooks CH, Callaghan JC, Dvorkin J: Experience with the radial artery graft for coronary artery bypass. Ann Thorac Surg 21:513,1976.

50. Forrester JS, Diamond G, Chatterjee K, Swan HJC: Medical therapy of acute myocardial infarction by application of hemodynamic subsets. N Engl J Med 295: 1356,1976.

51. Foster ED, Kranc MAT: Alternative conduits for aortocoronary bypass grafting. Circulation 79(Suppl I):I-34,1989.

52. Frye RL, Fisher L, Schaff HV, Gersh BJ, Viestra RE, Mock MB: Randomized trials in coronary artery bypass surgery. Prog Cardiovasc Dis 30:1,1987.

53. Gardner TJ, Stuart RS, Greene PS, Baumgartner WA: The risk of coronary bypass surgery for patients with postinfarction angina. Circulation 79(Suppl I): I-79,1989.

54. Gelbfish J, Jacobowitz IJ, Rose DM, Connolly MW, Acinapura AJ, Zisbrod Z, Lim KH, Cappabianca P, Cunningham JN: Cryopreserved homologous saphenous vein: early and late patency in coronary artery bypass. Ann Thorac Surg 42: 70,1986.

55. Gersh BJ, Califf RM, Loop FD, Akins CW, Pryor DB, Takaro TC: Coronary bypass surgery in chronic stable angina. Circulation 79(Suppl I):I-46,1989.

56. Gibbons RJ: Rest and exercise radionuclide angiography for diagnosis in chronic ischemic heart disease. Circulation 84(Suppl I):I-93,1991.

57. Goldman S, Tselos S, Cohn K: Marked depth of ST segment depression during treadmill exercise testing: indicator of severe coronary artery disease. Chest 69: 729,1976.

58. Gould KL: Clinical cardiac positron emission tomography: state of the art. Circulation 84(Suppl I):I-22,1991.

59. Green GE: Use of internal thoracic artery for coronary artery grafting. Circulation 79(Suppl I):I-30,1989.

60. Grondin CM, Campeau L, Thornton JC, Engle JC, Cross FS, Schreiber H: Coronary artery bypass grafting with saphenous vein. Circulation 79(Suppl I):I-24,1989.

61. Grondin CM, Vouhe P, Bourassa MG, Lesperance J, Bovier M, Campeau L: Optimal patency rates obtained in coronary artery grafting with circular vein grafts. J Thorac Cardiovasc Surg 75:161,1978.

62. Grossi EA, Esposito R, Harris LJ, Crooke GA, Galloway AC, Colvin SB, Culliford AT, Baumann FG, Yao K, Spencer FC: Sternal wound infections and use of internal mammary artery grafts. J Thorac Cardiovasc Surg 102:342,1991.

63. Gruentzig AR, Senning A, Siegenthaler WE: Nonoperative dilatation of coronary-artery stenosis. Percutaneous transluminal coronary angioplasty. N Engl J Med 301:61,1979.

64. Harlan BJ, Kyger ER, Reul FJ, Cooley DA: Needle suction of the aorta for left heart decompression during aortic cross-clamping. Ann Thorac Surg 23:259, 1977.

65. Hartman CW, Kong Y, Margolis JR, Warren SG, Peter RH, Behar VS, Oldham HN: Aortocoronary bypass surgery: correlation of angiographic, symptomatic and functional improvement at 1 year. Am J Cardiol 37:352,1976.

66. Heimbecker RO, McKenzie FN: A new approach to left heart decompression. Ann Thorac Surg 21:456,1976.

67. Helfant RH, Pine R, Meister SG, Feldman MS, Trout RG, Banka VS: Nitroglycerin to unmask reversible asynergy: correlation with postcoronary bypass ventriculography. Circulation 50:108,1974.

68. Holmes DR, Holubkov R, Vleitstra RE, Kelsey SF, Reeder GS, Dorros G, Williams DO, Cowley MJ, Faxon DP, Kent KM, Bentivoglio LG, Detre K: Comparison of complications during percutaneous transluminal coronary angioplasty from 1977 to 1981 and from 1985 to 1986: the National Heart, Lung, and Blood Institute Percutaneous Transluminal Coronary Angioplasty Registry. J Am Coll Cardiol 12:1149,1988.

69. Hurst JW, King SB III, Logue RB, Hatcher CR Jr, Jones EL, Craver JM, Douglas JS Jr, Franch RH, Dorney ER, Cobbs BW Jr, Robinson PH, Clements SD Jr, Kaplan JA, Bradford JM: Value of coronary bypass surgery. Am J Cardiol 42: 308,1978.

70. Hutchins GM, Bulkey BH, Ridolfi RL, Griffith LSC, Lohr FT, Piasio MA: Correlation of coronary arteriograms and left ventriculograms with postmortem strudies. Circulation 56:32,1977.

71. Irving JB, Bruce RA, DeRouen TA: Variations in and significance of systolic pressure during maximal exercise (treadmill) testing. Am J Cardiol 39:841,1977.

72. Isshiki T, Yamaguchi T, Nakamura M, Saeki F, Itaoka Y, Nagahara T, Furuta Y, Ikari Y, Wanibuchi Y, Suma H: Postoperative angiographic evaluation of gastroepiploic artery grafts: technical considerations and short-term patency. Cathet Cardiovasc Diagn 21:233,1990.

73. Johnson WD, Flemma RJ, Lepley D Jr, Ellison EH: Extended treatment of severe coronary artery disease: a total surgical approach. Ann Surg 170:460,1969.

74. Jones EL, Weintraub WS, Craver JM, Guyton RA, Cohen CL: Coronary bypass surgery: Is the operation different today? J Thorac Cardiovasc Surg 101:108,1991.

75. Judkins MP: Selective coronary arteriography: a percutaneous transfemoral technic. Radiology 89:815,1967.

76. Junod FL, Harlan BJ, Payne J, Smeloff EA, Miller GE Jr, Kelly PB, Ross KA, Shankar KG, McDermott JP: Preoperative risk assessment in cardiac surgery: comparison of predicted and observed results. Ann Thorac Surg 43:59,1987.

77. Kaiser GC, Schaff HV, Killip T: Myocardial revascularization for unstable angina pectoris. Circulation 79(Suppl I):I-60,1989.

78. Kennedy JW, Ivey TD, Misbach G, Allen MD, Maynard C, Dalquist JE, Kruse S, Stewart DK: Coronary artery bypass graft surgery early after acute myocardial infarction. Circulation 79(Suppl I):I-73,1989.

79. Kent KM, Borer JS, Green MV, Bacharach SL, McIntosh CL, Conkle DM, Epstein SE: Effects of coronary artery bypass operation on global and regional left ventricular function during exercise. N Engl J Med 298:1434,1978.

80. Killip T, Passamani E, Davis K: Coronary Artery Surgery Study (CASS): a randomized trial of coronary bypass surgery—eight years follow-up and survival in patients with reduced ejection fraction. Circulation 72(Suppl V):V-102,1985.

81. King SB III, Talley DJ: Coronary arteriography and percutaneous transluminal coronary angioplasty: changing patterns of use and results. Circulation 79(Suppl I):I-19,1989.

82. Kloster FE, Kremau EL, Ritzmann LW, Rahimtoola SH, Rosch J, Kanarek PH: Coronary bypass for stable angina: a prospective randomized study. N Engl J Med 300:149,1979.

83. Knoebel SB, McHenry PL, Phillips JF, Lowe DK: The effect of aortocoronary bypass grafts on myocardial blood flow reserve and treadmill exercise tolerance. Circulation 55:685,1974.

84. Kouchoukos NT, Murphy S, Phipott T, Pelate C, Marshall WG: Coronary artery bypass grafting for postinfarction angina pectoris. Circulation 79(Suppl I):I-68,1989.

85. Langou RA, Geha AS, Hammond GL, Cohen LS: Surgical approach for patients with unstable angina pectoris: intra-aortic balloon pumping in perioperative complications after aortocoronary bypass grafting. Am J Cardiol 42:629,1978.

86. Lapin ES, Murray JA, Bruce RA, Winterscheid L: Changes in maximal exercise performance in the evaluation of saphenous vein bypass surgery. Circulation 47: 1164,1973.

87. Laub GW, Muralidharan S, Clancy R, Eldredge J, Chen C, Adkins MS, Fernandez J, Anderson WA, McGrath LB: Cryopreserved allograft veins as alternative

coronary artery bypass conduits: early phase results. Ann Thorac Surg 54:
826,1992.

88. Lawrie GM, Lie JT, Morris GC, Beazley HL: Vein graft patency and intimal
proliferation after aortocoronary bypass: early and long-term angiopathologic
correlations. Am J Cardiol 38:856,1976.

89. Lawrie GM, Morris GC, Howell JF, Ogura JW, Spencer WH III, Cashion WR,
Winters WL, Beazley HL, Chapman DW, Peterson PK, Lie JT: Results of coronary bypass more than 5 years after operation in 434 patients. Am J Cardiol 40:
665,1977.

90. Lee L, Bates ER, Pitt B, Walton JA, Laufer N, O'Neill WW: Percutaneous transluminal coronary angioplasty improves survival in acute myocardial infarction
complicated by cardiogenic shock. Circulation 78:1345,1988.

91. Leinbach RC, Gold HK, Harper RW, Buckley MJ, Austen WG: Early intra-aortic
balloon pumping for anterior myocardial infarction without shock. Circulation
58:204,1978.

92. Lesperance J, Bourassa MG, Campeau L, Biron P, Saltiel J: Aorta to coronary
artery saphenous vein grafts: preoperative angiographic criteria for successful
surgery. Am J Cardiol 30:459,1972.

93. Lichtlen T, Morcetti T, Halter J: Postoperative evaluation of myocardial blood
flow in aorta to coronary artery vein bypass grafting using xenon-residue detection technique. Circulation 46:445,1972.

94. Linhart JW, Wheat MW: Myocardial dysfunction following aortic valve replacement: the significance of coronary artery disease. J Thorac Cardiovasc Surg 54:
259,1967.

95. Loop FD, Lytle BW, Cosgrove DM: Comment: new arteries for old. Circulation
79(Suppl I):I-40,1989.

96. Loop FD, Lytle BW, Cosgrove DM, Stewart RW, Goormastic M, Williams GW,
Golding LAR, Gill CC, Taylor PC, Sheldon WC, Proudfit WL: Influence of the
internal-mammary-artery graft on 10-year survival and other cardiac events. N
Engl J Med 314:1,1986.

97. Loop FD, Lytle BW, Cosgrove DM, Woods EL, Stewart RE, Golding LAR, Goormastic M, Taylor PC: Reoperation for coronary atherosclerosis: changing practice
in 2509 consecutive patients. Ann Surg 212:378,1990.

98. Lown B: Sudden cardiac death: the major challenge confronting contemporary
cardiology. Am J Cardiol 43:313,1979.

99. Lytle B, Cosgrove DM: Coronary artery bypass surgery. Curr Probl Surg 29:
737,1992.

100. Lytle BW, Cosgrove DM, Ratliff NB, Loop FD: Coronary artery bypass grafting
with the right gastroepiploic artery. J Thorac Cardiovasc Surg 97:826,1989.

101. Madigan NP, Rutherford BD, Barnhorst DA, Danielson GK: Early saphenous
vein grafting after subendocardial infarction: immediate surgical results and late
prognosis. Circulation 56(Suppl II):II-1,1977.

102. Madigan NP, Rutherford BD, Frye RL: The clinical course, early prognosis and
coronary anatomy of subendocardial infarction. Am J Med 60:634,1976.

103. Marco JD, Barner HB, Kaiser GC, Codd JE, Mudd JG, William V: Operative flow
measurements and coronary bypass graft patency. J Thorac Cardiovasc Surg 71:
545,1976.

104. Mathur VS, Guinn GA: Long-term follow-up (4–7 years) of a prospective randomized study to evaluate surgical vs medical treatment for stable angina pectoris: clinical status, exercise performance and survival. Am J Cardiol 43:382,1979.

105. Mathur VS, Guinn GA, Anastassiades LC, Chahine RA, Korompai FL, Montero
AC, Luchi RJ: Surgical treatment for stable angina pectoris: prospective randomized study. N Engl J Med 292:709,1975.

106. Matlof HJ, Alderman EL, Wexler L, Shumway NE, Harrison DC: What is the
relationship between the response of angina to coronary surgery and anatomical
success? Circulation 47(Suppl III):III-168,1973.

107. McAlpine WA: Heart and Coronary Arteries. Berlin, Heidelberg, New York,
Springer-Verlag, 1975.

108. Milgalter E, Pearl J, Laks H, Elami A, Louie HW, Baker ED, Buckberg GD: The
inferior epigastric arteries as coronary bypass conduits: size, preoperative duplex
scan assessment of suitability, and early clinical experience. J Thorac Cardiovasc
Surg 103:463,1992.

109. Mills NL, Everson CT: Technique for use of the inferior epigastric artery as a coronary bypass graft. Ann Thorac Surg 51:208,1991.
110. Moroko PR, Kjekshus JK, Sobel BE, Watanabe T, Covell JW, Ross J Jr, Braunwald E: Factors influencing infarct size following experimental coronary artery occlusion. Circulation 43:67,1971.
111. Moss AJ, Benhorin J: Prognosis and management after a first myocardial infarction. N Engl J Med 322:743,1990.
112. Mundth ED, Buckley MJ, Leinbach RC, DeSanctis RW, Sanders CA, Kantrowitz A, Austen WG: Myocardial revascularization for the treatment of cardiogenic shock complicating acute myocardial infarction. Surgery 70:78,1971.
113. Myers WO, Schaff HV, Gersh BJ, Fisher LD, Kosinski AS, Mock MB, Holmes DR, Ryan TJ, Kaiser GC: Improved survival of surgically treated patients with triple vessel coronary artery disease and severe angina pectoris: a report from the Coronary Artery Surgery Study (CASS) registry. J Thorac Cardiovasc Surg 97:487,1989.
114. Najafi H, Javid H, Hunter JA, Goldin MD, Serry C, Dye WS: Mitral insufficiency secondary to coronary heart disease. Ann Thorac Surg 20:529,1975.
115. National Cooperative Study Group: Unstable angina pectoris: National cooperative study group to compare surgical and medical therapy. II. In-hospital experience and initial follow-up results in patients with one, two and three vessel disease. Am J Cardiol 42:839,1978.
116. Naunheim KS, Fiore AC, Wadley JJ, McBride LR, Kanter KR, Pennington DG, Barner HB, Kaiser GC, Willman VL: The changing profile of the patient undergoing coronary artery bypass surgery. J Am Coll Cardiol 11:494,1988.
117. Oglietti J, Angelini P, Leachman RD, Cooley DA: Myocardial revascularization: early and late results after reoperation. J Thorac Cardiovasc Surg 71:732,1976.
118. Okies JE, Macmanus Q, Starr A: Myocardial revascularization and carotid endarterectomy: a combined approach. Ann Thorac Surg 23:560,1977.
119. Okies JE, Phillips SJ, Crenshaw R, Starr A: "No-vent" technique of coronary artery bypass. Ann Thorac Surg 19:191,1975.
120. Olinger GN, Bonchek LI, Keelan MH. Tresch DD, Siegel R, Bamrah V, Tristani FE: Unstable angina: the case for operation. Am J Cardiol 42:634,1978.
121. Ormand J, Piatt M, Mills L, Shapiro W, Pugh B, Blomgvist CG, Parkey RW, Willerson JT: Thallium 201 scintigraphy and exercise testing in evaluating the patients prior to and after coronary bypass surgery (abstr). Circulation 55, 56(Suppl III):III-131,1977.
122. Parsonnet V, Dean D, Bernstein AD: A method of uniform stratification of risk for evaluating the results of surgery in acquired adult heart disease. Circulation 79(Suppl I):I-3,1989.
123. Parsonnet V, Gilbert L, Gielchinsky I, Bahaktan EK: Endarterectomy of the left anterior descending and main stem coronary arteries: a technique for reconstruction of inoperable arteries. Surgery 80:662,1976.
124. Passamani E, Davis K, Gillespie MJ, Killip T: A randomized trial of coronary artery bypass surgery. N Engl J Med 312:1665,1985.
125. Peterson CR, Herr R, Crisera RV, Starr A, Bristow JD, Griswold HE: The failure of hemodynamic improvement after valve replacement surgery: etiology, diagnosis, and treatment. Ann Intern Med 66:1,1967.
126. Phillips SG, Kongtahworn C, Zeff RH, Iannone L, Brown T, Gordon DF: Emergency coronary artery revascularization: a possible therapy for acute myocardial infarction. Circulation 60:241,1979.
127. Pym J, Brown PM, Charrette EJP, Parker JO, West RO: Gastroepiploic-coronary anastomosis: a viable alternative bypass graft. J Thorac Cardiovasc Surg 94:256,1987.
128. Rees G, Bristow JD, Kremkau EL, Green GS, Herr RH, Griswold HE, Starr A: Influence of aortocoronary bypass surgery on left ventricular performance. N Engl J Med 284:1116,1971.
129. Richardson JV, Kouchoukos NT, Wright JO III, Karp RB: Combined aortic valve replacement and myocardial revascularization: results in 220 patients. Circulation 59:75,1979.
130. Ritchie JL, Narahara KA, Trobaugh GB, Williams DL, Hamilton GW: Thallium-201 myocardial imaging before and after coronary revascularization: assessment of regional myocardial blood flow and graft patency. Circulation 56:830,1977.

131. Rogers WJ, Baim DS, Gore JM, et al: Comparison of immediate invasive, delayed invasive, and conservative strategies after tissue-type plasminogen activator. Results of the Thrombolysis in Myocardial Infarction (TIMI) Phase II-A trial. Circulation 81:1457,1990.

132. Rosch J, Dotter CT, Antonovic R, Bonchek L, Starr A: Angiographic appraisal of distal vessel suitability for aortocoronary bypass graft surgery. Circulation 48:202,1973.

133. Salerno TA, Charrette EJP: Elimination of venting in coronary artery surgery. Ann Thorac Surg 27:340,1979.

134. Salerno TA, Charrette EJP: The short saphenous vein: an alternative to the long saphenous vein for aortocoronary bypass. Ann Thorac Surg 25:457,1978.

135. Schelbert HR: Positron emission tomography for the assessment of myocardial viability. Circulation 84(Suppl I):I-122,1991.

136. Selden R, Neill WA, Ritzmann LW, Okies JE, Anderson RP: Medical versus surgical therapy for acute coronary insufficiency: a randomized study. N Engl J Med 293:1329,1975.

137. Siderys H: The superior approach for operative decompression of the left side of the heart. Ann Thorac Surg 17:277,1974.

138. Sobel BE, Shell WE: Jeopardized, blighted, and necrotic myocardium. Circulation 47:215,1973.

139. Sones F, Shirey EK: Cine coronary angiography. Mod Conc Cardiovasc Dis 31:735,1962.

140. Sos TA, Baltaxe HA: Cranial and caudal angulation for coronary angiography revisited. Circulation 56:119,1977.

141. Stenson RE, Flamm MD Jr, Zaret BL, Killip T: Transient ST-segment elevation with postmyocardial infarction angina. Prognostic significance. Am Heart J 89:449,1975.

142. Stoney WS, Alford WC, Burrus GR, Glassford DM, Petracek MR, Thomas CS: The fate of arm veins used for aorta-coronary bypass grafts. J Thorac Cardiovasc Surg 88:522,1984.

143. Suma H, Fukumoto H, Takeuchi A: Coronary artery bypass grafting by utilizing in situ right gastroepiploic artery: basic study and clinical application. Ann Thorac Surg 44:394,1987.

144. Takaro T, Hultgren HN, Lipton MJ, Detre KM: The VA cooperative randomized study of surgery for coronary occlusive disease. II. Subgroup with significant left main lesions. Circulation 54(Suppl III):III-197,1976.

145. Talley JD, Weintraub WS, Roubin GS, Douglas JS, Anderson HV, Jones EL, Morris DC, Liberman HA, Craver JM, Guyton RA, King SB III: Failed elective percutaneous transluminal coronary angioplasty requiring coronary artery bypass surgery: in-hospital and late clinical outcome at 5 years. Circulation 82:1203,1990.

146. Tavilla G, van Son JAM, Verhagen AF, Smedts F: Retrogastric versus antegastric routing and histology of the right gastroepiploic artery. Ann Thorac Surg 53:1057,1992.

147. Thomson PD, Kelemen MH: Hypotension accompanying the onset of exertional angina: a sign of severe compromise of left ventricular blood supply. Circulation 52:28,1975.

148. Tyras DH, Ahmad N, Kaiser GC, Barner HB, Codd JE, Willman VL: Ventricular function and the native coronary circulation five years after myocardial revascularization. Ann Thorac Surg 27:547,1979.

149. Varnauskas E, the European Coronary Surgery Study Group: Twelve-year follow-up of survival in the randomized European Coronary Surgery Study. N Engl J Med 319:332,1988.

150. Vlodaver Z, Frech R, Van Tassel RA, Edwards JE: Correlation of the antemortem coronary arteriogram and the postmortem specimen. Circulation 47:162,1973.

151. Weaver FA, Barlow CR, Edwards WH, Mulherin JL, Jenkins JM: The lesser saphenous vein: autogenous tissue for lower extremity revascularization. J Vasc Surg 5:687,1987.

152. Weiner DA, Ryan TJ, McCabe CH, Chaitman BR, Sheffield LT, Ng G, Fisher LD, Tristini FE: Comparison of coronary artery bypass surgery and medical therapy in patients with exercise-induced silent myocardial ischemia: a report from the Coronary Artery Surgery Study (CASS) registry. J Am Coll Cardiol 12:595,1988.

153. Weiner DA, Ryan TJ, McCabe CH, Kennedy JW, Schloss M, Tristani F, Chaitman BR, Fisher LD: Exercise stress testing: correlations among history of angina, ST-segment response and prevalence of coronary-artery disease in the Coronary Artery Surgery Study (CASS). N Engl J Med 301:230, 1979.

154. Wijnberg DS, Boeve WJ, Ebels T, van Gelder IC, van den Toren EW, Lie KI, Homan van der Heide JN: Patency of arm vein grafts used in aorto-coronary bypass surgery. Eur J Cardio-thorac Surg 4:510, 1990.

155. Wolf NM, Kreulen TH, Bove AA, McDonough MT, Kessler KM, Strong M, LeMole G, Spann JF: Left ventricular function following coronary bypass surgery. Circulation 58:63, 1978.

156. Younis LT, Byers S, Shaw L, Barth G, Goodgold H, Chaitman BR: Prognostic importance of silent myocardial ischemia detected by intravenous dipyridamole thallium myocardial imaging in asymptomatic patients with coronary artery disease. J Am Coll Cardiol 14:1635, 1989.

157. Zir LM, Miller SE, Dinsmore RE, Gilbert JP, Harthorne JW: Interobserver variability in coronary angiography. Circulation 53:627, 1976.

10

Left Ventricular Aneurysm

Left ventricular aneurysm develops following myocardial infarction in 10%–38% of patients.[1,7,41] Since Cooley's report[9] in 1958 of resection utilizing cardiopulmonary bypass, the operation has become an established treatment for ventricular aneurysm causing congestive heart failure, intractable ventricular arrhythmia, or systemic emboli; resection of aneurysm in conjunction with coronary artery bypass for angina is also common.

This chapter concerns treatment of "true" ventricular aneurysm, as differentiated from "false" aneurysm. "True" left ventricular aneurysm is full-thickness scar of the wall of the ventricle, is discrete from the surrounding viable myocardium, and has paradoxical or outward motion during systole. "False" left ventricular aneurysm is a contained rupture of the left ventricle[30]; the rupture is contained by adhesions of epicardium and pericardium. "False" aneurysms or pseudoaneurysms typically expand and are at risk of rupture[16,18,19]; for this reason their existence is indication for surgical treatment. Diagnosis of pseudoaneurysm and differentiation from "true" aneurysm can often be made noninvasively by echocardiography[38] and radionuclide angiography.[5]

Ventricular aneurysm must also be differentiated from a large area of akinetic myocardium—an area of fibrosis interspersed with viable muscle. Excision of akinetic myocardium is generally not indicated. Excision is associated with high operative mortality, poor late survival, and little, if any, improvement in symptoms[26,45]

Resection

All aneurysms are opened and repaired. Plication—inversion or eversion of the aneurysm without opening it—is not performed. Plication has the definite hazard of dislodging mural thrombus and for this reason is not done. Using the open technique, little, if any, of the wall of a small aneurysm may be resected, but inclusion of the wall in the repair excludes the aneurysm from the functioning ventricle.

Indications

Congestive Heart Failure
Left ventricular aneurysm affects ventricular function adversely in a number of ways[25]: (1) the area of scar does not participate in contraction, (2) the

expansion of the aneurysm diminishes forward flow of blood and decreases the rate of development of tension in the viable muscle, and (3) the oxygen supply-demand balance in the viable myocardium can be upset, causing ischemic dysfunction of the ventricle. This increased myocardial oxygen demand is caused by the increased wall tension necessary to generate adequate chamber pressure as the ventricle enlarges (Laplace relationship).

Congestive heart failure is a common indication for surgery, being the primary indication in 23%–50% of patients.[6,11] Although congestive heart failure usually develops months after infarction, development of aneurysm may cause congestive heart failure as early as 3 weeks after infarction.[3,50]

Absolute contraindications to aneurysm resection have not been conclusively established, but a subset of patients in whom operative mortality is high and symptomatic improvements unlikely can be identified. Operative mortality and functional result following aneurysmectomy are best predicted by the contraction of the residual ventricle.[2,6,23,27,34,46,51] Qualitative analysis of residual ventricular function has been described by Burton and co-workers.[6] They found an operative mortality of 9.8% and 5-year survival of 80% in patients with "good" contraction of the residual ventricle, whereas patients with "poor" contraction had an operative mortality of 34% and a 5-year survival of 36%.

Quantitative analyses of the function of the residual ventricle have been described, including basilar fractional area reduction, contractile segment ejection fraction, and basilar half-ejection fraction.[23,27,51] Kapelanski and colleagues[23] found that patients undergoing urgent aneurysmectomy with a basilar half-ejection fraction below 30% had an 89% mortality, whereas patients with a basilar half-ejection over 30% had only 18% mortality. Watson and colleagues[51] found high operative mortality and poor functional improvement in patients with a contractile ejection fraction below 44%. Patients with a contractile ejection fraction over 45% all survived and had marked functional improvement.

Continued study of residual ventricular function is likely to improve selection of patients for surgery. Radionuclide studies will be an important component of such evaluation.[4,15,17,37,48,52]

Angina Pectoris

In the early years of cardiac surgery, angina was an infrequent indication for aneurysm resection. With the development of coronary artery surgery, unsuspected aneurysms were diagnosed in patients undergoing evaluation of angina. The increasing number of aneurysms being diagnosed has markedly increased the incidence of angina as a primary or associated indication for surgery. In a recent report from the Cleveland Clinic,[11] angina alone or angina with congestive heart failure was the indication for surgery in 63% of patients. Aneurysms discovered incidentally in the study of patients with angina pectoris should be resected in conjunction with the performance of coronary artery surgery.

Ventricular Arrhythmia

Ventricular aneurysms can be associated with serious ventricular arrhythmias. Medical management may not be successful in the management of these arrhythmias. Intractable ventricular arrhythmia is the primary indication for surgery in 8%–27% of patients.[6,11,39] Ventricular aneurysmectomy, however, is not always effective in controlling the arrhythmia, with failure rates approaching 50%.[6,11] The development of operative mapping and endocardial excision[22] or encircling ventriculotomy[20] in association with aneurysmectomy improves the results of surgery for arrhythmia, as does the use of implantable ventricular defibrillators.[32]

Systemic Embolism
Mural thrombi are commonly associated with ventricular aneurysms, found in approximately 60% of patients.[6,14,44] However, systemic emboli are rare, and systemic embolism is the least frequent indication for surgery, accounting for only 2%–5% of patients.[6,11,28] It does not appear that chronic anticoagulation has any effect on the frequency of preoperative systemic arterial embolization or the prevalence of left ventricular mural thrombus found at surgery.[44]

Surgical Strategy

Myocardial Preservation
Cold blood cardioplegia is the usual method of myocardial preservation (Chapter 6). Ischemic arrest at moderate hypothermia may also be used if the time of aneurysm repair is less than 15 minutes.

Management of Coexistent Conditions
Coronary artery disease: All patients undergoing study of ventricular aneurysm should also undergo coronary arteriography. We perform saphenous vein bypasses to vessels with 50% or more narrowing of luminal diameter and satisfactory distal vessels. Bypass is performed even if angina is not present. Our rationale for this practice is the strong suggestion that coexistent coronary artery surgery does not increase operative mortality,[11,43] may decrease operative mortality,[11] and appears to improve survival.[11,39] Patients who have had complete revascularization for multiple-vessel disease in association with aneurysmectomy have the same survival at 7 years as those patients who have only single-vessel disease to the area of aneurysm.[11]

Distal anastomoses are usually performed after resection of the aneurysm. Proximal anastomoses are performed over a partial occluding clamp while the vented, beating, nonworking heart recovers from the period of cardioplegic arrest.

Mitral regurgitation: Mitral valve replacement may be performed through the open aneurysm from the left ventricular side[10] or through the standard left atriotomy, with the latter being our preference.

Ventricular septal defect: The defect in the ventricular septum is closed in the standard fashion (Chapter 11) through the open aneurysm.

Surgical Anatomy

The vast majority of left ventricular aneurysms (approximately 90%[6,39]), are caused by infarction in the distribution of the left anterior descending coronary artery. Posterior aneurysms—aneurysms of the diaphragmatic wall occurring in the distribution of the right coronary artery—are rare, accounting for only 3%–5% of cases.[6,29] The rarity of posterior ventricular aneurysms may be due to frequent associated damage to the posterior papillary muscle and early death secondary to massive mitral regurgitation.[29]

Surgical Technique: Linear Repair

The area of the aneurysm is not dissected until bypass is initiated and the heart is arrested. This is to diminish the possibility of dislodging an intraventricular thrombus. Cardiopulmonary bypass is initiated with single atrial and ascending aortic cannulation. Systemic cooling is performed, the aorta is clamped, and cardioplegic solution is infused into the ascending aorta. If left heart decompression is necessary, it can be accomplished through the right superior pulmonary vein or by opening the aneurysm. Myocardial temperature is measured in an area of the left ventricle that is viable, and a temperature below 15°C is sought.

The middle of the aneurysm is incised and the incision is extended with scissors (Fig. 10–1). Intramural clot is carefully scooped out (Fig. 10–2), and

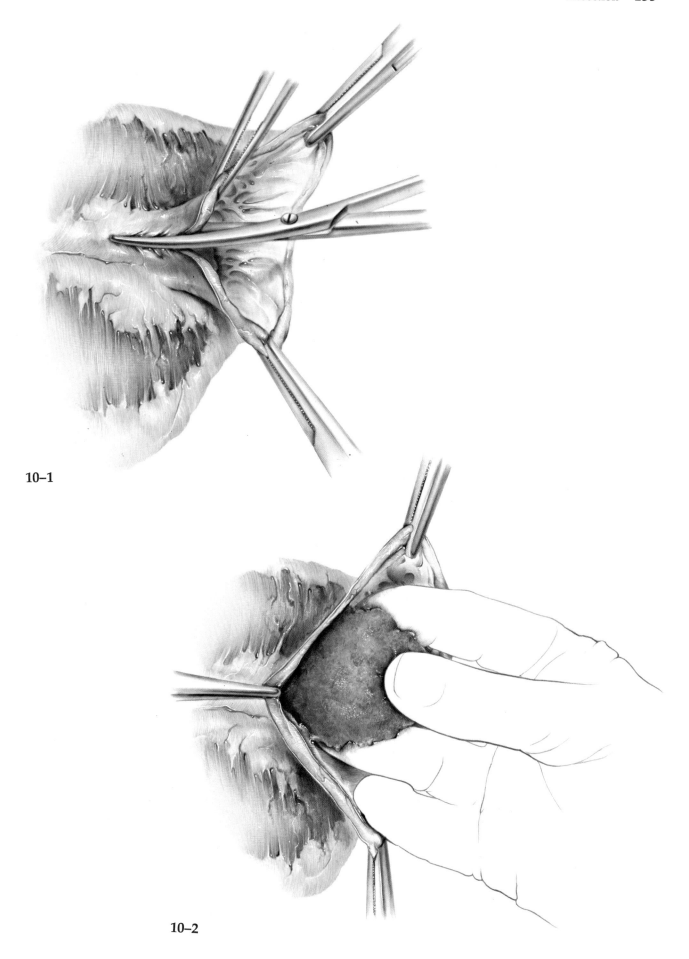

10–1

10–2

residual pieces are removed. Clamps placed on the edges of the aneurysm aid retraction and exposure.

At this point inspection of the interior of the left ventricle and assessment of the mitral apparatus can be done. The degree of involvement of the septum and the firmness of the septum can be determined. Although some have advocated exclusion of all infarcted septum by suturing the lateral edge of the aneurysm down to the viable septum[47,49] or buttressing of the infarcted septum with prosthetic material,[36] this has not been our general practice. Further evaluation of postoperative ventricular function and survival will be necessary to document the value of such technical modifications.[42]

Inspection of the mitral apparatus is important. Mild or moderate mitral regurgitation may be secondary to lateral "tethering" of the papillary muscles by a large aneurysm, rather than infarction of the papillary muscles or rupture of the chordae tendineae. Inspection in such an instance will show whether the disease process spares the papillary muscle and chordae. Repair of the aneurysm will usually cure the mitral regurgitation by bringing the papillary muscles back into more functional alignment.

Repair of the aneurysm is initiated by placing two wide strips of Teflon felt on each side of the aneurysm (Fig. 10–3). Horizontal mattress sutures of O polyester on a large (45-mm diameter) needle are taken through the felt strips and the fibrotic edges of the aneurysm. These are tied. A vent is left in the apex under the last stitch.

The edges of the aneurysm wall protruding over the Teflon strips are cut flush. A running up-and-back suture of the same O polyester is then taken. The aortic clamp is released as air is removed from the ascending aorta. The apex is elevated and the apical vent is partially removed to remove air and then repositioned. The heart is defibrillated if necessary, and recovery from cardioplegia is accomplished with a vented nonworking heart. The vent is then removed and several horizontal mattress sutures and simple interrupted sutures are taken at the apex to achieve complete hemostasis (Fig. 10–4). The

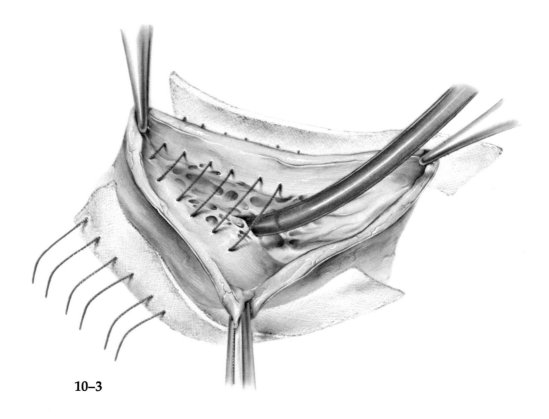

10–3

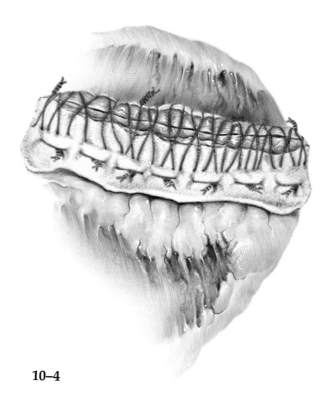

10–4

patient is then weaned from bypass. The suture line is checked prior to removing the venous cannula to assure hemostasis at normal systemic pressure.

Endoventricular Repair

Jatene[21] reported in 1985 his technique of sewing an oval Dacron patch in the orifice of the aneurysm. His theory is that this technique re-establishes more normal orientation and alignment of remaining viable myocardial fibers and thereby improves postoperative ventricular function. Cooley[10] has modified this technique and termed it "endoaneurysmorrhaphy." He repairs the aneurysm with a Dacron patch sutured to the opening and then uses the remaining aneurysmal wall to cover the Dacron patch, reinforcing this closure with polyester felt strips. Dor and colleagues[13] and Mills and colleagues[31] have also reported modifications of the Jatene technique.

Kesler and colleagues[24] did not find any difference in ventricular function postoperatively when they compared a group of patients who had linear closure with a group of patients who had endoventricular repair. Their patients were not randomized, and it is unlikely that any clear difference between the two techniques will be conclusively determined until a prospective randomized trial is performed. Endoventricular repair seems most appropriate when a linear repair would result in marked deformity of the left ventricle and a suture line with excessive tension.

Results

Operative Mortality
A compilation of series from 1976 to 1987 found operative mortality ranging from 2% to 19% with an average mortality of 9.9% in 3439 patients.[12]

Symptomatic Improvement
The vast majority of patients undergoing surgery have improvement in symptoms, usually achieving functional class I or II status.[23] A number of reports have documented 80% or more of patients in functional class I or II.[6,33,39,43]

Ventricular Function

The results of studies of ventricular function following aneurysm resection are conflicting.[17,46] This is probably caused by different patient variables (such as extent of coronary disease), different methods of evaluating ventricular function, and different methods of selection for postoperative study. Nevertheless, some general statements can be made regarding changes in ventricular function following aneurysmectomy.

A majority of patients appear to have improved diastolic function postoperatively, although function does not return to normal.[46,47] Stephens and co-workers,[46] in a study of 12 patients, showed that left ventricular aneurysmectomy reduced mean left ventricular filling pressure from 25 to 17 mm Hg at rest and from 39 to 32 mm Hg during exercise, after administration of isosorbide dinitrate. Both these changes were statistically significant.

There has been little evidence that aneurysmectomy improves systolic ventricular function, at least at rest. Froelich and colleagues,[17] studying ejection fraction by isotope ventriculogram, found an improvement of 5% or greater in only 3 of 15 patients. Stephens and colleagues,[46] measuring exercise hemodynamics by thermodilution, found no significant change in mean stroke volume index at rest or during exercise following aneurysmectomy. Functional class postoperatively appears to correlate better with ventricular filling pressure than with ventricular volume or ejection fraction.[43]

Ventricular Arrhythmia

Ventricular aneurysmectomy alone as treatment for ventricular tachyarrhythmias has had disappointing results, with persistence of arrhythmia requiring medical treatment in approximately 50% of patients.[6,11] The more rigorous the postoperative search for arrhythmias, the more arrhythmias are found. In a postoperative study of 8 patients using 24-hour ambulatory electrocardiogram, Sami and co-workers[40] found recurrent ventricular tachycardia in 5 and multifocal premature ventricular contractions in the other 3 patients.

Ventricular tachycardia is more effectively treated with endocardial excision. Intraoperative mapping is performed to localize the area of origin of the tachycardia, which is usually at the border of the aneurysm. Josephson and co-workers[22] have reported results with this technique in 12 patients. Ventricular tachycardia could not be initiated by repeat electrophysiologic study postoperatively in any patient. The 10 survivors remained free of sustained ventricular tachycardia for 9–20 months, with one late nonarrhythmic death.

Survival

Most studies of the natural history of ventricular aneurysm are retrospective studies of several decades ago using autopsy data. These studies give a grim picture of the natural history of the disease. Schlicter and co-workers[41] found a 3-year survival of 27% and a 5-year survival of 12%.

Survival data in surgically treated patients are quite good. Three-year survival calculated actuarially ranges from 71% to 81%.[35,39] Burton and colleagues[6] reported actuarial 5-year survival at 60%. Surgical treatment appears to enhance survival in symptomatic patients with ventricular aneurysm.

References

1. Applebaum E, Nicholson GHB: Occlusive disease of the coronary arteries: analysis of pathological anatomy in 168 cases. Am Heart J 10:662,1935.
2. Arthur A, Basta L, Kioschos M: Factors influencing prognosis in left ventricular aneurysmectomy. Circulation 46(Suppl II):II-127,1972.
3. Baudet M, Rigaud M, Rocha P, Bardet J, Bourdarias JP: Treatment of early postinfarction ventricular aneurysm by intra-aortic balloon pumping and surgery. J Thorac Cardiovasc Surg 78:445,1979.

4. Borer JS, Jacobstein JG, Bacharach SL, Green MV: Detection of left ventricular aneurysm and evaluation of effects of surgical repair: the role of radionuclide cineangiography. Am J Cardiol 45:1103,1980.

5. Botvinik EH, Shames D, Hutchinson JC, Roe BB, Fitzpatrick M: Noninvasive diagnosis of a false left ventricular aneurysm with a radioisotope gated cardiac blood pool imaging: differentiating from true aneurysm. Am J Cardiol 37:1089, 1976.

6. Burton NA, Stinson EB, Oyer PE, Shumway NE: Left ventricular aneurysm: preoperative risk factors and long-term postoperative results. J Thorac Cardiovasc Surg 77:65,1979.

7. Cheng TO: Incidence of ventricular aneurysm in coronary artery disease: an angiographic appraisal. Am J Med 50:340,1971.

8. Cooley, DA: Ventricular endoaneurysmorrhaphy: a simplified repair for extensive postinfarction aneurysm. J Card Surg 4:200,1989.

9. Cooley DA, Collins HA, Morris GC Jr, Chapman DW: Ventricular aneurysm after myocardial infarction: surgical excision with use of temporary cardiopulmonary bypass. JAMA 167:557,1958.

10. Cooley DA, Norman JC: Techniques in Cardiac Surgery. Houston, Texas Medical Press, 1975, p 165.

11. Cosgrove DM, Loop FD, Irarrazaval MJ, Groves LK, Taylor PC, Golding LA: Determinants of long-term survival after ventricular aneurysmectomy. Ann Thorac Surg 26:357,1978.

12. Cosgrove DM, Lytle BW, Taylor PC, Stewart RW, Golding LAR, Mahfood S, Goormastic M, Loop FD: Ventricular aneurysm resection: trends in surgical risk. Circulation 79(Suppl I);I-97,1989.

13. Dor V, Saab M, Kornaszewska M, Montiglio F: Left ventricular aneurysm: a new surgical approach. Thorac Cardiovasc Surg 37:11,1989.

14. Dubnow MH, Burchell HB, Titus JH: Postinfarction ventricular aneurysm: a clinico-morphologic and electrocardiographic study of 80 cases. Am Heart J 70:753, 1965.

15. Dymond DS, Jarritt PH, Britton KE, Spurrell RAJ: Detection of postinfarction left ventricular aneurysm by first pass radionuclide ventriculography using a multi-crystal gamma camera. Br Heart J 41:68,1979.

16. Ersek RA, Chesler E, Korns ME, Edwards JE: Spontaneous rupture of a false ventricular aneurysm following myocardial infarction. Am Heart J 77:677,1969.

17. Froehlich RT, Falsetti HL, Doty DB, Marcus ML: Prospective study of surgery for left ventricular aneurysm. Am J Cardiol 45:923,1980.

18. Gobel FL, Visudh-Arom K, Edwards JE: Pseudoaneurysm of the left ventricle leading to recurrent pericardial hemorrhage. Chest 59:23,1971.

19. Gueron M, Wanderman KL, Hirsch M, Borman J: Pseudoaneurysm of the left ventricle after myocardial infarction: a curable form of myocardial rupture. J Thorac Cardiovasc Surg 69:736,1975.

20. Guiraudon G, Fontaine G, Frank R, Escande G, Etievent P, Cabrol C: Encircling endocardial ventriculotomy: a new surgical treatment for life-threatening ventricular tachycardias resistant to medical treatment following myocardial infarction. Ann Thorac Surg 26:438,1978.

21. Jatene AD: Left ventricular aneurysmectomy. J Thorac Cardiovasc Surg 89: 321,1985.

22. Josephson ME, Harken AH, Horowitz LN: Endocardial excision: a new surgical technique for the treatment of recurrent ventricular tachycardia. Circulation 58: 1167,1978.

23. Kapelanski DP, Al-Sadir J, Lamberti JJ, Anagnostopoulos CE: Ventriculographic features predictive of surgical outcome for left ventricular aneurysm. Circulation 58:1167,1978.

24. Kesler KA, Fiore AC, Naunheim KS, Sharp TG, Mahomed Y, Zollinger TW, Sawada SG, Brown JW, Labovitz AJ, Barner HB: Anterior wall left ventricular aneurysm repair: a comparison of linear versus circular closure. J Thorac Cardiovasc Surg 103:841,1992.

25. Klein MD, Herman MV, Gorlin R: A hemodynamic study of left ventricular aneurysm. Circulation 35:614,1967.

26. Kouchoukos NT, Doty DB, Buettner LE, Kirklin JW: Treatment of postinfarction

cardiac failure by myocardial excision and revascularization. Circulation 45(Suppl I):I-72,1972.

27. Lee DC, Johnson RA, Boucher CA, Wexler LF, McEnany MT: Angiographic predictors of survival following left ventricular aneurysmectomy. Circulation 56(Suppl II):II-12,1977.

28. Loop FD, Effler DB, Navia JA, Sheldon WC, Groves LK: Aneurysms of the left ventricle: survival and results of a ten-year surgical experience. Ann Surg 178: 399,1973.

29. Loop FD, Effler DB, Webster JS, Groves LK: Posterior ventricular aneurysms: etiologic factors and results of surgical treatment. N Engl J Med 288:237,1973.

30. Malcolm ID, Fitchett DH, Stewart D, Marpole D, Symes J: Ventricular aneurysm: false or true? An important distinction. Ann Thorac Surg 29:474,1980.

31. Mills NL, Everson CT, Hockmuth DR: Technical advances in the treatment of left ventricular aneurysm. Ann Thorac Surg 55:792,1993.

32. Mirowski M, Reid PR, Mower MM, Watkins L, Gott V, Schauble JF, Langer A, Heilman MS, Kolenik SA, Fischell RE, Weisfeldt ML: Termination of malignant ventricular arrhythmias with an implanted automatic defibrillator in human beings. N Engl J Med 303:322,1980.

33. Moran JM, Scanlon PJ, Nemickus R, Pifarre R: Surgical treatment of post-infarction ventricular aneurysm. Ann Thorac Surg 21:107,1976.

34. Mullen DC, Posey L, Gabriel R, Singh HM, Flemma RJ, Lepley D: Prognostic considerations in the management of left ventricular aneurysms. Ann Thorac Surg 23:455,1977.

35. Okies JE, Dietl C, Garrison HB, Starr A: Early and late results of resection of ventricular aneurysm. J Thorac Cardiovasc Surg 75:255,1978.

36. Reul GJ: Discussion of Walker et al. J Thorac Cardiovasc Surg 76:830,1978.

37. Rigo P, Murray M, Strauss HW, Pitt B: Scintiphotographic evaluation of patients with suspected left ventricular aneurysm. Circulation 50:985,1974.

38. Roelandt J, Van den Brand M, Vletter WB: Echocardiographic diagnosis of pseudoaneurysm of the left ventricle. Circulation 52:466,1975.

39. Rogers WJ, Oberman A, Kouchoukos NT: Left ventricular aneurysmectomy in patients with single vs multivessel coronary artery disease. Circulation 58(Suppl I):I-50,1978.

40. Sami M, Charpin D, Chabot M, Bourassa MG: Long-term follow-up of aneurysmectomy for recurrent ventricular tachycardia or fibrillation (abstr). Am J Cardiol 39:269,1977.

41. Schlicter J, Hellerstein HK, Katz LN: Aneurysm of the heart. Correlative study of 102 proved cases. Medicine 33:43,1954.

42. Schmidt CA, Bailey LL, Wareham EE: Septal wall motion: its significance in outcome of left ventricular scar resection. Arch Surg 115:624,1980.

43. Shaw RC, Connors JP, Hieb BR, Ludbrook PA, Krone R, Kleigher RE, Ferguson TB, Weldon CS: Postoperative investigation of left ventricular aneurysm resection. Circulation 56(Suppl II):II-7,1977.

44. Simpson MT, Oberman A, Kouchoukos NT, Rogers WJ: Prevalence of mural thrombi and systemic embolization with left ventricular aneurysm: effect of anticoagulation therapy. Chest 77:4,1980.

45. Spencer FC, Green GE, Tice DA, Walsh E, Mills NL, Glassman E: Coronary artery bypass grafts for congestive heart failure: a report of experience with 40 patients. J Thorac Cardiovasc Surg 62:529,1971.

46. Stephens JD, Dymond DS, Stone DL, Rees GM, Spurrell RAJ: Left ventricular aneurysm and congestive heart failure: value of exercise stress and isosorbide dinitrate in predicting hemodynamic results of aneurysmectomy. Am J Cardiol 45: 932,1980.

47. Stoney WS, Alford WC, Burrus GR, Thomas CS: Repair of anteroseptal ventricular aneurysm. Ann Thorac Surg 15:394,1973.

48. Strauss HW, Zaret BL, Hurley PJ, Natarajan TK, Pitt B: A scintiphotographic method for measuring left ventricular ejection fraction in man without cardiac catheterization. Am J Cardiol 28:575,1971.

49. Walker WE, Stoney WS, Alford WC Jr, Burrus GR, Frist RA, Glassford DM, Thomas CS Jr: Techniques and results of ventricular aneurysmectomy with emphasis on anteroseptal repair. J Thorac Cardiovasc Surg 76:824,1978.

50. Walker WE, Stoney WS, Alford WC Jr, Burrus GR, Glassford DM, Thomas CS Jr: Results of surgical management of acute left ventricular aneurysms. Circulation 62(Suppl I):I-75,1980.
51. Watson LE, Dickhaus DW, Martin RH: Left ventricular aneurysm: preoperative hemodynamics, chamber volume, and results of aneurysmectomy. Circulation 52: 868,1975.
52. Zaret BL, Strauss HW, Hurley PJ, Natarajan TK, Pitt B: A noninvasive scintiphotographic method for detecting regional ventricular dysfunction in man. N Engl J Med 284:1165,1971.

11

Postinfarction Ventricular Septal Defect

Rupture of the ventricular septum is a rare but devastating complication of myocardial infarction. Advances in perioperative support, myocardial preservation, and technique of repair have improved surgical results in a lesion that was almost always lethal prior to the advent of surgical therapy.

Indications for Surgery

Ventricular septal defect (VSD) is found in only 1%–2% of patients dying from acute myocardial infarction.[11,17] Septal rupture usually occurs from 2 to 4 days after infarction.[16,24] The natural history of the lesion is grim: approximately 25% of patients die within 24 hours and 60%–70% within 2 weeks, with only 10%–20% surviving 2 months.[21,22]

The lethal nature of postinfarction VSD stimulated the development of surgical treatment.[4] The early results indicated a lower mortality if repair was performed 6 or more weeks after infarction.[2] The defect rim at that stage is fibrotic and easier to repair,[18] seeming to suggest that a strategy of delay would be desirable.

However, the good results in patients operated upon weeks after infarction most likely reflect a selected group of patients with small defects and a relatively smaller amount of myocardial necrosis. The vast majority of patients die before 6 weeks. Therefore, delay should not be a goal. If a patient has no serious hemodynamic compromise from the development of a VSD, operation may be delayed. The vast majority of patients will require institution of circulatory support, proper study, and prompt surgery within hours or days of developing septal rupture.[5,6,16]

Surgical Strategy

Indications for Intraaortic Balloon Pump

Mechanical circulatory support with the intraaortic balloon pump (IABP) is a valuable advance in the management of low cardiac output secondary to septal rupture. IABP results in significant clinical and hemodynamic improvement in all cases, with a fall in the pulmonary capillary wedge pressure, a rise in mean arterial pressure, and a fall in the pulmonic/systemic flow ratio.[3,8] Pharmacologic manipulation with nitroprusside may also help to improve hemodynamics.[27]

142

It is our practice to institute IABP at the first sign of depressed cardiac output and to maintain it through catheterization and the immediate postoperative period.

Myocardial Preservation

Our method of myocardial preservation is cold blood cardioplegia (Chapter 6).

Management of Associated Conditions

Coronary Artery Disease
The value of bypassing diseased coronary arteries supplying the viable myocardium is controversial.[6] The study by Muerhrcke, Daggett, and colleagues[19] supports our feeling that it is likely to be beneficial and should not add any risk to the operation. They found that patients who had bypass for multivessel disease had the same long-term survival as those patients with single-vessel disease who did not have any coronary disease in vessels supplying the viable myocardium. We recommend grafting any major coronary arteries that supply viable myocardium and have stenosis of 50% or more of the luminal diameter.

Mitral Regurgitation
Rupture or dysfunction of the papillary muscle is associated with posterior infarction in the distribution of the right coronary artery.[6,16] Replacement of the mitral valve can be performed through the ventriculotomy.[16]

Surgical Anatomy

Approximately 70% of defects are anterior, at or near the apex.[26] Posterior defects are usually more extensive, may extend from the atrioventricular groove to the apex, and do not have as well-defined borders as anterior defects.[6,16]

Surgical Technique

Closure of Anteroapical Defect

The earliest reported repair of postinfarction VSD using cardiopulmonary bypass, by Cooley in 1957,[4] was through a right ventriculotomy. Many early repairs utilized the same approach.[1,9] The left ventricular approach, through the infarct, was increasingly advocated[7,10,13,14] and has become the preferred approach. There are several distinct advantages of the left ventricular approach over the right: (1) There are better exposure and delineation of the defect; (2) The patch is placed on the left ventricular side of the septum, with broader distribution of forces over the septum; (3) Right ventricular function is preserved.

The incision is usually made through the middle of the infarct. The loose edges of the defect are trimmed and the margins defined. A woven Dacron patch, considerably larger than the defect, is cut.

We use a modification of the double-patch technique described by Iben and colleagues.[9] This method employs broad pledgets on the right ventricular side and the patch on the left ventricular side. This is technically easier than the double-patch technique, but incorporates the same principles: broad distribution of suture force and buttressing of both sides of the septum.

Broad horizontal mattress sutures are placed with Teflon pledgets on the right ventricular side (Fig. 11–1). These are placed away from the border of the defect, in as viable muscle as is available. After all the sutures are placed, the patch is seated and tied. An additional suture line can be placed around the edge of the patch (Fig. 11–2). Closure of the ventricle is accomplished using Teflon strips, as for ventricular aneurysmectomy (Chapter 10).

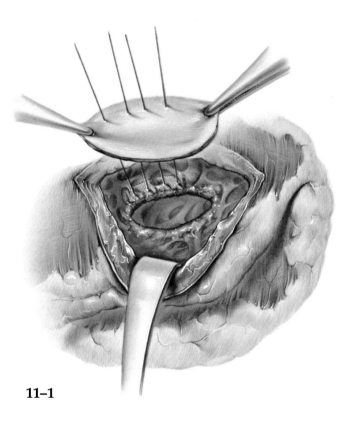

11–1

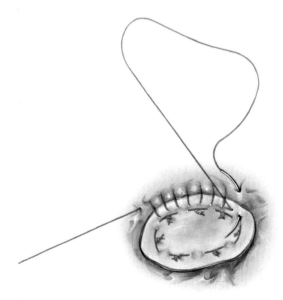

11–2

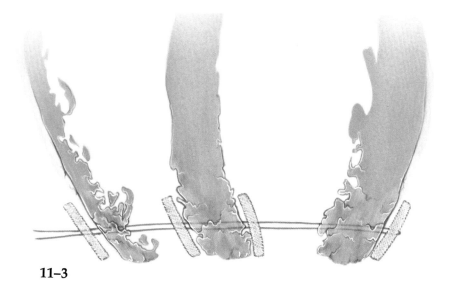

11–3

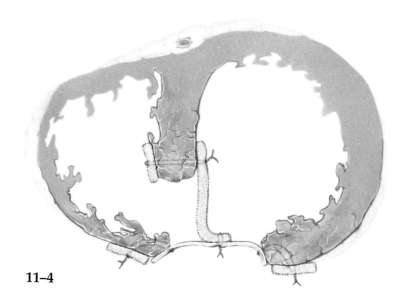

11–4

Alternate Methods of Repair

Modifications in repair should be made to suit the wide variety of pathologic anatomy. Repair of an anterior defect may require incorporation of part of the patch in the ventriculotomy closure. Amputation of the apex can be performed with closure of the ventricles incorporating four Teflon strips (Fig. 11–3).

Posterior defects may require extensive patching of the septum and the wall of the ventricle (Fig. 11–4), as advocated by Daggett and colleagues.[6]

Results

Operative Mortality

Overall operative mortality is in the range of 20%–50%.[6,12,15,16,20,23,25] Subgroups with higher operative mortality include those with inferior defects, those requiring valve replacement, and those in refractory cardiogenic shock.

The mortality of patients with inferior defects is two to three times that of patients with anterior defects.[12,25]

Late Survival

The prognosis for operative survivors, at least for several years, is good. Late survival is 80%–90% 2 to 3 years postoperatively,[6,16] and at 5 years it is 72% in patients receiving concomitant coronary artery bypass.[19]

References

1. Boicourt OW, Ritzmann L, Starr A, McCord CW: Rupture of the infarcted interventricular septum. Circulation 26:1321,1962.
2. Brandt B III, Wright CB, Ehrenhaft JL: Ventricular septal defect following myocardial infarction. Ann Thorac Surg 27:589,1979.
3. Buckley MJ, Mundth ED, Daggett WM, Gold HK, Leinbach RC, Austen WG: Surgical management of ventricular septal defect and mitral regurgitation complicating acute myocardial infarction. Ann Thorac Surg 16:598,1973.
4. Cooley DA, Belmonte BA, Seis LB, Schnur S: Surgical repair of ruptured interventricular septum following acute myocardial infarction. Surgery 41:930,1957.
5. Daggett WM, Buckley MJ, Akins CW, Leinbach RC, Gold HK, Block PC, Austen WG: Improved results of surgical management of postinfarction ventricular septal rupture. Ann Surg 196:269,1982.
6. Daggett WM, Guyton RA, Mundth ED, Buckley MJ, McEnany MT, Gold HK, Leinbach RC, Buckley MJ, Austen WG: Early repair of ventricular septal defect complicating inferior myocardial infarction. Circulation 50(Suppl III):III-112,1974.
7. Dubost C: Discussion of Iben AB, et al: Surgical treatment of post-infarction ventricular septal defects. Ann Thorac Surg 8:252,1969.
8. Gold HK, Leinbach RC, Sanders CA, Buckley MJ, Mundth ED, Austen WG: Intraaortic balloon pumping for ventricular septal defect or mitral regurgitation complicating acute myocardial infarction. Circulation 47:1191,1973.
9. Iben AB, Puppello DF, Stinson EB, Shumway NE: Surgical treatment of postinfarction ventricular septal defects. Ann Thorac Surg 8:252,1969.
10. Javid H, Hunter JA, Najafi H, Dye WS, Julian OC: Left ventricular approach for the repair of ventricular septal perforation and infarctectomy. J Thorac Cardiovasc Surg 63:14,1972.
11. Jonas V, Hyncik V, Chlumsky J, Chlumska A: Eight year survival after perforation of ventricular septum in myocardial infarction. Acta Univ Carol (Med) 16: 133,1970.
12. Jones MT, Schofield PM, Dark JF, Moussalli H, Deiraniya AK, Lawson RAM, Ward C, Bray CL: Surgical repair of acquired ventricular septal defects; determinants of early and late outcome. J Thorac Cardiovasc Surg 93:680,1987.
13. Kay JH: Discussion of Iben AB, et al: Surgical treatment of post-infarction ventricular septal defects. Ann Thorac Surg 8:252,1969.
14. Kitamura S, Mendez A, Kay JH: Ventricular septal defect following myocardial infarction. Experience with surgical repair through a left ventriculotomy and review of the literature. J Thorac Cardiovasc Surg 61:186,1971.
15. Komeda M, Fremes SE, David TE: Surgical repair of postinfarction ventricular septal defect. Circulation 82(Suppl IV):IV-243,1990.
16. Loisance DY, Cachera JP, Poulain H, Aubry P, Juvin AM, Galey JJ: Ventricular septal defect after acute myocardial infarction. J Thorac Cardiovasc Surg 80: 61,1980.
17. Lundberg S, Soderstrom J: Perforation of the interventricular septum in myocardial infarction: a study based upon autopsy material. Acta Med Scand 172: 413,1980.
18. Mallory GK, White PD: The speed of healing of myocardial infarction: a study of the pathologic anatomy in 72 cases. Am Heart J 18:647,1939.
19. Muehrcke DD, Daggett WM, Buckley MJ, Akins CW, Hilgenberg AD, Austen WG: Postinfarct ventricular septal defect repair: effect of coronary artery bypass grafting. Ann Thorac Surg 54:876,1992.

20. Naifeh JG, Grehl TM, Hurley EJ: Surgical treatment of postmyocardial infarction ventricular septal defects. J Thorac Cardiovasc Surg 79:483,1980.

21. Oyamada A, Queen FB: Spontaneous rupture of the interventricular septum following acute myocardial infarction with some clinicopathological observations on survival in five cases. Presented at Pan Pacific Pathology Congress, Tripler US Army Hospital, 1961.

22. Sanders RJ, Kern WH, Blount SG Jr: Perforation of the interventricular septum complicating myocardial infarction: a report of eight cases, one with cardiac catheterization. Am Heart J 51:736,1956.

23. Scanlon PJ, Montoya A, Johnson SA, McKeever LS, Sullivan HJ, Bakhos M, Pifarre R: Urgent surgery for ventricular septal rupture complicating acute myocardial infarction. Circulation 72(Suppl II):II-185,1985.

24. Selzer A, Gerbode F, Kerth WJ: Clinical, hemodynamic, and surgical considerations of rupture of the ventricular septum after myocardial infarction. Am Heart J 78:598,1969.

25. Skillington PD, Davies RH, Luff AJ, Williams JD, Dawkins KD, Conway N, Lamb RK, Shore DF, Monro JL, Ross JK: Surgical treatment for infarct-related ventricular septal defects: improved results combined with analysis of late function. J Thorac Cardiovasc Surg 99:798,1990.

26. Swithinbank JM: Perforation of the interventricular septum in myocardial infarction. Br Heart J 21:562,1959.

27. Tecklenberg PL, Fitzgerald J, Allaire BI, Alderman EL, Harrison DC: Afterload reduction in the management of postinfarction ventricular septal defect. Am J Cardiol 38:956,1976.

12

Mitral Valve Surgery

The earliest operations on the mitral valve, by Souttar,[81] Cutler,[23] Bailey,[6] and others, were bold surgical feats. Since this pioneering surgery, great advances have been made. The early closed operations have been replaced by open procedures with full visualization of the valve, allowing precise repair or replacement.

Improvements in perioperative care, myocardial preservation, and valvular prostheses have lowered the risks of mitral valvular surgery and improved the likelihood of long-term hemodynamic and symptomatic improvement. In this chapter, we describe the indications for and techniques of both conservative and replacement surgery of the mitral valve and the results that can be expected.

Commissurotomy

Percutaneous Balloon Commissurotomy

Percutaneous transseptal balloon commissurotomy evolved during the 1980s into an effective and safe therapy for properly selected patients with rheumatic mitral stenosis, the selection hinging almost entirely on precise echocardiographic assessment of the mitral valve. Early studies of in vitro dilatation[72] and early clinical application through a cutdown on the saphenous vein[44] led to increasing clinical application of percutaneous balloon commissurotomy with good early results.[1,57,88]

Percutaneous balloon commissurotomy has the best results in patients with mobile leaflets and minimal chordal thickening or chordal fusion.[1,53] It is the appropriate initial procedure of choice in this subset of patients. The prevalence of this subset varies enormously with geography, and it is uncommon in the United States. Abascal and colleagues[1] have used an echocardiographic score to predict which patients are most likely to benefit from percutaneous balloon commissurotomy.

Patients with less leaflet mobility, more leaflet thickening, chordal thickening and fusion, and some calcification are more appropriately treated by open commissurotomy, since this group can still have good long-term results with open commissurotomy.[39,64]

Indications for Surgical Commissurotomy

The rheumatic process leading to stenosis of the mitral valve begins with fusion of the leaflets at the commissures. The area of fusion enlarges; fibrosis and constriction of the chordae occur. Later, the leaflets thicken and calcify. Prior to leaflet thickening and calcification, a conservative surgical procedure can open the commissures and free the subvalvular mechanism. This procedure can result in normal hemodynamics if adequate leaflet mobility is present.

Mitral commissurotomy is a low-risk operation with few late complications. Therefore, patient variables favoring commissurotomy instead of valve replacement influence early recommendation of surgery, even in the patient who has not reached functional class III status. The classical signs favoring commissurotomy instead of valve replacement are (1) a loud opening snap on auscultation, (2) good leaflet mobility on the ventriculogram and echocardiogram, and (3) absence of valvular calcification on x-ray. Echocardiographic assessment of mitral valve calcification and mobility also appears to be of value in planning the surgical approach in patients with mitral stenosis.[65] The degree of mitral subvalvular fibrosis, assessed radiographically, can also be a predictive factor in conservative versus replacement surgical therapy.[2]

We recommend operation for patients with catheterization-proven severe mitral stenosis (mitral valve areas less than 1.5 cm^2) even if the patient is in functional class II. Patients with small resting gradients which markedly increase with exercise should also be offered operation. There are convincing arguments for early, open commissurotomy,[83] among them the possibility that early commissurotomy, by maintaining leaflet mobility, may prevent progressive leaflet fibrosis from turbulent flow of blood.[80] This is suggested by our studies from the University of Oregon[43] which show that the incidence of reoperation following mitral commissurotomy is lowest in those patients with good leaflet mobility. Also, adequate commissurotomy is highly protective against thromboembolism.

Surgical Anatomy

The functional components of the mitral apparatus include the left atrial wall, anulus, leaflets, chordae tendineae, papillary muscles, and left ventricular wall.[68] Those components that have most relevance to mitral commissurotomy are the leaflets and chordae. The mitral valve (Fig. 12–1) has two leaf-

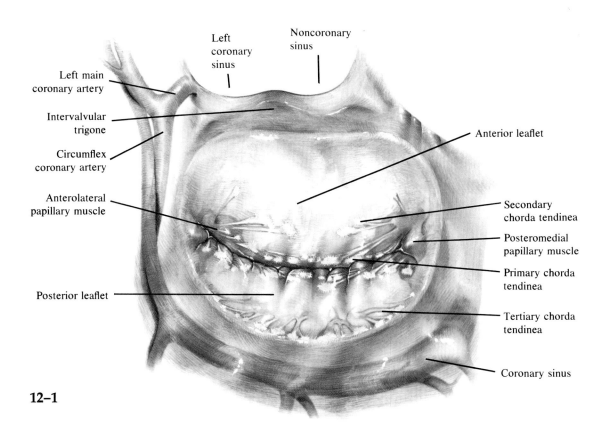

12–1

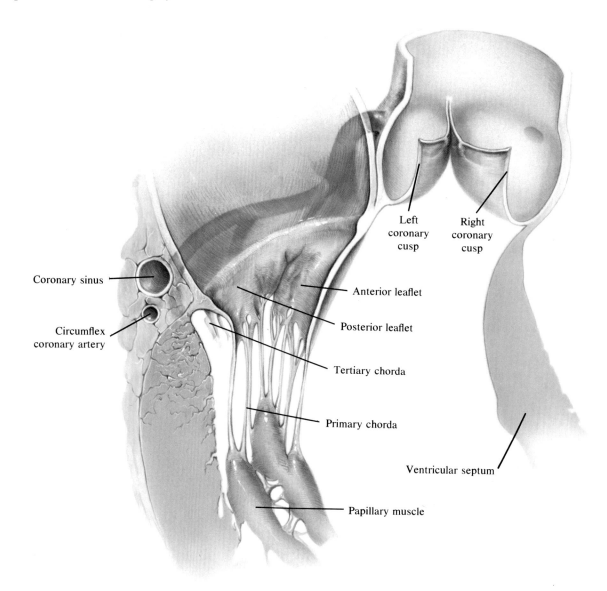

Coronary sinus

Circumflex
coronary artery

Left
coronary
cusp

Right
coronary
cusp

Anterior leaflet

Posterior leaflet

Tertiary chorda

Primary chorda

Ventricular septum

Papillary muscle

12–2

lets—a large anterior leaflet and a small posterior leaflet. The posterior leaflet is usually triscalloped, with a large middle scallop between two smaller commissural scallops.[71] The anterior leaflet has also been termed the aortic leaflet and the posterior, the mural leaflet. The leaflets join at two commissures—lateral and medial—and are supported by a subvalvular mechanism (Fig. 12-2) consisting of two papillary muscles—the anterolateral and posteromedial—and chordae tendineae.

Tandler[87] has divided the chordae into three classifications: primary, secondary, and tertiary. The primary and secondary chordae arise from the papillary muscles. The primary chordae insert into the leaflet edges; the secondary chordae insert into the leaflet undersurface. The tertiary chordae arise from the posterior left ventricular wall and insert into the underside of the base of the posterior leaflet (Fig. 12-1). These tertiary chordae have also been termed mural[60] or basal[55] chordae.

The chordae divide and subdivide so that as many as 120 chordae can insert into the two leaflets.[74] Commissural chordae[55] insert into the leaflets at the commissures between the anterior and posterior leaflets.

Surgical Technique

We have used the open technique of mitral commissurotomy exclusively since 1960. Although the mitral valve may be approached from a left thoracotomy, right thoracotomy, or median sternotomy, we prefer the midline approach. A median sternotomy allows easy access to all cardiac valves, provides for easy cannulation of the ascending aorta, permits (with elevation of the apex of the left ventricle) reliable removal of air, and results in the least pulmonary impairment postoperatively.

Bicaval and ascending aorta cannulation is performed, and the patient is placed on high-flow cardiopulmonary bypass and cooled to 26°–28°C. The interatrial groove is developed. The aorta is clamped, and cold blood cardioplegic solution is infused into the ascending aorta. The left atrium is opened (Fig. 12–3). Cardioplegic arrest causes relaxation of the left ventricle, resulting in improved exposure of the valve. If 10 minutes or less of ischemia is anticipated, hypothermia alone is a satisfactory alternative to cardioplegia.

The atrial incision can be extended behind the inferior cava to improve exposure of the valve (Fig. 12–4). A retractor is applied and traction sutures

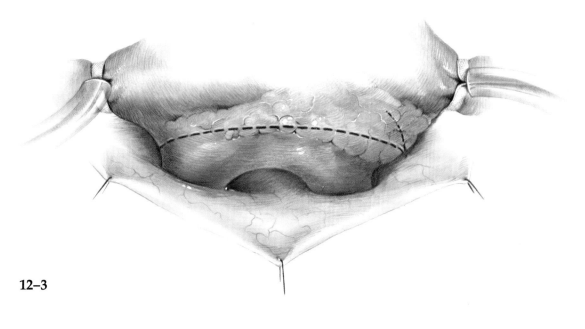

12–3

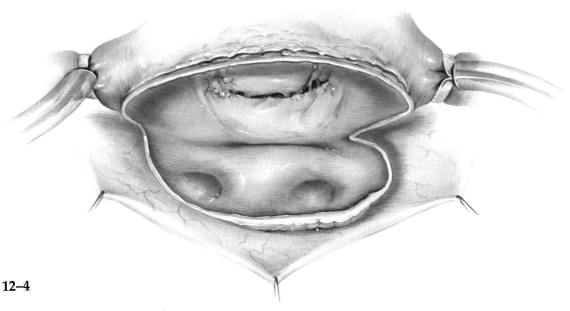

12–4

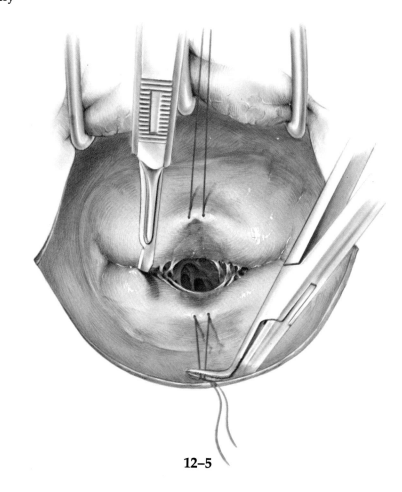

12–5

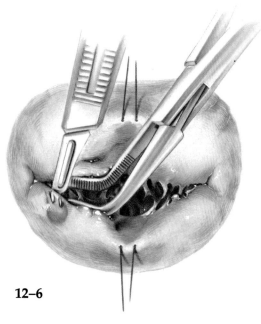

12–6

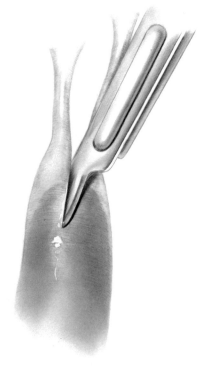

12–7

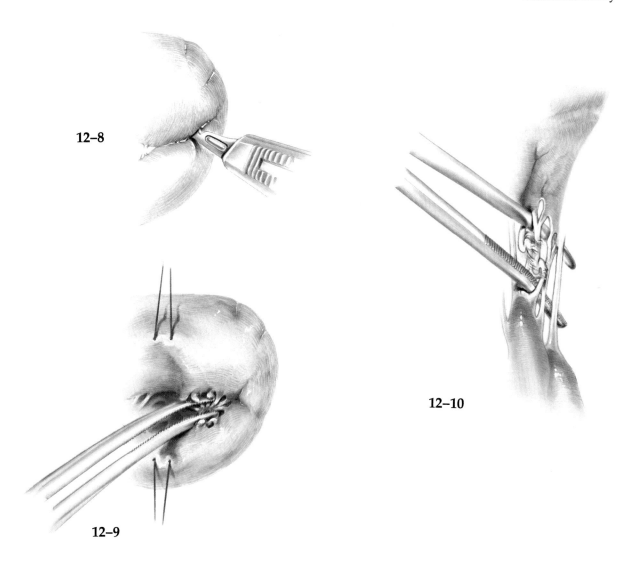

12–8

12–9

12–10

are placed in the middle of the anterior and posterior leaflets. Traction on these sutures brings the fused area at the lateral commissure into view. The lateral commissure is then sharply incised (Fig. 12–5), with careful avoidance of injury to the commissural chordae inserting into the edge of each leaflet.

The commissural chordae are assessed. If the chordae are foreshortened, an incision is made into the tip of the papillary muscle (Figs. 12–6, 12–7), improving leaflet mobility. The medial commissure is incised close to the anulus (Fig. 12–8). This incision lets in some light, improving visualization of the medial commissural chordae, which are usually quite close together. The commissural incision is then completed.

The chordae may be fused. They can be teased apart by blunt dissection (Fig. 12–9). If the chordae are folded on themselves, and adherent to each other, they can often be freed by stretching them between the papillary muscle tips and leaflet edge (Fig. 12–10).

The left atrium is partially closed around a vent catheter. The aortic clamp is removed and air is removed from the left ventricle. The vent catheter is removed after the heart is beating.

Results

Open mitral commissurotomy can be accomplished with an operative risk of 1% or less.[30,39,43,63] Almost all patients will be in functional class I or II postoperatively for at least 5 years. Significant restenosis increases at 5 years,

and 50% of patients will require reoperation 8 years following initial commissurotomy.[43] Open mitral commissurotomy is a safe, effective, predictable procedure with good results lasting 5 to 10 years.

Valvuloplasty/Anuloplasty

Coauthored by Alain Carpentier

Mitral valve repair for patients with mitral regurgitation can be performed
with the same operative mortality as valve replacement and is associated with
less thromboembolism, endocarditis, and anticoagulant-related hemorrhage.[12,15,20,22,29,77] Repair results in better early and late ventricular function
than replacement.[10,26] For these reasons mitral valve repair became much
more widely applied in the 1980s, especially in the United States.[20,29,84]

The first mitral valve repair with a prosthetic ring was performed in 1968 at
the Broussais Hospital, Paris, France.[13] Since that time over 7000 mitral valve
repairs have been performed at the Broussais Hospital. This section describes
the techniques developed by Carpentier and his associates of the Broussais
Hospital over more than 20 years of evolution. When properly applied, without alteration, these techniques provide the most reliable and stable long-
term results.[27]

Indications

Patients with mitral regurgitation should usually be symptomatic to be candidates for surgical treatment. If mitral valve repair seems likely from clinical,
angiographic, and echocardiographic evaluation, surgery can be recommended before functional class III is reached. Asymptomatic patients should
be offered surgery if they have deteriorating ventricular function or at the
first onset of atrial fibrillation.[15,27]

Surgical Anatomy

Anatomic abnormalities of the anulus, leaflets, chordae, and papillary muscles are complex and often occur together. These abnormalities are often
amenable to surgical repair. A simplified functional approach to valve analysis has been developed, determined by whether the motion of each leaflet is
normal (Type I), prolapsed (Type II), or restricted (Type III).[12] Lesions that
produce regurgitation with normal leaflet motion include anular dilatation
and leaflet perforation. Lesions that produce regurgitation with prolapsed
leaflet motion include chordal rupture, chordal elongation, papillary muscle
rupture, and papillary muscle elongation. Lesions that produce regurgitation
with restricted leaflet motion include chordal fusion or thickening, leaflet
thickening, and commissure fusion. This classification will be used in describing the various steps of the operation and the techniques used.

Surgical Technique

Valve Exposure and Analysis
Adequate exposure is a fundamental condition for mitral valve repair, and a
tonic heart that is not yet arrested by cardioplegia is a fundamental condition
for mitral valve analysis. As soon as the heart fibrillates, as a result of either
core cooling or induced electrical fibrillation under normothermia, a left atriotomy is performed before cross-clamping the aorta. The left atriotomy extends
posteriorly beneath both venae cavae. A self-retaining retractor improves
exposure of the mitral valve. The papillary muscles can be exposed better by
placing a laparotomy pad in the pericardial sac. A pad placed in front of the
heart will help expose the anterolateral papillary muscle. A pad placed in the
diaphragmatic portion of the pericardial sac will help expose the posterome-

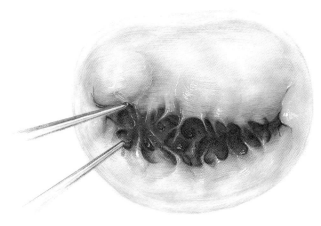

12–11

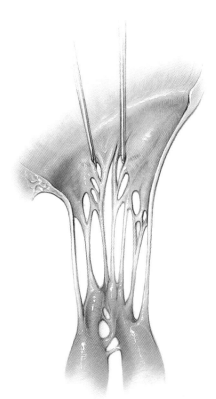

12–12

dial papillary muscle. An alternative approach is a thorough intraoperative transesophageal echocardiographic evaluation of the mitral valve prior to bypass and administration of cardioplegia prior to left atriotomy.

Valve analysis begins by examining the left atrium for a jet lesion, which would indicate a prolapse of the opposing leaflet. The anulus is evaluated for dilatation and/or deformation. The leaflets and leaflet motion are examined. Nerve hooks are used to assess leaflet pliability and to assess leaflet prolapse or restricted leaflet motion (Figs. 12–11, 12–12). Leaflet prolapse can be measured by the "reference point" method. A nonprolapsed area can usually be found on the mural leaflet at the anterolateral commissure. This can be used to measure the degree of prolapse of the rest of the mural leaflet and the anterior leaflet. Once valve analysis is complete, cold blood cardioplegic solution is administered.

Prosthetic Ring Anuloplasty

Early techniques of reducing a dilated anulus involved figure-of-eight sutures at the commissures, placed in such a manner that the anulus was constricted and the posterior leaflet was advanced toward the anterior leaflet.[51] The use of a semirigid ring anuloplasty has the advantages of selectively reducing the anulus yet maintaining an optimal orifice area and reshaping the anulus to its normal elliptical configuration. Unlike flexible—and therefore deformable—rings, the Carpentier ring has selective rigidity and produces a stable remodeling and repair. Deformation does not take place once the heart restores its contraction, nor does deformation occur in the long term as a result of progressive disease. For these reasons ring anuloplasty is used in almost all cases of mitral valve insufficiency.

The size of the ring is chosen by measurement of the surface area of the anterior leaflet. This is performed by placing a right-angled clamp around the chordae to the anterior leaflet and measuring the stretched leaflet with sized obturators (Fig. 12–13).

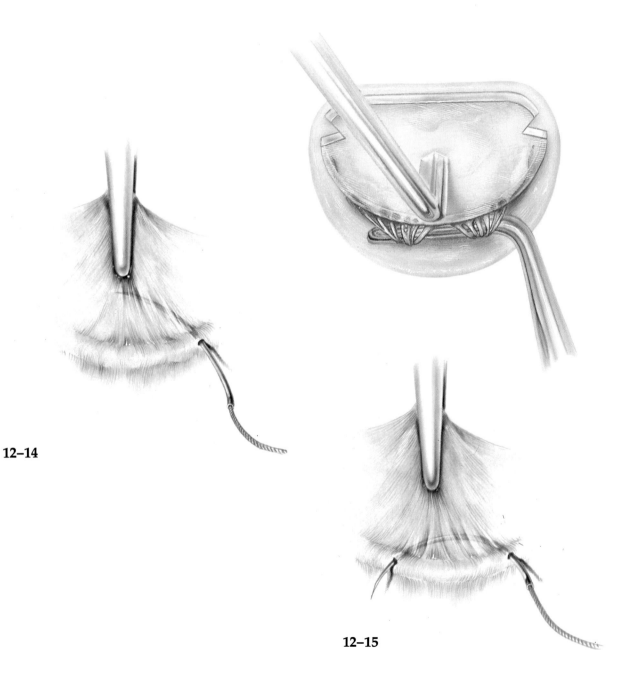

12–14

12–15

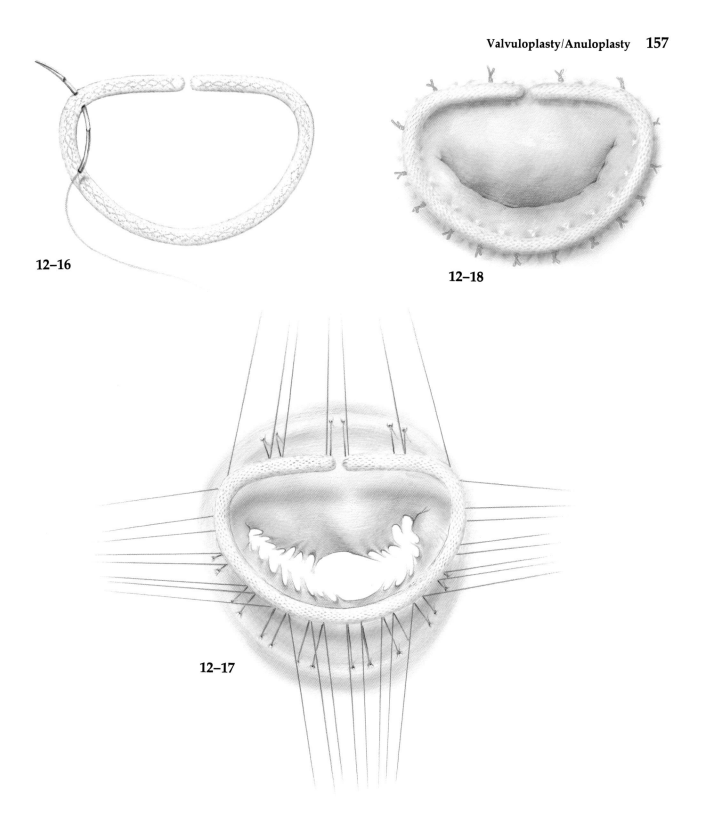

12–16

12–18

12–17

Sutures of 2–0 polyester are then placed through the anulus (Figs. 12–14, 12–15) and through the ring (Fig. 12–16). The sutures at the base of the anterior leaflet are placed so there is no gathering of this portion of the anulus. The sutures at the commissures and along the posterior anulus are placed more narrowly on the ring than they are on the anulus (Fig. 12–17). The ring is then seated and the valve is tested by injecting saline into the ventricular cavity with a bulb syringe. The aortic root should be vented to prevent air embolism to the coronary arteries. The sutures are then tied, gathering in the commissures and posterior portion of the anulus (Fig. 12–18)

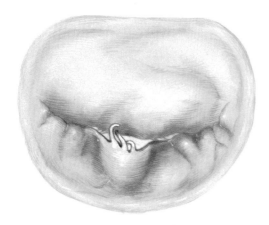

12–19

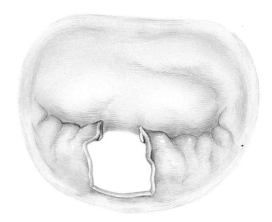

12–20

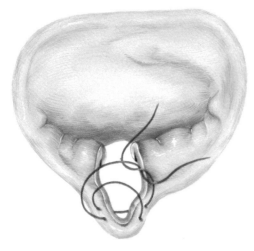

12–21

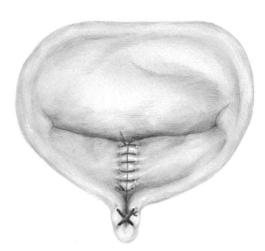

12–22

to produce a competent valve. Leaflet closure and symmetrical line of closure may be retested by injecting saline into the left ventricle with a large bulb syringe.

Rectangular Excision of Flail Portion of Posterior Leaflet

Prolapse of the midportion of the posterior leaflet can be caused by ruptured chordae (Fig. 12–19) or elongated chordae. Repair is achieved by rectangular excision of a portion of the posterior leaflet (Fig. 12–20). Stay sutures are placed around the normal chordae adjacent to the prolapsed portion of the leaflet. The leaflet is incised perpendicular to the anulus and a rectangular portion is excised. A figure-of-eight suture is taken in the anulus (Fig. 12–21). The leaflet is repaired with interrupted sutures of 5–0 polyester with the sutures being tied so the knots are on the ventricular side (Fig. 12–22). A ring anuloplasty is performed to remodel the anulus, reinforce the repair, and avoid further dilatation of the anulus.

Rectangular Excision of Posterior Leaflet and Sliding Leaflet Repair

The sliding leaflet repair is used whenever a large leaflet resection is necessary, such as with Barlow's syndrome.[7] A large plication of the posterior

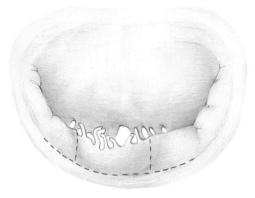

12–23

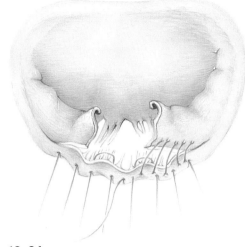

12–24

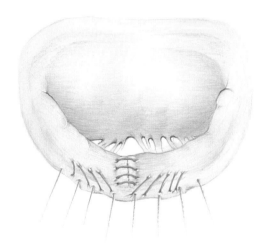

12–25

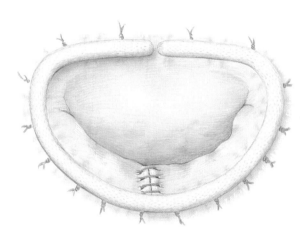

12–26

leaflet can displace the mitral valve orifice toward the left ventricular outflow tract, causing obstruction. If there is excess tissue of the posterior leaflet, a reduction of the height of the leaflet must be carried out in order to avoid left ventricular outflow tract obstruction.

The quadrangular resection is performed in the usual manner. Two additional incisions are made transversely at the anulus (Fig. 12–23). If excess posterior leaflet tissue is present, this is excised by removing a triangular piece of tissue at the base of each of the two leaflet remnants. Mattress sutures of 2–0 polyester are placed through the anulus in the area of resection and detachment (Fig. 12–24). The detached leaflets are sutured to the anulus with 5–0 polyester, gathering a correspondingly larger portion of anular tissue than leaflet tissue (Fig. 12–25). This brings the two edges of the posterior leaflet into contact. They are sutured together with interrupted sutures of 5–0 polyester with the knots on the ventricular side (Fig. 12–25). A prosthetic ring is inserted, using the measurements of the anterior leaflet as well as the measurement of the reduced orifice. The previously placed mattress sutures in the posterior anulus are placed at reduced intervals on the ring, creating a purse-string effect (Fig. 12–26).

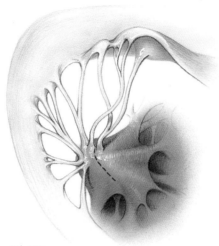

12–27

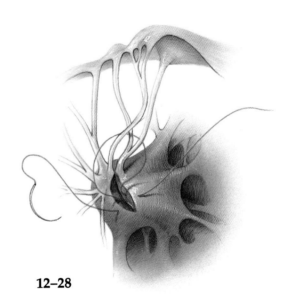

12–28

12–29

Shortening Plastic Repair of the Chordae
Chordal elongation can be corrected by invaginating the excess length of chordae into a trench made in the papillary muscle. The tip of the papillary muscle is incised (Fig. 12–27). A 5–0 polyester suture is placed through half of the trench, then around the chordae, and then through the other half of the trench (Fig. 12–28). Traction on this suture pulls the excess length of chordae into the trench in the papillary muscle (Fig. 12–29). The trench is closed using a figure-of-eight suture, avoiding contact between the suture and the chordae, since contact can lead to chordal abrasion (Figs. 12–30, 12–31, 12–32).

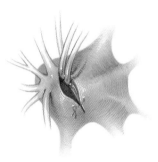

12–30

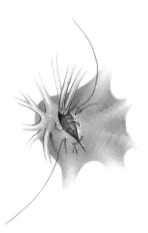

12–31

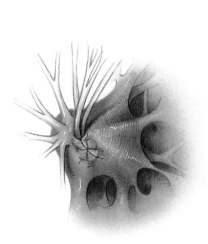

12–32

Transposition of Chordae

Rupture of chordae of the anterior leaflet can be repaired using transposition of chordae from the posterior leaflet. A 2- to 3-mm-wide and up to 10-mm-long piece of posterior leaflet is excised (Fig. 12–33). The supporting papillary muscle can be mobilized toward the anterior leaflet by cutting muscular bands attaching the base of the papillary muscle to the posterior wall of the ventricle. The strip of posterior leaflet is sutured to the free edge of the anterior leaflet using interrupted sutures of 5–0 polyester (Figs. 12–34, 12–35). If a 6-mm or longer piece of posterior leaflet has been used, a quadrangular resection is performed and a ring inserted (Fig. 12–36).

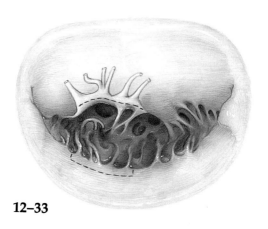

12–33

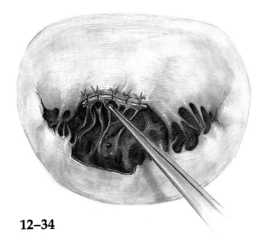

12–34

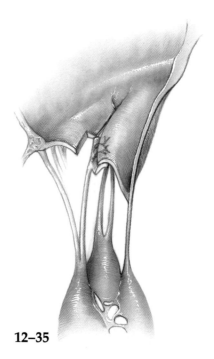

12–35

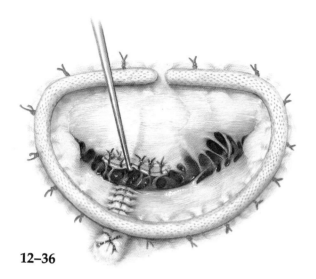

12–36

Results

Properly performed valvuloplasty/anuloplasty results in low operative mortality, improvement in ventricular function, low incidence of thromboembolism, low incidence of reoperation, and lasting improvement in hemodynamics and symptomatic state. Reports of operative mortality have ranged from 0% to 4.3%.[17,20,21,25,77,84] Bonchek and colleagues[10] have reported a significant fall in left ventricular end-diastolic volume index and end-systolic volume index. Preservation of the papillary muscle apparatus appears to result in better ventricular function following mitral valve repair than following mitral valve replacement.[26,36] The incidence of thromboembolism is low, ranging from 0% to 1.6% per patient-year.[17,20] Deloche and colleagues[27] reported 93.9% of patients were free of thromboembolism at 15 years. The incidence of reoperation is low. Cohn and co-workers[15] reported a freedom from reoperation at 48 months of 85% ± 5%, and Deloche and co-workers[27] reported 92.7% of patients with degenerative disease were free from reoperation at 15 years. They also reported that at 15 years 74% of patients were in New York Heart Association class I or II, normal ventricular contractility was present in 84.5%, and 91% had either no mitral regurgitation or trivial mitral regurgitation. It is clear that the techniques of mitral valve repair are widely applicable to the North American population.[14,84]

Replacement

Indications

Mitral Stenosis

Isolated mitral stenosis is the only left-sided valvular lesion that does not place an increased hemodynamic burden on the left ventricle; it does place a progressive burden on the pulmonary vasculature, right ventricle, and tricuspid valve. Valve replacement of an irreparably damaged stenotic mitral valve should be performed before irreversible changes occur in the pulmonary vasculature, right ventricle, or tricuspid valve.

Patients who are likely to require valve replacement for mitral stenosis should be experiencing moderate interference (NYHA FC III) with their normal activity before surgery is recommended. Valve replacement may be indicated in less symptomatic patients for recurrent emboli unresponsive to anti-coagulant therapy. Valve replacement in patients who are functional class IV often gives good results; for this reason pulmonary hypertension is never a contraindication to surgery for mitral stenosis.

Mitral Regurgitation

Chronic mitral regurgitation results in a combination of hemodynamic abnormalities and compensatory mechanisms that require special consideration in order to determine proper timing of valve replacement. It has long been known that valve replacement for congestive heart failure caused by chronic mitral regurgitation is associated with a higher operative mortality and worse long-term results than valve replacement for congestive heart failure caused by mitral stenosis.[52,54] The physiologic reasons for this difference are becoming increasingly clear.

Mitral regurgitation results in the left ventricle ejecting into a low-resistance system (left atrium and pulmonary venous bed) and a high-resistance system (the systemic arterial bed). As the regurgitant volume increases, the ventricle dilates and hypertrophies to maintain adequate forward cardiac output to the body.

The increasing amount of regurgitation may or may not cause early development of symptoms, depending upon the response of the left atrium. If the left atrium does not dilate, pulmonary venous pressure rises and symptoms occur. However, if the left atrium is compliant and dilates, atrial and pulmonary venous pressure may not rise—severe mitral regurgitation may occur with normal left atrial pressure.[11] So symptoms may not accurately indicate the severity of chronic mitral regurgitation. Symptomatic state may also be a poor indication of the level and reversibility of ventricular function.

Progressive dilatation of the left ventricle can occur in chronic mitral regurgitation with a lower "cost" in myocardial energetics than occurs with dilatation in response to pressure overload. The lower energetics result from a more rapid decrease in left ventricular volume because of the low-impedance (left atrial) leak. This results in a lower systolic wall tension (afterload).[40,89]

It appears, however, that the price of the temporary "advantage" of the low-impedance leak may be extremely high: irreversible deterioration in ventricular function may occur in spite of the presence of a normal ejection fraction. Schuler and co-workers[79] have shown that, after a certain level of ventricular dilatation, valve replacement and the resultant elimination of the low-impedance leak do not result in diminution of left ventricular size: rather, there is no change in chamber size, no regression of myocardial hypertrophy, and progressive deterioration in ventricular function occurs with a fall in ejection fraction.

Patients with chronic mitral regurgitation should undergo valve repair or replacement before congestive heart failure occurs and before ejection fraction becomes abnormal, probably before ejection fraction reaches the low-normal range. Echocardiographic[90] and nuclear[73] studies are likely to aid in assessment of ventricular function and timing of surgery. Evaluation of the patient with mitral regurgitation must be more sophisticated than simple assessment of symptoms and response to medical therapy. Evaluation must involve careful assessment of ventricular function and the degree to which pathologic compensatory changes have occurred.

Choice of Prosthesis

The current choice, for the most part, is between three widely used types of mechanical prostheses—ball valve (Starr-Edwards), tilting disc (Medtronic-Hall), and bileaflet (St. Jude)—and the porcine xenograft bioprostheses.

Mechanical and xenograft prostheses are similar in hemodynamic function in the commonly used sizes, removing hemodynamics as a basis of choice in most instances. However, the porcine xenografts are more likely to produce a "prosthesis-patient mismatch" in the smaller sizes.[70]

The main factors affecting choice of prosthesis are anticoagulation, and the attitude of the patient and surgeon regarding reoperation. Porcine valves have the advantage of a low embolic rate in the absence of anticoagulant therapy if sinus rhythm is present; they have the disadvantage of lower durability. Porcine valves over time require reoperation due to degeneration and structural failure. Twenty to forty percent of porcine mitral valves fail by 10 years.[34] Structural deterioration is rare, however, in the elderly patient. Jamieson and colleagues[47] and Louagie and colleagues[58] found no structural valve deterioration in patients who were 70 years or older when they received a porcine bioprosthesis. We feel the possibility of eventual reoperation should be understood and accepted by the patient before a porcine xenograft is implanted.

All mechanical prostheses require continuous anticoagulants; therefore, patient factors weighing against anticoagulation (previous bleeding history, inability or unwillingness to conform to daily medication and periodic blood tests) favor use of a xenograft valve. However, mitral valve disease frequently results in a condition favoring continuous anticoagulation—atrial fibrillation, a thrombogenic state often requiring anticoagulation regardless of type of prosthesis used.

Many groups placing bioprostheses in the mitral position continue anticoagulants indefinitely.[18] Use of a bioprosthesis when continuous anticoagulation is planned appears paradoxical, since the presence of anticoagulation seems to negate the major advantage a bioprosthesis has over a mechanical prosthesis.

In the presence of long-standing atrial fibrillation and in the absence of any contraindication to anticoagulation, we recommend a mechanical prosthesis. If the patient is in sinus rhythm, the patient's attitude toward anticoagulant therapy and reoperation is determined. If the patient prefers not to take anticoagulants and has few qualms about the possibility of reoperation, a bioprosthesis is used.

The variables influencing valve selection between mechanical and tissue valves are as follows:

1. What is the risk of anticoagulant therapy in a particular patient?
2. Is the patient a reasonable risk for reoperation? How does the patient view that possibility?
3. Is there a pregnancy planned?
4. What is the anticipated life expectancy of the patient? Is it shorter than the known durability of the bioprosthesis?
5. Will the sound of the mechanical prosthesis bother the patient?
6. Having made a tentative selection, are there anatomic conditions at surgery favoring one prosthesis over the other?
7. Is the patient over 70 years of age with a very low risk of structural failure with a bioprosthesis?

Surgical Strategy

Myocardial Preservation
Cold blood cardioplegic arrest is used for mitral valve replacement (Chapter 6). Cold blood cardioplegia results in excellent myocardial preservation and good exposure of the mitral valve.

Associated Cardiac Procedures
1. *Coronary artery bypass:* Distal anastomoses are done after injecting cardioplegic solution in the aortic root and often in the coronary sinus and after opening the left atrium. The mitral valve is then replaced and the left atrium

partially closed, leaving a vent in the left atrium. Proximal vein anastomoses are done over a partial occluding clamp after release of the aortic cross-clamp, while the heart is beating and rewarming.

2. *Aortic valve replacement:* The mitral valve and aortic valves are excised. Sutures are placed in the mitral anulus and through the prosthetic valve. The valve can be seated and tied at this time or after placement of the aortic anular sutures: the latter may give better exposure of the aortic anulus. Sutures are placed through the aortic anulus and prosthetic valve. The mitral valve is then seated and tied, followed by the aortic valve.

3. *Tricuspid valve surgery:* Tricuspid surgery is performed after the mitral valve is replaced.

Preservation of Chordae Tendineae

Experiments in dogs in 1956 by Rushmer[76] demonstrated the integrity of the mitral apparatus was important in left ventricular function. Chordal sparing during mitral valve replacement was described by Lillihei in 1964[56] but did not become widely used, with most mitral valve replacements involving complete excision of the valve and chordae.

The depression of left ventricular function that was seen following mitral valve replacement for mitral regurgitation was initially thought to be due to the increase in afterload caused by the elimination of flow into the left atrium.[69] However, a drop in left ventricular function was usually not found after mitral valve repair,[10,32] focusing attention once again on the contribution of the chordal apparatus to ventricular function.

Experiments in the 1980s by Spence,[82] Hansen,[35,36] and Sarris[78] all demonstrated that division of the chordae tendineae in association with mitral valve replacement resulted in profound deterioration of left ventricular function. Hansen and colleagues[35] found that the anterior and posterior mitral leaflets have an additive influence upon global left ventricular systolic performance, with the anterior chordae tending to be more important.

Clinical studies have confirmed the importance of preserving some or all of the chordae tendineae during mitral valve replacement to avoid postoperative impairment in left ventricular function.[26,38] Preservation of the posterior leaflet and its chordae also probably prevents rupture of the left ventricle following mitral valve replacement.[22,49,85] David and Ho[24] found that in patients undergoing mitral valve replacement for mitral regurgitation secondary to myocardial infarction, only cardiogenic shock and complete excision of the native valve were predictive of operative mortality, and only complete excision of the mitral valve and ejection fraction lower than 35% were predictive of late mortality. Goor and co-workers[33] found that in patients undergoing mitral valve replacement for ischemic mitral insufficiency, preservation of the posterior leaflet resulted in an operative mortality of 0%, whereas excision of the posterior leaflet resulted in an operative mortality of 73%. Okita and colleagues[66] studied postoperative ventricular function following mitral valve replacement and found better left ventricular function in patients who had preservation of chordae tendineae. Hennein and co-workers[37] studied patients undergoing mitral valve replacement for isolated mitral regurgitation before and 6 months after operation by treadmill testing, catheterization, echocardiography, and radionuclide angiography. In patients in whom the chordae were excised, exercise capacity, left ventricular systolic dimensions, and cardiac index did not improve after mitral valve replacement, and left ventricular function deteriorated. In contrast, exercise capacity improved and left ventricular function was maintained or improved in patients in whom the chordae were preserved. They found no difference between posterior chordal preservation only and preservation of the entire apparatus.

Several methods of preserving the chordae have been described. The anterior leaflet with its chordae can be excised, preserving the posterior leaflet and its chordae.[33,37] Miki[62] and Okita[66] describe a technique of preserving all the chordal apparatus by incising the anterior leaflet near the anulus from commissure to commissure, excising the midportion of the anterior leaflet which is free of any chordal insertion, and then fixing the remaining portions of the anterior leaflet to the mitral ring near the lateral and medial commissures and retaining but splitting the posterior leaflet. Feikes and co-workers[28] have described a technique of preserving all chordae by incising the anterior leaflet near the anulus from commissure to commissure, splitting and trimming the anterior leaflet, and fixing the trimmed anterior leaflet portions directly posteriorly to the posterior leaflet.

The anterior leaflet should probably not be left completely intact when inserting a mitral prosthesis. It can be pushed anteriorly and cause left ventricular outflow tract obstruction, particularly with the use of bioprosthetic valves.[19]

Suture Technique

Suture techniques applicable to the mitral valve include simple interrupted, interrupted vertical mattress, interrupted horizontal mattress with or without pledgets (pledgets on atrial or ventricular side of anulus), and continuous. Our standard technique for use with the Starr-Edwards mitral prosthesis is interrupted vertical mattress sutures. If the anulus is thin, horizontal mattress sutures with pledgets may be used (pledgets on the atrial side); this technique is also well suited for use with porcine prostheses.

Surgical Anatomy

Detailed knowledge of the mitral valve is essential to excise the valve properly and place the anular sutures properly. While posterior left ventricular wall rupture—one of the most disastrous and highly fatal complications of cardiac surgery[8,50,91]—may occur spontaneously after mitral valve replacement, it also can be caused by improper valve excision or suture placement.

The left ventricle, unlike the right ventricle, has a common outlet and inlet, thereby creating continuity between the mitral and aortic valves.[75,92] The mitral valve is shown from the atrial view in Figure 12–1. Figure 12–2 demonstrates the close relationship between the mitral valve and the aortic valve as well as the thin atrioventricular junction at the base of the posterior leaflet.

Surgical Technique

Left atriotomy is performed within the interatrial groove after its dissection (Fig. 12–3) and extended behind the inferior vena cava (Fig. 12–4) to facilitate exposure of the valve.

A retraction suture is placed through the midportion of the anterior leaflet (Fig. 12–37). This suture is clamped and retracted posteriorly. An incision is made in the anterior leaflet, leaving about 5 mm of subaortic curtain (Fig. 12–38). An Allis clamp is then placed on the valve and the incision extended medially, then posteriorly, across the medial commissure, without entering the valve orifice (Fig. 12–39).

The incision is carried laterally under the aortic valve and then posteriorly, exposing the papillary muscles. The papillary muscles are transected at their tips, where the white fibrous tissue meets the muscular tissue (Fig. 12–40). Transection of too much papillary muscle will weaken the ventricular wall, predisposing to rupture.

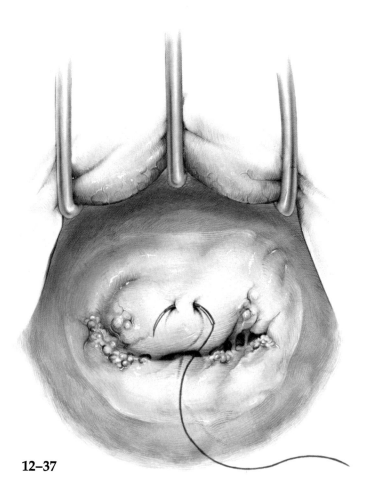

12–37

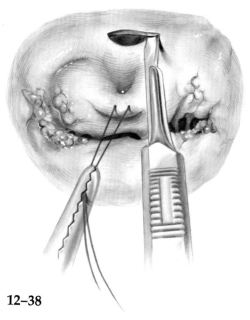

12–38

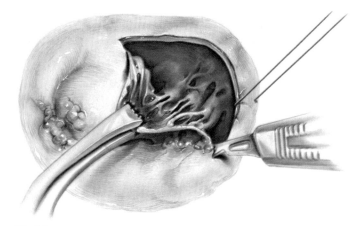

12–39

Every effort is made to preserve the posterior leaflet and its chordae. If the posterior leaflet is extremely fibrotic and the chordae are markedly foreshortened, the valve is then prolapsed into the left atrium. The mural leaflet is cut, taking extreme care to leave good anular tissue (Fig. 12–41). The tertiary chordae are not cut; their support of the posterior anulus is important. Improper excision posteriorly (Fig. 12–42) will result in deficient tissue for suture placement or complete detachment of the atrium from the ventricle—with disastrous consequences.

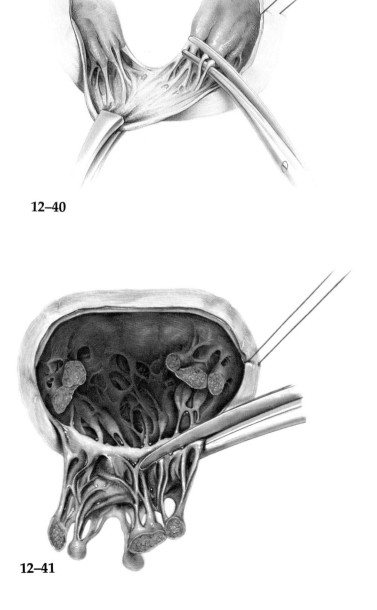

12–40

12–41

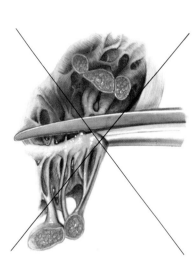

Figure 12–42 *What not to do.* This is excessive excision posteriorly and can result in detachment of the atrium from the ventricle.

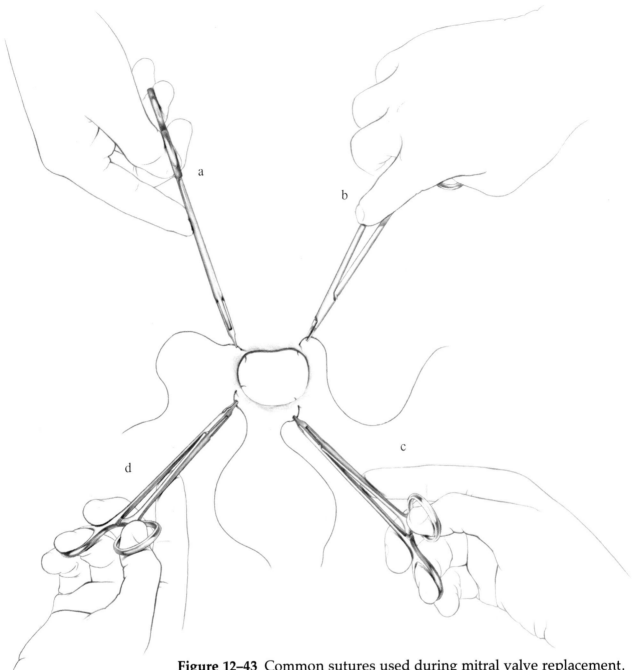

Figure 12–43 Common sutures used during mitral valve replacement. a. Forehand down, elbow out. b. Backhand down. c. Backhand up. d. Forehand down, elbow in.

The most commonly used suture motions are shown in Figure 12–43. Backhand-up sutures are placed in the posteromedial quadrant (Fig. 12–44). These sutures should come out the fibrous portion of the anulus (Fig. 12–45), *not* out the muscular posterior wall underlying the fibrous anulus (Fig. 12–46). Sutures placed through the muscle will tear the muscle as they are tied, creating an area of weakness where dissection of the wall can begin, resulting in posterior left ventricular rupture.

Sutures are carried laterally (Fig. 12–47). If exposure is good, sutures can be placed in the valve sewing ring at the same time. If exposure is poor, all anular sutures are placed and tagged and then placed in the valve sewing ring.

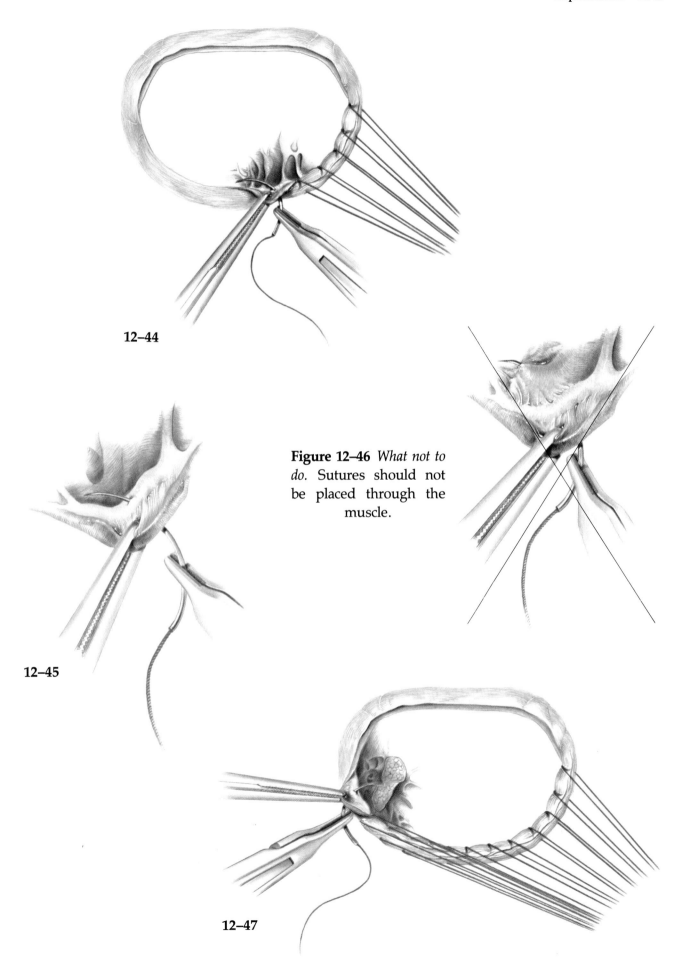

12–44

12–45

Figure 12–46 *What not to do*. Sutures should not be placed through the muscle.

12–47

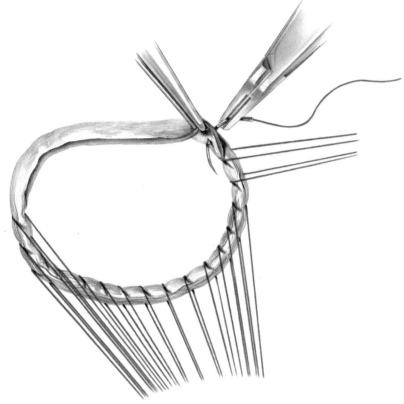

12–48

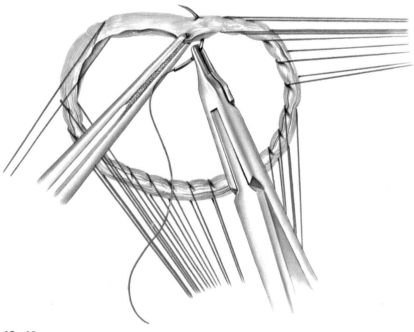

12–49

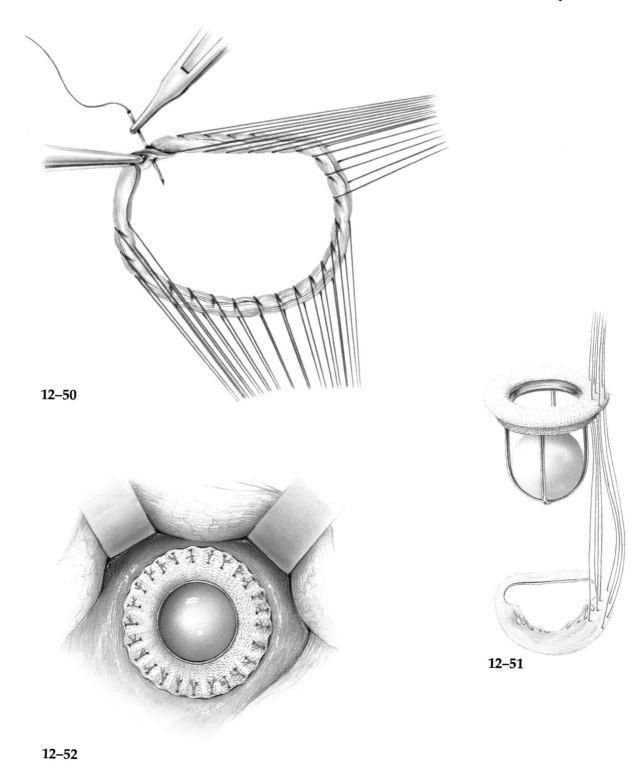

12–50

12–51

12–52

Backhand-down sutures are then placed in the anteromedial quadrant (Fig. 12–48). Exposure of the subaortic curtain can be improved by placing a retraction suture anterolaterally. Backhand-up sutures are placed in the subaortic curtain (Fig. 12–49). Forehand sutures can be used anterolaterally (Fig. 12–50). The technique for placing sutures through the posterior leaflet is shown in Figure 12–51. The valve is seated and sutures are tied (Fig. 12–52).

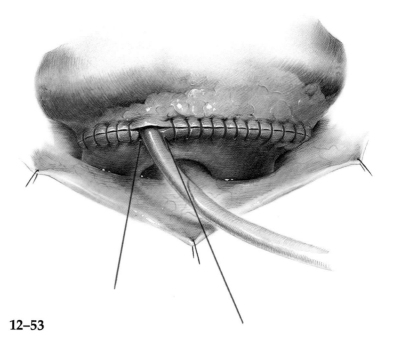

12–53

A vent is placed into the left atrium, sometimes through the valve, and the atriotomy is closed (Fig. 12–53). The aortic clamp is released as air is removed from the ascending aorta. Suction on an aortic needle vent may improve air removal. The heart can then be resuscitated for several minutes in a beating, vented state. The vent is removed, and air is expelled from the left atrium as the atrial suture is tied. The apex of the left ventricle is elevated, and air is removed with a needle. If the apex of the ventricle cannot be elevated because of dense adhesions, suction can be applied to an aortic needle with compression of the left ventricle and intermittent unclamping and clamping of the aorta as the heart begins to beat. The adequacy of air removal can be assessed by watching the suction line for air or echocardiographic evaluation of the cardiac chambers.

Results

Operative Mortality
Elective mitral valve replacement in patients who are in functional class III can be performed with an operative mortality of 2% or less.[4,9,48] Mortality can be as high as 25% in patients who are in functional class IV, many of whom have end-stage mitral regurgitation.[4] It appears that the preoperative state of the myocardium and the method of operative myocardial protection are the strongest determinants of operative risk. Valve replacement earlier in the course of disease, improving techniques of myocardial protection, and methods of chordal preservation will likely continue to lower the overall risk of mitral valve replacement.[16]

Late Mortality
Excluding operative deaths, the 5-year survival following mitral valve replacement is approximately 80%–85%, and this survival is found for ball valves, tilting disc valves, bileaflet valves, and porcine heterografts.[5,18,59,86] The majority of late deaths are not caused by prosthesis-related complications, but by myocardial factors—emphasizing again that the most critical factor relating to the success of valvular surgery is the functional and structural status of the myocardium preoperatively.

Hemodynamics

The Starr-Edwards, Medtronic-Hall, and porcine prostheses have similar hemodynamics in the commonly used sizes (30–32 mm). There is usually a small resting transvalvular gradient of 4–6 mm Hg, which increases 2–4 mm Hg with exercise.[31,41,42,46,61] Horstkotte and colleagues[42] have reported an average transvalvular gradient in 29-mm St. Jude valves of 2.3 mm Hg.

Prosthesis-Related Complications

Thromboembolism: Most reports show a rate of thromboembolism for the ball valve, the tilting-disc valve, and the bileaflet valve, in patients maintained on continuous anticoagulation, of 2%–4%/year.[34] Approximately half of these thromboembolic episodes are minor—there is no residual neurologic deficit or peripheral or coronary embolic complications.

Overall, thromboembolism rates for the porcine heterografts are 1%–3%/year.[18,34,67] This indicates that a large proportion of emboli following mitral valve replacement probably come from the fibrillating atrium rather than the prosthesis. Most centers using porcine valves for mitral valve replacement maintain anticoagulation indefinitely if atrial fibrillation is present; anticoagulants are given for 6–12 weeks to patients in sinus rhythm and then slowly discontinued. The thromboembolic rate in patients in sinus rhythm who do not require anticoagulants is extremely low; Cohn and co-workers[18] reported no embolic episodes in a series of patients followed for a mean of 3 years.

Anticoagulant-related morbidity and mortality: Patients on continuous anticoagulation have a constant and continuing risk of hemorrhagic complications. The probability of a major hemorrhage is approximately 1.5%/year, and the risk of minor bleeding is about the same.[3,45] The risk of fatal hemorrhage is approximately 0.5%/year.

Structural failure: Structural failure is almost unheard of in the Starr-Edwards Silastic ball valve, the Medtronic tilting disc valve, and the St. Jude bileaflet valve.[34] The Bjork-Shiley Convexo-Concave valve has had structural failure due to fracture of the welded outflow strut and has been withdrawn from the market. Structural failure is also rare in porcine prostheses followed to 5 years,[18,67] but begins to accelerate after 5 years and has occurred in 20%–40% by 10 years.[34] Structural failure is extremely rare in patients 70 years or older at the time they receive a porcine mitral valve.[47,58]

References

1. Abascal VM, Wilkins GT, O'Shea JP, Choong CY, Palacios IF, Thomas JD, Rosas E, Newell JB, Block PC, Weyman AE: Prediction of successful outcome in 130 patients undergoing percutaneous balloon mitral valvotomy. Circulation 82:448, 1990.

2. Akins CW, Kirklin JK, Block PC, Buckley MJ, Austen MG: Preoperative evaluation of subvalvular fibrosis in mitral stenosis: a predictive factor in conservative vs replacement surgical therapy. Circulation 60(Suppl I):I-71, 1979.

3. Allen WB, Karp RB, Kouchoukos NT: Mitral valve replacement: Starr-Edwards cloth-covered composite-seat prosthesis. Arch Surg 109:642, 1975.

4. Appelbaum A, Kouchoukos NT, Blackstone EH, Kirklin JW: Early risks of open heart surgery for mitral valve disease. Am J Cardiol 37:201, 1976.

5. Arom KV, Nicoloff DM, Kersten TE, Northrup WF III, Lindsay WG, Emery RW: Ten years' experience with the St. Jude medical valve prosthesis. Ann Thorac Surg 47:831, 1989.

6. Bailey CP: The surgical treatment of mitral stenosis (mitral commissurotomy). Dis Chest 15:377, 1949.

7. Barlow JB, Pocock WA: Billowing, floppy, prolapsing or flail mitral valves? Am J Cardiol 55:501, 1985.

8. Bjork VO, Henze A, Rodriguez L: Left ventricular rupture as a complication of mitral valve replacement: surgical experience with eight cases and a review of the literature. J Thorac Cardiovasc Surg 73:14, 1977.

9. Bonchek LI, Anderson RP, Starr A: Mitral valve replacement with cloth-covered composite-seat prostheses. J Thorac Cardiovasc Surg 67:93,1974.

10. Bonchek LI, Olinger GN, Siegel R, Tresch DD, Keelan MH: Left ventricular performance after mitral reconstruction for mitral regurgitation. J Thorac Cardiovasc Surg 88:122,1984.

11. Braunwald E, Awe NC: The syndrome of severe mitral regurgitation with normal left atrial pressure. Circulation 27:29,1963.

12. Carpentier A: Cardiac valve surgery—the "French correction." J Thorac Cardiovasc Surg 86:323,1983.

13. Carpentier A, Deloche A, Dauptain J, Soyer R, Prigent CL, Blondeau P, Piwnica A, Dubost C, McGoon DC: A new reconstructive operation for correction of mitral and tricuspid insufficiency. J Thorac Cardiovasc Surg 61:1,1971.

14. Chavez AM, Cosgrove DM III, Lytle BW, Gill CC, Loop FD, Stewart RW, Golding LR, Taylor PC: Applicability of mitral valvuloplasty techniques in a North American population. Am J Cardiol 62:253,1988.

15. Cohn L: Surgery for mitral regurgitation. JAMA 260:2883,1988.

16. Cohn LH, Couper GS, Kinchla NM, Collins JJ Jr: Decreased operative risk of surgical treatment of mitral regurgitation with or without coronary artery disease. J Am Coll Cardiol 16:1575,1990.

17. Cohn LH, DiSesa VJ, Couper GS, Peigh PS, Kowalker W, Collins JJ Jr: Mitral valve repair for myxomatous degeneration and prolapse of the mitral valve. J Thorac Cardiovasc Surg 98:987,1989.

18. Cohn LH, Koster JK, Mee RBB, Collins JJ: Long-term follow-up of the Hancock bioprosthetic heart valve: a 6-year review. Circulation 60:(Suppl I):I-87,1979.

19. Come PC, Riley MF, Weintraub RM, Wei JY, Markis JE, Lorell BH, Grossman W: Dynamic left ventricular outflow tract obstruction when the anterior leaflet is retained at prosthetic mitral valve replacement. Ann Thorac Surg 43:561,1987.

20. Cosgrove DM, Chavez AM, Lytle BW, Gill CC, Stewart RW, Taylor PC, Goormastic M, Borsh JA, Loop FD: Results of mitral valve reconstruction. Circulation 74(Suppl I):I-82,1986.

21. Craver JM, Cohen C, Weintraub WS: Case-matched comparison of mitral valve replacement and repair. Ann Thorac Surg 49:964,1990.

22. Craver JM, Jones EL, Guyton RA, Cobbs BW Jr, Hatcher CR Jr: Avoidance of transverse midventricular disruption following mitral valve replacement. Ann Thorac Surg 40:163,1985.

23. Cutler EC, Beck CS: The present status of surgical procedures in chronic valvular disease of the heart. Arch Surg 18:403,1929.

24. David TE, Ho WC: The effect of preservation of chordae tendineae on mitral valve replacement for postinfarction mitral regurgitation. Circulation 74(Suppl I):I-116,1986.

25. David TE, Komeda M, Pollick C, Burns RJ: Mitral valve annuloplasty: the effect of the type on left ventricular function. Ann Thorac Surg 47:524,1989.

26. David TE, Uden DE, Strauss HD: The importance of the mitral apparatus in left ventricular function after correction of mitral regurgitation. Circulation 68(Suppl II):II-76,1983.

27. Deloche A, Jebara VA, Relland JYM, Chauvaud S, Fabiani JN, Perier P, Dreyfus G, Mihaileanu S, Carpentier A: Valve repair with Carpentier techniques: the second decade. J Thorac Cardiovasc Surg 99:990,1990.

28. Feikes HL, Daugharthy JB, Perry JE, Bell JH, Hieb RE, Johnson GH: Preservation of all chordae tendineae and papillary muscle during mitral valve replacement with a tilting disc valve. J Card Surg 5:81,1990.

29. Galloway AC, Colvin SB, Baumann FG, Harty S, Spencer FC: Current concepts of mitral valve reconstruction for mitral insufficiency. Circulation 78:1087,1988.

30. Gerami S, Messner BJ, Hallman GL, Cooley DA: Open mitral commissurotomy. J Thorac Cardiovasc Surg 62:366,1971.

31. Glancy DL, O'Brien KP, Reis RL, Epstein SE, Morrow AG: Hemodynamic studies in patients with 2M and 3M Starr-Edwards prostheses: evidence of obstruction to left atrial emptying. Circulation 39(Suppl I):I-113,1969.

32. Goldman ME, Mora F, Guarino T, Fuster V, Mindich BC: Mitral valvuloplasty is superior to valve replacement for preservation of left ventricular function: an intraoperative two-dimensional echocardiographic study. J Am Coll Cardiol 10:568,1987.

33. Goor DA, Mohr R, Lavee J, Serraf A, Smolinsky A: Preservation of the posterior leaflet during mechanical valve replacement for ischemic mitral regurgitation and complete myocardial revascularization. J Thorac Cardiovasc Surg 96:253,1988.

34. Grunkemeier GL, Starr A, Rahimtoola S: Prosthetic heart valve performance: long-term follow-up. Curr Probl Cardiol 17:333,1992.

35. Hansen DE, Cahill PD, Derby GC, Miller DC: Relative contributions of the anterior and posterior mitral chordae tendineae to canine global left ventricular function. J Thorac Cardiovasc Surg 93:45,1987.

36. Hansen DE, Sarris GE, Niczyporuk MA, Derby GC, Cahill PD, Miller DC: Physiologic role of the mitral apparatus in left ventricular regional mechanics, contraction synergy, and global systolic performance. J Thorac Cardiovasc Surg 97:521, 1989.

37. Hennein HA, Swain JA, McIntosh CL, Bonow RO, Stone CD, Clark RE: Comparative assessment of chordal preservation versus chordal resection during mitral valve replacement. J Thorac Cardiovasc Surg 99:828,1990.

38. Hetzer R, Bougioukas G, Frenz M, Borst HG: Mitral valve replacement with preservation of papillary muscles and chordae tendineae—revival of a seemingly forgotten concept. Thorac Cardiovasc Surg 31:291,1983.

39. Hickey MSJ, Blackstone EH, Kirklin JW, Dean LS: Outcome probabilities and life history after surgical mitral commissurotomy: implications for balloon commissurotomy. J Am Coll Cardiol 17:29,1991.

40. Hood WP Jr, Rackley CE, Rolett EL: Wall stress in the normal and hypertrophied human left ventricle. Am J Cardiol 22:550,1968.

41. Horowitz MS, Goodman DJ, Fogarty TJ, Harrison DC: Mitral valve replacement with glutaraldehyde-preserved porcine heterograft: clinical, hemodynamic, and pathological correlations. J Thorac Cardiovas Surg 67:885,1974.

42. Horstkotte D, Haerten K, Seipel L, Korfer R, Budde T, Bircks W, Loogen F: Central hemodynamics at rest and during exercise after mitral valve replacement with different prostheses. Circulation 68(Suppl II):II-161,1983.

43. Housman L, Bonchek LI, Lambert LE, Grunkemeier GL, Starr A: Prognosis of patients after open mitral commissurotomy: actuarial analysis of late results in 100 patients. J Thorac Cardiovasc Surg 73:742,1977.

44. Inoue K, Owaki T, Nakamura T, Kitamura F, Miyamoto N: Clinical application of transvenous mitral commissurotomy by a new balloon catheter. J Thorac Cardiovasc Surg 87:394,1984.

45. Isom OW, Spencer FC, Glassman E, Teiko P, Boyd AD, Cunningham JN: Long-term results in 1,375 patients undergoing valve replacement with the Starr-Edwards cloth-covered composite-seat prostheses: a six-year appraisal. Ann Surg 186:310,1977.

46. Isom OW, Williams CD, Falk EA, Glassman E, Spencer FC: Long-term evaluation of cloth-covered metallic ball prostheses. J Thorac Cardiovasc Surg 64:354,1972.

47. Jamieson WRE, Burr LH, Munro I, Miyagishima RT, Gerein AN: Cardiac valve replacement in the elderly: clinical performance of biological prostheses. Ann Thorac Surg 48:173,1989.

48. Junod FL, Harlan BJ, Payne J, Smeloff EA, Miller GE Jr, Kelly PB Jr, Ross KA, Shankar KG, McDermott JP: Preoperative risk assessment in cardiac surgery: comparison of predicted and observed results. Ann Thorac Surg 43:59,1987.

49. Karlson KJ, Ashraf MM, Berger RL: Rupture of left ventricle following mitral valve replacement. Ann Thorac Surg 46:590,1988.

50. Katske G, Golding LR, Tubbs RR, Loop FD: Posterior midventricular rupture after mitral valve replacement. Ann Thorac Surg 27:130,1979.

51. Kay JH, Zubiate P, Mendez AM, Carpena C, Watanabe K, Magidson O: Mitral valve repair for patients with pure mitral insufficiency. JAMA 236:1584,1976.

52. Kirklin JW: Replacement of the mitral valve for mitral incompetence. Surgery 77: 827,1972.

53. Kirklin JW: Percutaneous balloon versus surgical closed commissurotomy for mitral stenosis. Circulation 83:1450,1991.

54. Kirklin JW, Pacifico AD: Surgery for acquired valvular heart disease. Part 2. N Engl J Med 288:194,1973.

55. Lam JHC, Ranganathan N, Wigle ED, Silver MD: Morphology of the human mitral valve. I. Chordae tendineae: a new classification. Circulation 41:449,1970.

56. Lillihei CW, Levy MJ, Bonnabeau RC Jr: Mitral valve replacement with preserva-

tion of papillary muscles and chordae tendineae. J Thorac Cardiovasc Surg 47: 532,1964.

57. Lock JE, Khalilullah M, Shrivastava S, Bahl V, Keane JF: Percutaneous catheter commissurotomy in rheumatic mitral stenosis. N Engl J Med 313:1515,1985.

58. Louagie Y, Noirhomme P, Aranguis E, Eucher P, Vanruyssevelt P, Buche M, Dion R, Jaumin P, Schoevaerdts JC: Use of the Carpentier-Edwards porcine bioprosthesis: assessment of patient selection policy. J Thorac Cardiovasc Surg 104: 1013,1992.

59. Lytle BW, Cosgrove DM, Gill CC, Stewart RW, Golding LAR, Goormastic M, Taylor PC, Loop FD: Mitral valve replacement combined with myocardial revascularization: early and late results for 300 patients, 1970 to 1983. Circulation 71: 1179,1985.

60. McAlpine WA: Heart and Coronary Arteries. New York, Springer-Verlag, 1975.

61. McAnulty JH, Morton M, Rahimtoola SH, Kloster FE, Ahuja N, Starr A: Hemodynamic characteristics of the composite strut ball valve prostheses (Starr-Edwards Track Valves) in patients on anticoagulants. Circulation 59(Suppl I):I-159,1978.

62. Miki S, Kusuhara K, Ueda Y, Komeda M, Ohkita Y, Tahata T: Mitral valve replacement with preservation of chordae tendineae and papillary muscles. Ann Thorac Surg 45:28,1988.

63. Mullin MJ, Engelman RM, Isom OW, Boyd AD, Glassman E, Spencer FC: Experience with open mitral commissurotomy in 100 consecutive patients. Surgery 76: 974,1974.

64. Nakano S, Kawashima Y, Hirose H, Matsuda H, Shirakura R, Sato S, Taniguchi K, Kawamoto T, Sakaki S, Ohyama C: Reconsiderations of indications for open mitral commissurotomy based on pathologic features of the stenosed mitral valve: a fourteen-year follow-up study in 347 consecutive patients. J Thorac Cardiovasc Surg 94:335,1987.

65. Nanda NC, Gramiak R, Shah PM, DeWeese JA: Mitral commissurotomy versus replacement: preoperative evaluation by echocardiography. Circulation 51:262, 1975.

66. Okita Y, Miki S, Kusuhara K, Ueda Y, Tahata T, Yamanaka K, Higa T: Analysis of left ventricular motion after mitral valve replacement with a technique of preservation of all chordae tendineae: comparison with conventional mitral valve replacement or mitral valve repair. J Thorac Cardiovasc Surg 104:786,1992.

67. Oyer PE, Stinson EB, Reitz BA, Miller DO, Rossiter S, Shumway NE: Long-term evaluation of the porcine xenograft bioprosthesis. J Thorac Cardiovasc Surg 78: 343,1979.

68. Perloff JK, Roberts WC: The mitral apparatus: functional anatomy of mitral regurgitation. Circulation 46:227,1972.

69. Peter CA, Austin EH, Jones RH: Effect of valve replacement for chronic mitral insufficiency on left ventricular function during rest and exercise. J Thorac Cardiovasc Surg 82:127,1981.

70. Rahimtoola SH: The problem of valve prosthesis-patient mismatch. Circulation 58:20,1978.

71. Ranganathan N, Lam JHC, Wigle ED, Silver MD: Morphology of the human mitral valve. II. The valve leaflets. Circulation 41:459,1970.

72. Reifart N, Nowak B, Baykut D, Bussman WD, Kaltenbach M: Experimental mitral valvuloplasty of fibrotic and calcified valves with balloon catheters (abstr). J Am Coll Cardiol 4:448,1985.

73. Rigo P, Alderson PO, Robertson RM, Becker LC, Wagner HN Jr: Measurement of aortic and mitral regurgitation by gated cardiac blood pool scans. Circulation 60: 306,1979.

74. Roberts CW, Cohen LS: Left ventricular papillary muscle. Description of the normal and a survey of conditions causing them to be abnormal. Circulation 46: 138,1972.

75. Rosenquist GC, Clark EB, Sweeney LJ, McAllister HA: The normal spectrum of mitral and aortic valve discontinuity. Circulation 54:298,1976.

76. Rushmer RF: Initial phase of ventricular systole: asynchronous contraction. Am J Physiol 184:188,1956.

77. Sand ME, Naftel DC, Blackstone EH, Kirklin JW, Karp JW: A comparison of repair and replacement for mitral valve incompetence. J Thorac Cardiovasc Surg 94: 208,1987.

78. Sarris GE, Cahill PD, Hansen DE, Derby GC, Miller DC: Restoration of left ventricular systolic performance after reattachment of the mitral chordae tendineae: the importance of valvular-ventricular interaction. J Thorac Cardiovasc Surg 95: 969,1989.

79. Schuler G, Peterson KL, Johnson A, Francis G, Dennish G, Utley J, Daily PO, Ashburn W, Ross J Jr: Temporal response of left ventricular performance to mitral valve surgery. Circulation 59:1218,1979.

80. Selzer A, Cohn KE: Natural history of mitral stenosis: a review. Circulation 45: 878,1972.

81. Souttar HS: The surgical treatment of mitral stenosis. Br Med J 2:603,1925.

82. Spence PA, Peniston CM, David TE, Mihic N, Jabr AK, Narini P, Salerno TA: Toward a better understanding of the etiology of left ventricular dysfunction after mitral valve replacement: an experimental study with possible clinical implications. Ann Thorac Surg 41:363,1986.

83. Spencer FC: A plea for early, open mitral commissurotomy. Am Heart J 95: 668,1978.

84. Spencer FC, Colvin SB, Culliford AT, Isom OW: Experiences with the Carpentier techniques of mitral valve reconstruction in 103 patients (1980–1985). J Thorac Cardiovasc Surg 90:341,1985.

85. Spencer FC, Galloway AC, Colvin SB: A clinical evaluation of the hypothesis that rupture of the left ventricle following mitral valve replacement can be prevented by preservation of the chordae of the mural leaflet. Ann Surg 202:673,1985.

86. Starr A, Grunkemeier G, Lambert L, Okies JE, Thomas D: Mitral valve replacement: a 10-year follow-up of noncloth-covered vs cloth-covered caged-ball prostheses. Circulation 54(Suppl III):III-47,1976.

87. Tandler J: Anatomie des Herzens. Jena, G. Fischer, 1913.

88. Turi ZG, Reyes VP, Raju S, Raju R, Kumar DN, Rajagopal P, Sathyanarayana PV, Rao P, Srinath K, Peters P, Connors B, Fromm B, Farkas P, Wynne J: Percutaneous balloon versus surgical closed commissurotomy for mitral stenosis: a prospective, randomized trial. Circulation 83:1179,1991.

89. Urschel CW, Covell JW, Sonnenblick EH, Ross J Jr, Braunwald E: Myocardial mechanics in aortic and mitral regurgitation. The concept of instantaneous impedance as a determinant of the performance of the intact heart. J Clin Invest 47: 867,1968.

90. Wanderman KL, Goldberg MJ, Stack RS, Weissler AM: Left ventricular performance in mitral regurgitation assessed with systolic time intervals and echocardiography. Am J Cardiol 38:831,1976.

91. Wolpowitz A, Barnard MS, Sanchez H, Barnard CN: Intraoperative posterior left ventricular wall rupture associated with mitral valve replacement. Ann Thorac Surg 25:551,1978.

92. Zimmerman J, Bailey CP: The surgical significance of the fibrous skeleton of the heart. J Thorac Cardiovasc Surg 44:701,1962.

13

Aortic Valve Surgery

Surgery of the aortic valve spans all age groups and encompasses a broad spectrum of pathologic anatomy and surgical technique. In this chapter we will illustrate aortic valvotomy and replacement and briefly review surgical relief of other forms of left ventricular outflow obstruction.

Valvotomy

Indications for Surgery

The indications for aortic valvotomy differ according to age group. Congestive heart failure is the main indication for surgery in infancy, whereas prevention of sudden death and relief of symptoms are the main indications in childhood.[10,55,89] Valvotomy should be performed in any infant in congestive failure and should be performed in any child with critical aortic stenosis, regardless of symptoms. Selection of neonates for aortic valvotomy rather than heart transplantation or a Norwood procedure is based on left ventricular size and other measurements of left ventricular outflow dimensions. Leung and co-workers[93] found that echocardiographic dimensions of the left ventricle, the subaortic region, the ventriculoaortic junction, the ascending aorta, and the mitral valve orifice all correlated with a good result from aortic valvotomy. Rhodes and colleagues[125] found they were able to predict outcome after aortic valvotomy based on mitral valve area, long-axis dimension of the left ventricle relative to the long-axis dimension of the heart, diameter of the aortic root, and body surface area.

In children, surgery is usually indicated when the gradient is over 50 mm Hg in the presence of normal cardiac output or a valve area index less than $0.5 \text{ cm}^2/\text{m}^2$.[81]

Surgical Anatomy

Congenital aortic stenosis occurs most commonly as a relative underdevelopment of the right coronary cusp and fusion with the adjacent cusps at the commissures. The orifice is usually a slit between the left and noncoronary cusps, and the commissure between these two cusps is usually well developed, whereas the other commissure can vary in degree of development and may be only a primitive raphe. A safe incision can usually be made in at least one commissure of the right coronary cusp. Incision of the other commissure depends upon its degree of development and the development and depth of the right coronary cusp.

Surgical Technique

A transverse aortotomy is made and the valve is exposed with small leaflet retractors. With forceps holding the leaflets, the well-developed commissure is incised back to the anulus (Figs. 13–1, 13–2). The depth of support and degree of development of the right coronary cusp are then assessed. If it is clear that the right coronary cusp will coapt with the other cusps rather than prolapse, the other commissure is incised. Following valvotomy the subvalvular area should be inspected to ensure the absence of any subvalvular stenosis.

Results

Although valvotomy has been associated with high operative mortality in the neonate,[49] recent reports[78,153] have shown much better results in properly selected patients, with Turley and colleagues[153] reporting an operative mortality of 13% in neonates undergoing open valvotomy. Survivors have good relief of congestive heart failure and good late survival.[49] A large proportion of patients who die constitute an intermediate group between patients with hypoplastic left heart syndrome and normals.[49,93,125]

Valvotomy in children has low operative risk (operative mortality around 2%), produces excellent symptomatic improvement, but does not usually eliminate the valvular gradient entirely.[35,75,90,139] Conkle and co-workers[35] reported 38 patients operated upon between 1 and 21 years of age. Ninety percent were asymptomatic. The average mean gradient was reduced from 91 to 27 mm Hg. Lawson and colleagues[90] from the University of Oregon reported 44 patients, with a mean age at surgery of 10 years. Ninety-two percent survived 10 years and 82% were reoperation-free at 10 years. After 10 years, reoperation becomes increasingly common, being performed for either restenosis or progressive regurgitation. Wheller and colleagues[155] found that 70% of patients were free of reoperation at 10 years.

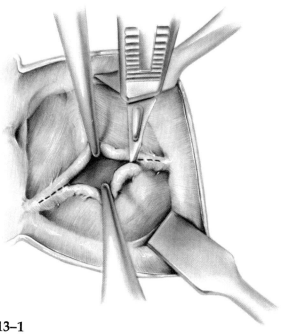

13–1

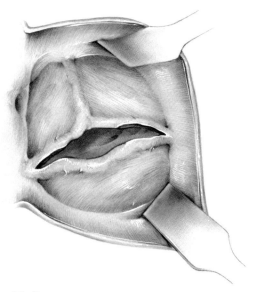

13–2

Percutaneous Balloon Valvotomy in Infants and Children

Lababidi[87] reported in 1984 a series of children who underwent percutaneous balloon aortic valvuloplasty. Their ages ranged from 2 to 17 years. The mean of the gradients decreased from 113 ± 48 mm Hg before valvotomy to 32 ± 15 mm Hg following valvotomy. Mild aortic regurgitation followed valvotomy in 43% of patients. Balloon valvotomy has also been advocated for neonates.[79,158] More studies will be needed, particularly long-term follow-up studies, to determine the role of balloon valvotomy.

Replacement

Indications for Surgery

Aortic Stenosis

The natural history of severe aortic stenosis in the adult is markedly unfavorable, with a mortality of 8%–9% per year.[53,122] With the onset of angina the life expectancy is 5 years, and with syncope it is 3 years. Kelly and colleagues[83] reported 39 symptomatic patients who were not treated surgically because of their physician's decision. The group had a mean age of 72 years and a mean doppler peak gradient of 68 mm Hg. The 1-year mortality was 38%. The onset of congestive heart failure carries the worst prognosis, with average life expectancy of less than 2 years.[73,132] Proper timing of aortic valve replacement prevents early and late death, results in normal functional status, and preserves normal ventricular function or returns abnormal function to normal. Knowledge of how the natural course is altered by properly timed and properly performed valve replacement forms the basis for decision regarding surgical intervention.

Aortic stenosis is usually a progressive disease. The increasing resistance to left ventricular outflow caused by progressive stenosis of the aortic valve is compensated by the generation of increasingly higher left ventricular pressure in order to maintain adequate systemic pressure and cardiac output. This increased left ventricular pressure is achieved by concentric ventricular hypertrophy, with thickening of the left ventricular wall and increase in mass of the left ventricle.[51,67,116] Such hypertrophy normalizes wall stress and initially maintains normal left ventricular systolic pump function.[64,66]

However, the ventricle may reach a limit of concentric hypertrophy and begin to dilate, using the Frank-Starling mechanism in order to maintain left ventricular pump function. The dilatation and change in shape are critical developments in the decompensation of ventricular function. Parameters of systolic pump function such as ejection fraction and mean velocity of circumferential fiber shortening may be maintained initially in the normal range,[134] but subsequently are reduced in all, and eventually congestive heart failure results.

Hemodynamic and metabolic alterations are the consequence of these progressive stages of left ventricular compensation and then decompensation; the hemodynamic and metabolic changes cause the symptoms and events characteristic of aortic stenosis. As the ventricular compliance falls with increasing hypertrophy, the end-diastolic pressure and pulmonary venous pressure rise. This can cause increasing shortness of breath. As the myocardial wall tension increases and the oxygen demand rises, an imbalance between oxygen supply and demand may occur, resulting in myocardial ischemia and the symptom of angina pectoris. The presence of coronary artery disease will cause myocardial ischemia earlier in the course of the disease.

Transient periods of systemic hypotension may occur, resulting in dizziness or syncope. Sudden death may occur, probably most commonly caused by ventricular arrhythmias secondary to myocardial ischemia. Chronic congestive heart failure develops as decompensation progresses, with the alteration in ventricular shape and dynamics creating a vicious cycle, terminating in death if surgical treatment does not ensue.

Surgical intervention in aortic stenosis should be timed to relieve symptoms, prevent or reverse ventricular dysfunction, and prevent cardiac death. This timing can be determined with assurance, since the results for surgical treatment of severe aortic stenosis are clearly superior to the natural history.[6,116,144,146] Valve replacement for aortic stenosis results in alleviation of symptoms and improvement in ventricular function in the vast majority of patients. Even those patients with congestive heart failure and marked deterioration of ventricular function usually have marked improvement in symptoms and ventricular function,[144] illustrating the reversibility of the ventricular dysfunction occurring from aortic stenosis. However, in this group late death following successful valve replacement is more common.

Because of the poor prognosis of severe aortic stenosis and the excellent results of surgical treatment, surgery should be performed if severe stenosis is documented by catheterization, regardless of the symptomatic state. Hemodynamic evaluation in our institutions involves determination of the valvular gradient and calculation of the aortic valve area and the aortic valve area index. In the presence of a normal ejection fraction and cardiac output, a gradient of 50 mm Hg or more usually correlates with severe aortic stenosis (aortic valve area index less than 0.75 cm^2/m^2). If cardiac output is low, severe aortic stenosis may exist without a high gradient.[31] It is for this reason that valve area index is calculated. Aortic valve replacement should be performed for severe aortic stenosis even in the presence of a left ventricular ejection fraction of less than 25%.[135]

Aortic valve replacement should be strongly considered for symptomatic patients with moderate aortic stenosis (aortic valve area 0.7–1.2 cm^2). Kennedy and co-workers[85] reported a series of 66 patients with moderate aortic stenosis. During a mean follow-up period of 35 months, 14 patients died of causes attributed to aortic stenosis. The estimated probability for remaining free of any complication of aortic stenosis at the end of the first 4 years was only 59%.

Percutaneous Balloon Valvuloplasty for Aortic Stenosis in Adults

Balloon valvuloplasty for aortic stenosis was reported by Cribier and colleagues[41] in 1986. This procedure has been most widely applied in elderly patients, many of whom are considered poor risks for aortic valve replacement. The procedure results in a decrease in the aortic valve gradient and a small increase in the aortic valve area.[42,92,113,137] However, there is a rapid development of restenosis, and mortality at 6 months of follow-up is as high as 22%.[137] In addition, most patients have valve areas that are still in the range of severe stenosis.[121]

We do not feel balloon valvuloplasty is appropriate for the vast majority of elderly patients with aortic stenosis if a surgical mortality of less than 15% can be achieved.[94,152,157] Age alone, even over age 85, should not be a contraindication to surgery, since the mortality of surgery in this age group is acceptably low.[5] Balloon valvuloplasty may be of some benefit in those patients with severe coexistent medical problems, patients in urgent need of noncardiac surgical procedures, patients in whom other organ system function may improve after valvuloplasty, making them acceptable candidates for valve replacement, and patients with severe depression of left ventricular function in whom there is a question about reversibility.[121]

Aortic Regurgitation

Acute aortic regurgitation, as can occur with endocarditis or dissection of the ascending aorta, can present as sudden hemodynamic deterioration,[122,151,156] requiring urgent surgery. The hemodynamic indications in the face of sudden hemodynamic deterioration are clear and uncontroversial.

However, there is still some controversy regarding the indications for surgical intervention in chronic aortic regurgitation.[15,22,120,121,136] This reflects both recognition of the inadequacy of the older indications—development of severe symptoms, congestive heart failure, or marked cardiomegaly—and realization that a predictable and widely acceptable new set of indications is still evolving.

Aortic valve replacement for chronic aortic regurgitation has generally been less satisfactory than replacement for aortic stenosis, in terms of improvement in symptoms, improvement in ventricular function, and late survival.[6,21,34,57] It appears that there are several reasons for this disparity in results: (1) aortic regurgitation usually does not cause symptoms until considerable ventricular dysfunction has developed[51,60]; (2) the ventricular dysfunction present at the time symptoms develop seldom improves completely to normal following successful valve replacement[21,57]; (3) severe ventricular dysfunction often progresses in spite of successful valve replacement, resulting in late death.[16,68,69,71]

The major compensatory changes caused by aortic regurgitation are left ventricular hypertrophy and ventricular dilatation.[116] Such compensation can maintain normal ejection fraction and normal end-diastolic pressure for a long period of time, by increasing stroke volume in response to volume overload. Eventually the ejection fraction begins to fall, first only during exercise,[20] then at rest. The left ventricular end-diastolic pressure rises and pulmonary venous hypertension ensues, causing dyspnea and orthopnea. Therefore, with aortic regurgitation, in contrast to aortic stenosis, symptoms usually do not occur until considerable ventricular dysfunction has occurred.[51] Also, the ventricular structural and functional changes occurring with volume overload are more severe and much less reversible than the changes occurring with pressure overload.[101,116,133]

Maron and colleagues[101] have described cardiac muscle degeneration in the left ventricle of patients with pure aortic regurgitation or combined aortic stenosis and regurgitation. These morphologic features are decreased size of cells; loss of myofibrils; preferential loss of thick (myosin) filaments; streaking, streaming, and clumping of Z-band material; markedly increased amounts of interstitial fibrous tissue; loss of contact between adjacent cells; dilatation or proliferation of sarcoplasmic reticulum; and thickening of the basement membrane. Although their series is small, including only 16 patients, they did not observe any such degeneration in the 6 patients with predominant aortic stenosis.

Experimental work by Ross and colleagues[133] has shown that chronic left ventricular volume overload results in slippage between myofibrils, reflected by a loss of normal alignment of the Z lines. It has been suggested that such a fundamental qualitative change in the microarchitecture of the ventricle with chronic volume overloading may be partially or totally irreversible.[51]

Dissatisfaction with the traditional indications for valve replacement in aortic regurgitation has stimulated the search for better parameters upon which to base the timing of surgery.[30] These have involved invasive and noninvasive evaluation of ventricular size and function, at rest and during stress.

Afterload stress with angiotensin has resulted in a fall in ejection fraction in approximately 50% of patients with aortic regurgitation.[12] The stress-induced dysfunction correlated with a regurgitant fraction over 0.50 and a left ventricular end-diastolic volume index over 160 ml/m^2. Radionuclide cineangiography has demonstrated an abnormal ejection fraction during exercise in almost all patients with aortic regurgitation and in approximately 50% of asymptomatic patients.[20]

Echocardiographic studies of left ventricular dimensions have been correlated with postoperative results.[32,68] Patients with left ventricular end-systolic dimensions below 55 mm usually have good results. It has been recommended that asymptomatic patients with end-systolic dimensions of 50–54 mm be followed with serial echocardiograms every 4 to 6 months, and that operation be performed at an end-systolic dimension of 55 mm or greater, in spite of absence of symptoms.[69]

Bonow and colleagues[17-19] have shown that the duration of preoperative left ventricular dysfunction in patients with aortic regurgitation is an important determinant of the reversibility of left ventricular function and survival after aortic valve replacement. They found that patients who had a period of subnormal left ventricular function of less than 14 months had excellent postoperative survival and a high likelihood of normal postoperative ventricular function.

We recommend valve replacement in severe aortic regurgitation and impaired resting left ventricular ejection fraction or left ventricular end-systolic dimension over 55 mm, regardless of symptomatic state. Asymptomatic patients with normal left ventricular function at rest should be followed carefully and undergo valve replacement when left ventricular function at rest becomes subnormal.[15,19] All symptomatic patients with severe aortic regurgitation should undergo valve replacement.

Combined Stenosis and Regurgitation

Patients with aortic stenosis and regurgitation cover a broad spectrum of physiologic conditions and must be evaluated carefully, since they can have a more rapidly progressive and malignant course, probably due to the early loss of ventricular shape in the presence of outflow obstruction. Patients with symptoms and normal ventricular function should undergo surgery, as should asymptomatic patients with resting left ventricular dysfunction.

Endocarditis

The treatment of endocarditis is primarily medical. The indications for operation in endocarditis are many and varied, depending on the organism, its response to antibiotic treatment, hemodynamic abnormalities, and other factors.[23,106,126,143,154] Surgery should be undertaken if there is persistent infection, development of congestive heart failure, septic embolus, or heart block. Echocardiography can be helpful in defining pathology and predicting the risk of complications.[140,148]

Surgery should also be influenced by the type of organism. Fungal endocarditis and most gram-negative infections should indicate early surgery regardless of the hemodynamic state.[23,126,154] Infection with *Staphylococcus aureus* is prone to cause heart failure, anular and myocardial abscesses, heart block, and coronary embolism. Early surgery for staphylococcal endocarditis, regardless of hemodynamic state, has also been recommended.[126] Surgical excision of the focus of infection prior to extension or abscess formation is an advantage of early surgical intervention in medically recalcitrant situations.

Combined with Coronary Artery Surgery

Valvular replacement in the presence of untreated coronary disease is associated with higher early and late mortality than valvular replacement in the absence of coronary disease,[39,95,97,118] as discussed in Chapter 9. Copeland and co-workers[39] found a 3-year survival of 60% in 129 patients with isolated aortic valve replacement who had untreated coronary disease. The 3-year survival following isolated aortic valve replacement in 213 patients without coronary artery disease was 85%, a statistically significant difference.

There is good evidence that performing coronary bypass for coronary artery disease at the time of valve replacement improves survival in patients with combined disease if the operative mortality is low (below 6%).[110,127] It is our policy to perform coronary arteriography in all patients over 40 years of age who have valvular disease.[4,13] Coronary artery bypass is performed to major vessels with over 50% narrowing of luminal diameter. Bypass is done even if angina is not present.

Choice of Prosthesis or Valve

Mechanical Prosthesis Versus Porcine Prosthesis

The reasoning underlying our choice of mechanical valve versus porcine heterograft for aortic valve replacement is essentially the same as for mitral valve replacement as outlined in Chapter 12. As with the mitral porcine prosthesis, the aortic porcine prosthesis has excellent durability in the elderly patient. Two reports[76,96] have shown no structural deterioration of Carpentier-Edwards porcine valves implanted in patients 70 years and older.

Homograft

The use of homografts for replacement of the aortic valve was pioneered by Ross[129] and Barratt-Boyes[7,8] in the 1960s. Their early results showed a very low incidence of valve-related complications other than valve degeneration and an almost complete freedom from thromboembolism.[9,104] The use of homografts never spread beyond a small number of centers until the report by O'Brien[114] in 1987 describing the excellent results obtained by using a cryopreserved valve stored at −196°C. O'Brien found that freedom from reoperation for valve degeneration at 10 years was 100% and freedom from thromboembolism at 10 years was 97%. Concomitant with this report was the growing availability of cryopreserved aortic homografts from commercial sources.

The aortic homograft is particularly suitable for children, women of childbearing age, and patients with active endocarditis, and is an excellent valve when the anatomic conditions are appropriate and the surgeon is familiar with the technical details of implantation.[72]

Pulmonary Valve Autograft

Ross[130] reported the replacement of the aortic valve with the patient's pulmonary valve in 1967. The pulmonary valve was replaced with a pulmonary valve homograft. His experience with this technique has been good and long-term results have been similar to those with homografts.[58,59] The operation is technically demanding, requiring attention to important details.[50] If the growth potential of the autograft is realized, this method would be particularly attractive for use in children. Larger numbers of patients and longer follow-up will be necessary to determine the proper place of the pulmonary autograft in patients requiring replacement of the aortic valve.

Surgical Strategy

Myocardial Preservation

Cold blood cardioplegic arrest is used for aortic valve replacement (Chapter 6). In patients with aortic insufficiency, initial infusion is directly into the coronary ostia with hand-held cannulas, with subsequent infusions either directly into the coronary ostia or into the coronary sinus. Initial infusion in patients with pure aortic stenosis is given in the aortic root and subsequent infusions either directly into the coronary ostia or into the coronary sinus.

Venting

The left ventricle is usually vented through the right superior pulmonary vein.

Associated Cardiac Procedures

1. *Coronary artery bypass:* Distal anastomoses are done after opening the aorta and injecting cardioplegic solution into the coronary ostia via hand-held cannulas. Incisions in the epicardium over the sites of planned coronary arteriotomy prior to infusion of cardioplegic solution can help in assuring accurate incision in the coronary arteries. Following all the distal vein anastomoses, the aortic anular sutures are placed, the valve inserted, and the aortotomy closed. If an internal mammary anastomosis is to be performed, it is done.

Proximal vein anastomoses are done over a partial occluding clamp after release of the aortic cross-clamp, while the vented heart is beating and rewarming.

2. *Mitral valve replacement:* The mitral valve and aortic valve are excised. Sutures are placed in the mitral anulus and through the prosthetic valve. The valve can be seated and tied at this time or after placement of the aortic anular sutures; the latter may give better exposure of the aortic anulus. Sutures are placed through the aortic anulus and prosthetic valve. The mitral valve is then seated and tied, followed by the aortic valve.

Suture Technique
Suture techniques applicable to replacement of the aortic valve with a mechanical valve or porcine bioprosthesis include: (1) simple interrupted, (2) interrupted vertical mattress, (3) interrupted mattress with pledgets, and (4) continuous. Our standard technique for use with the Starr-Edwards aortic prosthesis is interrupted vertical mattress. The porcine bioprosthesis is inserted with simple interrupted sutures.

Management of the Small Aortic Anulus
There are two main methods of managing a small aortic anulus: (1) if a moderate increase in anular diameter is required (2–6 mm), the aortic anulus can be divided at the base of the anterior leaflet of the mitral valve and patch reconstruction performed in conjunction with aortic valve replacement. (2) If a marked increase in anular diameter is desired, the aortic anulus can be divided through the right coronary cusp and into the muscular ventricular septum and right ventricular outflow tract, with patch repair of the ventricular and right ventricular outflow defects performed in conjunction with aortic valve replacement.

Anular enlargement through the anulus at the base of the mitral leaflet involves several variables: (1) location of the anular incision, (2) depth of the anular incision (whether there is extension onto the mitral leaflet and, if so, its depth), (3) whether incision is made into the left atrium, (4) level of valve ring placement, and others.[11,77,100,119,128] Our preferred methods are illlustrated in the technique section which follows.

A more radical method of anular enlargement may be required, especially in the child undergoing surgery for congenital aortic stenosis with hypoplastic anulus. A method that permits as much as doubling of the anular diameter has been described by Konno.[86] This procedure involves incising the aortic anulus through the right coronary cusp to the left of the right coronary orifice. The incision is carried into the ventricular septum and into the right ventricular outflow tract. A two-layered Dacron patch is then used to close the ventricular defect. The valve is then inserted and fixed to the patch. One layer of patch is sutured to the right ventricular outflow tract and the other layer is sutured to the aortotomy. This technique of aortoventriculoplasty is an effective and safe operation for a difficult anatomic problem.[123]

Management of Anular Erosion or Abscess
Destruction of tissue of the aortic root can present one of the most formidable challenges encountered by the cardiac surgeon. Such destruction usually occurs secondary to *Staph. aureus* endocarditis. The effect is similar to that of a mycotic aneurysm.[61] Erosion or abscess formation can occur into the ventricular septum under the right coronary cusp, between the left or noncoronary cusp and the mitral leaflet, as well as at the junction of the left atrial wall. Erosions can perforate into the right ventricle, right atrium, or pericardium.[27,33]

A number of methods have been described to deal with this serious problem. Closure of the erosions with Teflon strips for buttressing, with pulling together of the erosion as the valve is seated, has been recommended.[29,142,154]

Danielson and colleagues[46] have described implantation of an aortic valve prosthesis into the ascending aorta, anastomosis of saphenous vein grafts to the right and left coronary systems, with proximal anastomoses placed above the aortic valve, and closure of the coronary ostia. Frantz and co-workers[54] reported two patients with left ventricular-aortic discontinuity complicating bacterial endocarditis who underwent composite prosthetic valve–Dacron tube graft reconstruction of the aortic root. The prosthetic valve was sutured into the remaining aortic anulus, ventricular muscle, and base of the aortic leaflet of the mitral valve. The coronary arteries were sutured to openings in the side of the graft.

We have not encountered a case of anular erosion that appeared to require as extensive an operation as those described by Danielson or Frantz. Our usual technique has been either to take deep bites with large sutures through each lip of the erosions and then through the valve sewing ring, or to use Teflon strips to buttress the closure of the erosion and incorporate these sutures in the valve ring. Solid mooring of the sutures in this condition is essential: this may involve deep bites into the mitral valve or into the septum, and occasionally the conduction system must be sacrificed knowingly in order to accomplish a secure valve implantation. In the face of active infection and destruction of the aortic root, homograft conduit replacement can be effective treatment. If abscesses have been sterilized and have a good fibrotic margin, but primary closure of the opening would result in excessive tension, glutaraldehyde-treated autologous pericardial patches can be used to close the openings and a valve then placed in the usual subcoronary position.

Aortic Valve Repair for Regurgitation

Aortic valve repair has been described by Duran[48] and Cosgrove,[40] using anular and leaflet plasties, leaflet resection, and leaflet extension. Short-term results are satisfactory, but more follow-up will be necessary to determine the role of aortic valve repair over the long term. If the primary goal is to preserve left ventricular function over the short term, then this goal is already achievable with aortic valve repair.

Surgical Anatomy

The anatomy of the aortic valve is shown in Figures 13–3 and 13–4. Figure 13–3 shows the valve from above, with the orientation as usually seen through a standard transverse aortotomy.

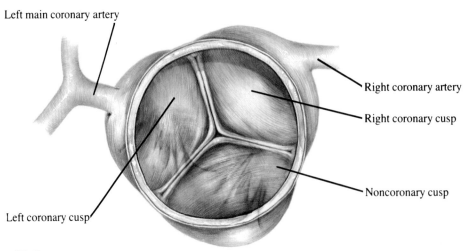

Left main coronary artery

Right coronary artery

Right coronary cusp

Noncoronary cusp

Left coronary cusp

13–3

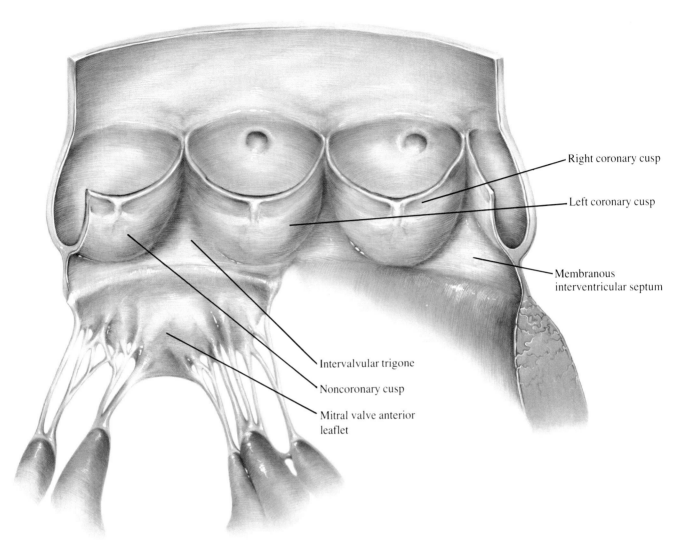

Right coronary cusp

Left coronary cusp

Membranous
interventricular septum

Intervalvular trigone

Noncoronary cusp

Mitral valve anterior
leaflet

13–4

Figure 13–4 is an opened-out view of the aortic valve to illustrate the sub-valvular anatomy. With the exception of the nomenclature of the cusps, the nomenclature is that of McAlpine.[105] Because the left ventricle has a common inlet and outlet, the anatomy of the aortic valve and mitral valve is intimately related.

Surgical Technique

A transverse aortotomy is made (Figs. 13–5, 13–6). The incision should be made approximately 15 mm above the level of the right coronary artery. The incision should not be too low, since this can jeopardize the right coronary artery and create technical difficulties in valve seating and aortotomy closure. Erring on the high side is of little consequence, since the aortotomy can quickly be angled downward, and the anterior ''lip'' created by a high incision can be easily retracted. The aortotomy should be extended to approximately 10 mm above the commissure between the left coronary cusp and right coronary cusp and to a similar distance above the commissure between the left coronary cusp and the noncoronary cusp. Cold cardioplegic solution is injected into the coronary ostia via hand-held cannulas.

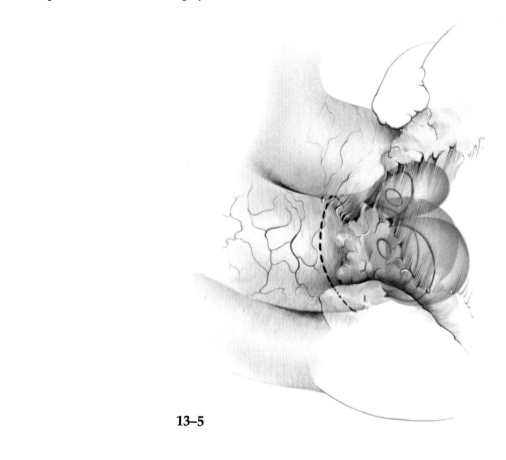

13–5

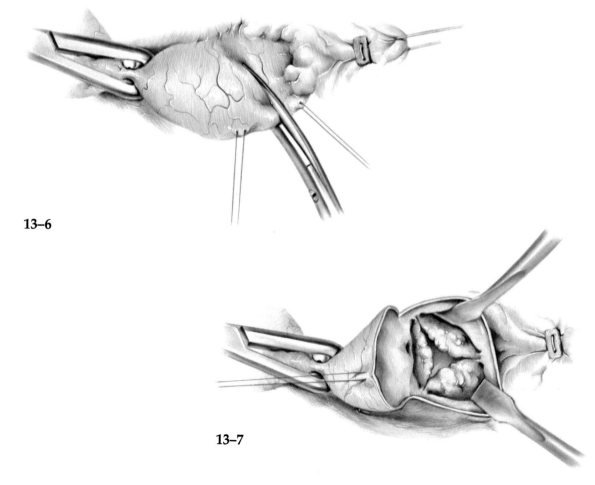

13–6

13–7

Retractors are placed, the valve is exposed (Fig. 13–7), and a strategy for excision is determined. The goal of excision is to establish a bed as free of calcium as is consistent with avoidance of injury to the aortic wall and the bundle of His. Many heavily calcified valves have calcification that stops prior to the anulus, leaving a thin zone of noncalcified attachment. In these instances, advantage may be taken of this morphologic feature by starting the incision with a scalpel in the calcium-free area near the anulus. This incision increases leaflet mobility, allowing more light under the leaflet, and more clearly indicates the area of subsequent incision. The incision can be completed with scissors.

If the valve does not contain a clear zone for incision, excision can be started with heavy scissors (Fig. 13–8). Incision is *not* made close to the anulus, since such heavy calcification can obscure landmarks and a portion of the anulus can be inadvertently excised.

Debridement of the calcium is then performed with rongeurs (Fig. 13–9).

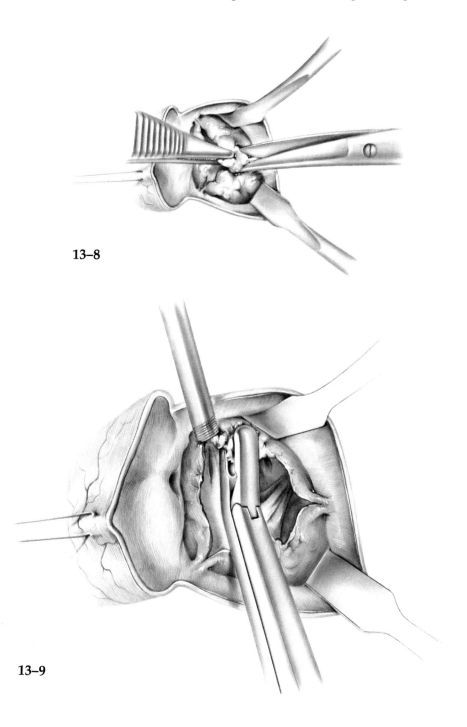

13–8

13–9

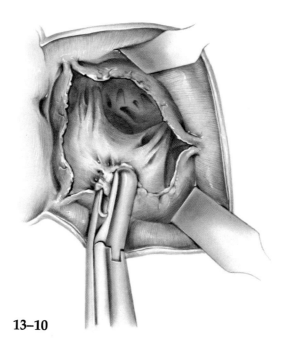

13–10

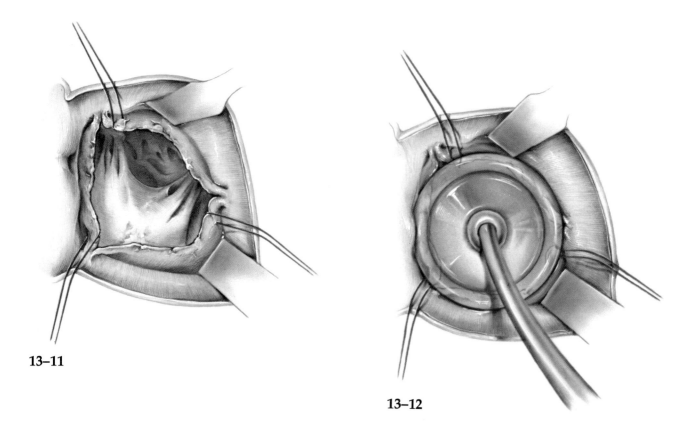

13–11

13–12

The top is removed from the wall sucker to provide a vacuuming instrument to suction small fragments of calcium if they break off. The calcium can be crushed with the rongeur and then teased or peeled away from the anulus. Again, it is important to proceed cautiously to prevent removal of any of the anulus.

Calcification will sometimes extend down onto the base of the anterior leaflet of the mitral valve. A plane can usually be located between the calcium

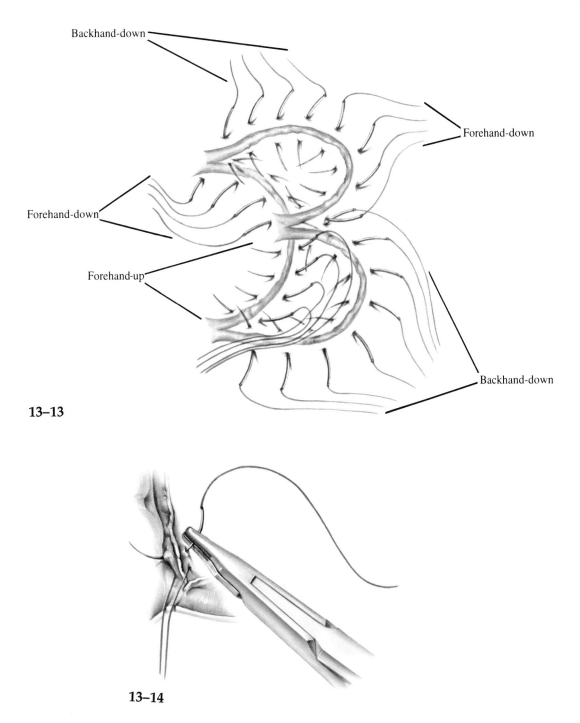

Backhand-down

Forehand-down

Forehand-down

Forehand-up

Backhand-down

13–13

13–14

and the leaflet, and the calcium is peeled off (Fig. 13–10). The debrided anulus is flexible, accepts sutures easily, and coapts to the valve ring tightly and completely.

Sutures of 2–0 Teflon-coated Dacron are placed near each commissure for retraction (Fig. 13–11). These sutures will also be prosthesis sutures. They may be placed during debridement as needed for retraction and exposure.

The anulus is then sized (Fig. 13–12). Progressively larger sizers are used. The proper fit for a Starr-Edwards valve is shown in Figure 13–12. Trying to "stuff in" a valve that is too large can cause disaster, such as coronary ostial impingement or tearing of the anulus.

The standard sutures for aortic valve replacement are shown in Figure 13–13. The sutures are started on the left coronary cusp near the commissure with the noncoronary cusp, with forehand-up sutures (Fig. 13–14). The su-

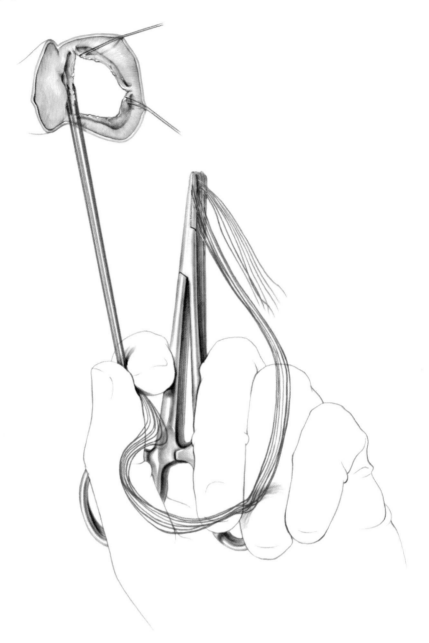

13–15

tures may then be placed directly in the valve sewing ring or they may be clamped and held (Fig. 13–15) for later placement in the valve. Retraction of the sutures toward the patient's right facilitates exposure of the cusp.

As the left coronary cusp reaches its nadir and begins to come up to the commissure with the right coronary cusp, the easiest suture is usually a forehand-down (Fig. 13–16), either with the elbow in tight toward the body or with the elbow across the table.

The beginning sutures in the right coronary cusp are backhand-down with the elbow out (Fig. 13–17). As the cusp rises from its deepest point, forehand sutures are taken (Fig. 13–18).

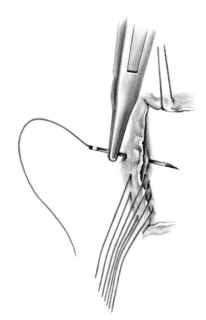

13–16

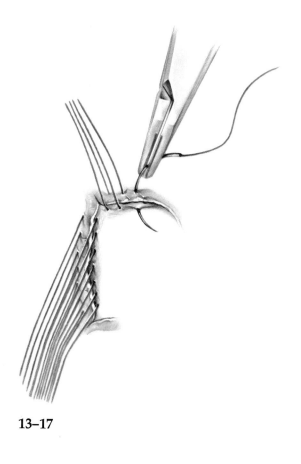

13–17

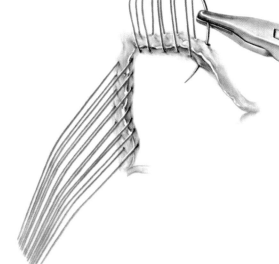

13–18

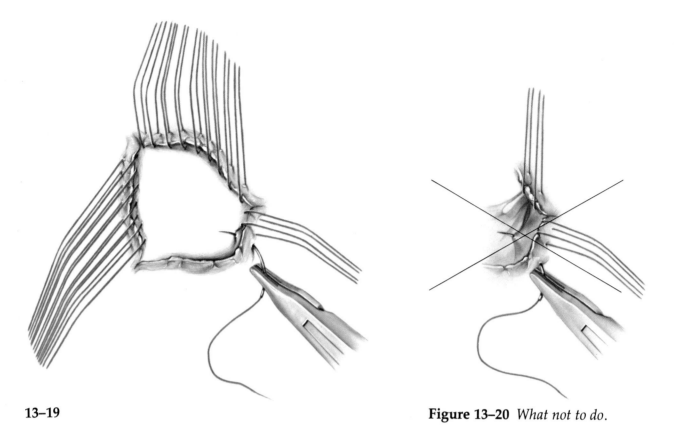

13–19

Figure 13–20 *What not to do.*

The noncoronary cusp is sutured backhand-down (Fig. 13–19). Underneath the commissure with the right coronary cusp is the membranous septum. A deep suture in this area *should not* be taken (Fig. 13–20), since such a suture can injure the conduction system. Retraction of the noncoronary cusp sutures toward the patient's right groin facilitates exposure.

Sutures are placed in the sewing ring in a vertical mattress fashion, with the suture coming out the ventricular side taking a broad bite through the sewing ring, and the suture on the aortic side taking a smaller bite in the lip (Fig. 13–21). This technique pulls the anulus into the compressible ring as the sutures are tied, for good sewing ring-anulus coaptation. The sutures are tied with slight compression of the sewing ring (Fig. 13–22).

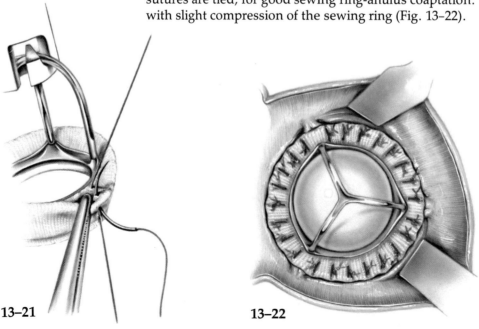

13–21   **13–22**

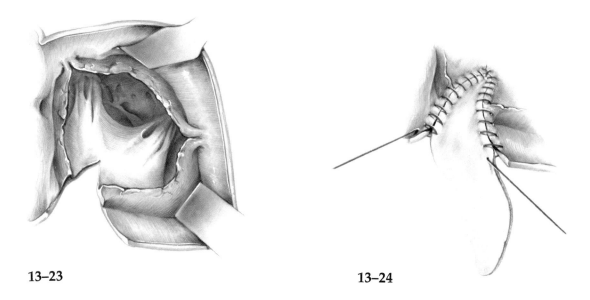

13–23

13–24

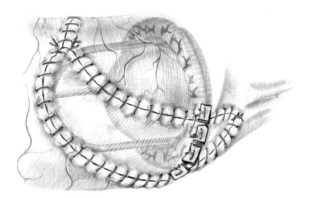

13–25

Anular Enlargement

The aortotomy is extended through the commissure between the left coronary cusp and the noncoronary cusp, onto the mitral valve for 10–15 mm (Fig. 13-23). The left atrium is not usually entered. A woven Dacron graft is then sewn to the mitral leaflet, across the incised anulus, and up onto the aortotomy (Fig. 13-24). The valve is placed at the normal anular level. At the area of the patch, horizontal mattress sutures are taken through the valve ring, brought through the patch, and tied over Teflon pledgets. The patch is carried up and incorporated in the aortotomy closure (Fig. 13-25).

Implantation of a Cryopreserved Homograft

The aortic homograft is implanted at St. Vincent/Portland using the interrupted and running technique of Ross[131] and at Sutter/Sacramento using the entirely running technique of Barratt-Boyes,[8] which will be shown here. When the use of a homograft is planned, the aortotomy is kept higher on the side of the pulmonary artery, well above the commissure between the right coronary cusp and the left coronary cusp, and is carried down into the noncoronary sinus. This provides both adequate exposure and room to accommodate the commissural posts of the homograft.

A cryopreserved aortic homograft is chosen which is 2 mm smaller in diameter than the measured diameter of the recipient anulus, and the homograft

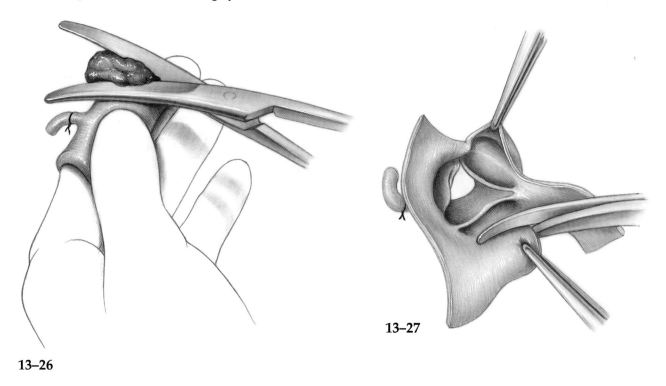

13–26

13–27

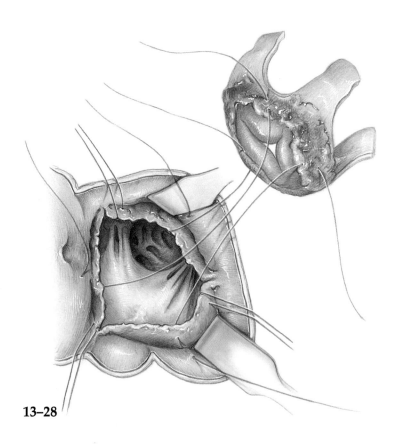

13–28

is thawed. The excess muscle below the right coronary cusp is carefully trimmed (Fig. 13–26). The sinuses are removed, leaving a rim of aortic wall above the leaflets (Fig. 13–27). Three sutures of 4–0 polypropylene are placed through the homograft and the recipient anulus (Fig. 13–28). The right coronary cusp of the homograft is oriented to the left coronary cusp anulus of the

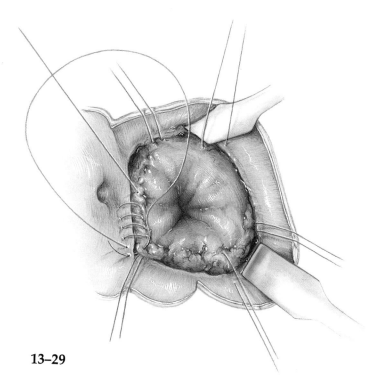

13–29

recipient so the muscular ridge of the homograft is least likely to cause any obstruction. The homograft is then lowered into the recipient's anulus and the homograft is inverted into the ventricle (Fig. 13–29).

The polypropylene sutures are then run toward each commissure and tied. The suture line is kept at or slightly below the recipient's anulus, with special care to avoid the conduction tissue under the commissure between the right coronary cusp and noncoronary cusp. The homograft is then everted and 4–0 polypropylene sutures begin at the low points of the sinuses and are brought up to the commissures (Fig. 13–30). The commissural posts can be buttressed with horizontal pledgetted mattress sutures.

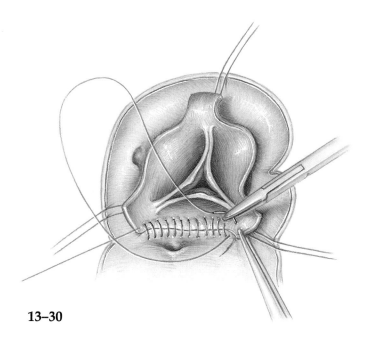

13–30

Results

Operative Mortality

Isolated aortic valve replacement can be performed with an operative mortality of 0%–2%.[1,62,141] Similarly excellent results can be achieved with combined valve replacement and coronary artery bypass.[127] Valve replacement earlier in the course of disease and improving techniques of myocardial protection are both likely to continue to lower the overall risk of aortic valve replacement.[98]

Ventricular Function

Aortic stenosis: Successful, uncomplicated valve replacement results in maintenance of ejection fraction that is normal preoperatively.[84,116,117,150] In addition, left ventricular mass decreases[108] and mean velocity of fiber shortening increases.[116] Marked reversal of impaired left ventricular function usually occurs.[32,43,144] Smith and co-workers[144] reported 10 patients with an increase of mean ejection fraction from 34% to 63%. Croke and colleagues[43] reported 7 patients with an increase in average ejection fraction from 13% to 45%. Ejection fractions improve in all patients in congestive heart failure if there is no perioperative myocardial infarction.[144]

The reversibility of impaired ventricular function may occur because the impaired cardiac performance preoperatively is due to inappropriately high wall stress—"afterload mismatch"—rather than depressed contractility.[30,66,132] Contractile function, as characterized by the isovolumic rate of stress development, is not necessarily impaired in chronic pressure-overload hypertrophy. The rate of stress development was nearly identical in patients with aortic stenosis and in normal subjects. Gunther and co-workers[66] have shown that left ventricular wall thickness and geometry are closely correlated with ventricular performance in patients with pressure-overload hypertrophy due to aortic stenosis. They suggest that poor cardiac performance may often be due to hypertrophy (or inappropriate geometry) rather than to depression of myocardial contractility.

Aortic regurgitation: As in aortic stenosis, ejection fraction that is normal preoperatively remains normal.[84,116,150] Unfortunately, impaired ventricular function does not always improve. Clark and colleagues[34] reported a series of patients with an average preoperative left ventricular ejection fraction of 0.43. Left ventricular systolic pump function improved in only 50% of patients. Regardless of preoperative systolic pump function, successful valve replacement usually results in decreases in left ventricular mass, diastolic and systolic volumes, and end-diastolic pressure.[34,108,116]

Late Survival

The major determinant of late survival after aortic valve replacement is preoperative left ventricular function.[14,17,68,71,138] Large series of patients, with varied valvular pathology and types of prosthesis, have shown 5-year survival (excluding operative death) of approximately 75%–85%, and this survival is for ball valves, tilting disc valves, bileaflet valves, and porcine heterografts.[44,99,115,146] The majority of late deaths are not caused by prosthesis-related complications, but by myocardial factors—emphasizing again that the most critical factor relating to the success of valvular surgery is the functional and structural status of the myocardium preoperatively. Greves and colleagues,[62] from the University of Oregon reported early and late survival for patients undergoing aortic valve replacement for severe, isolated aortic regurgitation from 1973 to 1978. In patients with ejection fractions over 0.50, there were no operative deaths and no late deaths at an average follow-up of 5 years.

Prosthesis Hemodynamics

The three most commonly used mechanical valves in the United States in 1993 were the Starr-Edwards Silastic ball valve, the St. Jude bileaflet valve, and the Medtronic-Hall tilting disc valve. None of the models of the Bjork-

Shiley valve were available in the United States. The Starr-Edwards, St. Jude, and Medtronic-Hall mechanical valves and the porcine bioprostheses have similar hemodynamics in the commonly used sizes (23–25 mm). There is usually a small resting transvalvular gradient of 10–20 mm Hg, which increases to 20–30 mm Hg with exercise.[25,26,77] The St. Jude valve has superior hemodynamic performance in the smaller sizes.[45]

Prosthesis-Related Complications

Thromboembolism: The rate of thromboembolism for the Starr-Edwards, St. Jude, and Medronic-Hall aortic valves is approximately 2%/patient-year in patients maintained on continuous anticoagulation.[3,65] The rate of thromboembolism for the Carpentier-Edwards and Hancock porcine bioprostheses is approximately 1%/patient-year in patients on no anticoagulation.[65] Approximately half of the thromboembolic episodes are minor—there is no residual neurologic deficit or peripheral or coronary embolic complications. Thromboembolism is extremely rare with the cryopreserved homograft, with 97% of patients remaining free of thromboembolism at 10 years.[114]

Anticoagulant-related morbidity and mortality: Patients on continuous anticoagulation have a constant and continuing risk of hemorrhagic complications. The probability of a major hemorrhage is approximately 1.5%/patient-year, and the risk of minor bleeding is about the same.[74] The risk of fatal hemorrhage is approximately 0.1%/patient-year in our experience.

Structural failure: Structural failure is almost nonexistent with the Starr-Edwards, St. Jude, and Medtronic-Hall mechanical valves. The freedom from structural failure of porcine valves is approximately 85% at 10 years, and structural failure is extremely rare in patients receiving a porcine valve when 70 years of age or older.[65,76] O'Brien and colleagues[114] reported that 92% of their patients receiving cryopreserved homografts were free of reoperation at 10 years, with no patients requiring reoperation because of valve degeneration.

Surgical Relief of Other Forms of Left Ventricular Outflow Obstruction

Supravalvular Stenosis

Supravalvular aortic stenosis is a rare condition. The most common anatomy is narrowing just above the commissures.[124] Surgical treatment has consisted of patch enlargement into the noncoronary sinus.[107,124,145] Our preferred technique is patch enlargement by incision into the right and noncoronary sinuses and use of a pantaloon patch as described by Doty.[47] Brom[28] has described a technique of transecting the aorta above the area of stenosis and making incisions down into all three sinuses. Each sinus is patched with a separate patch and then anastomosed to the distal aorta. Myers and colleagues[111] have described a modification of Brom's technique in which the use of prosthetic material is avoided by incising the distal aorta in three places and advancing these flaps into the incisions in the sinuses. In the case of diffuse narrowing of the ascending aorta, a left ventricle-to-aorta conduit can be performed,[38] or a radical aortic root enlargement extending into the aortic arch.

Subaortic Membrane

Membranous subvalvular aortic stenosis is usually caused by a discrete membrane immediately beneath and unattached to the aortic valve.[80,82,112] It is usually circumferential and has continuity with the anterior leaflet of the mitral valve. Membranous subvalvular aortic stenosis is a progressive disease.[91]

Surgical excision is straightforward, provided the bases of the aortic leaflets are not attached to the membranous ring. The aortic valve cusps are retracted and the membrane grasped and retracted posteriorly. The initial incision is made anteriorly under the right coronary cusp with a sharp-pointed blade. The incision is carried clockwise with careful assessment of the contiguous structures. Particular care is necessary near the bundle of His and the anterior leaflet of the mitral valve. The membrane can frequently be excised in one piece. In some cases, after the initial incision is made, blunt dissection with traction can remove the rest of the ring. A myectomy is frequently added to membrane resection.

Recurrence of stenosis is a problem following surgical treatment, with recurrence rates 4 years after surgery ranging from 15% to 25%.[56,147]

Idiopathic Hypertrophic Subaortic Stenosis

Idiopathic hypertrophic subaortic stenosis (IHSS) presents a broad spectrum of anatomy, physiology, and clinical course.[24,70,102] The treatment of IHSS is primarily medical.[52] Patients with large resting or provoked gradients are candidates for surgical therapy.[109]

Several operations have been proposed for treatment of IHSS, including (1) left ventriculomyotomy and myectomy through the aortic valve,[109,149] (2) myectomy with a combined approach through the aorta and left ventricle,[2] (3) septal myectomy via right ventriculotomy,[36] and (4) mitral valve replacement.[37] Our surgical procedure of choice is transaortic myectomy as described by Morrow.[109] Intraoperative transesophageal echocardiography can be helpful in planning the extent of the resection, assessing the immediate result, and excluding important complications.[63] This operation results in long-lasting clinical improvement in most patients.[103]

References

1. Adams PX, Cunningham JN, Trehan NK, Brazier JR, Reed GE, Spencer FC: Clinical experience using potassium-induced cardioplegia with hypothermia in aortic valve replacement. J Thorac Cardiovasc Surg 75:564,1978.
2. Agnew TM, Barratt-Boyes BG, Brandt PWT, Roche AHG, Lowe JB, O'Brien KP: Surgical resection in idiopathic hypertrophic subaortic stenosis with a combined approach through aorta and left ventricle. J Thorac Cardiovasc Surg 74:307,1977.
3. Akins CW: Mechanical cardiac valvular prostheses. Ann Thorac Surg 52:161,1991.
4. Anderson RP, Bonchek LI, Wood JA, Chapman RP, Starr A: The safety of combined aortic valve replacement and coronary bypass grafting. Ann Thorac Surg 15:249,1973.
5. Azariades M, Fessler C, Ahmad A, Starr A: Aortic valve replacement in patients over eighty years of age: a comparative standard for balloon valvoplasty. Eur J Cardiothorac Surg 5:373,1991.
6. Barnhorst DA, Oxman HA, Connolly DC, Pluth JR, Danielson GK, Wallace RB, McGoon DC: Long-term follow-up of isolated replacement of the aortic or mitral valve with the Starr-Edwards prosthesis. Am J Cardiol 35:228,1975.
7. Barratt-Boyes BG: Homograft aortic valve replacement in aortic incompetence and stenosis. Thorax 19:131,1964.
8. Barratt-Boyes BG: A method for preparing and inserting a homograft aortic valve. Br J Surg 52:847,1965.
9. Barratt-Boyes BG, Roche AHG, Subramanyan R, Pemberton JR, Whitlock RML: Long-term follow-up of patients with the antibiotic-sterilized aortic homograft valve inserted freehand in the aortic position. Circulation 75:768,1987.
10. Bernhard WF, Keane JF, Fellows KE, Litwin SB, Gross RE: Progress and problems in the surgical management of congenital aortic stenosis. J Thorac Cardiovasc Surg 66:404,1973.
11. Blank RH, Pupello DF, Bessone LN, Harrison EE, Sbar S: Method of managing the small aortic annulus during valve replacement. Ann Thorac Surg 22:356,1976.
12. Bolen JL, Holloway EL, Zener JC, Harrison DC, Alderman EL: Evaluation of left

ventricular function in patients with aortic regurgitation using afterload stress. Circulation 53:132,1976.

13. Bonchek LI, Anderson RP, Rosch J: Should coronary arteriography be performed routinely before valve replacement? Am J Cardiol 31:462,1973.

14. Bonchek LI, Starr A: Ball valve prostheses: current appraisal of late results. Am J Cardiol 35:843,1975.

15. Bonow RO, Epstein SE: Is preoperative left ventricular function predictive of survival and functional results after aortic valve replacement for chronic aortic regurgitation? J Am Coll Cardiol 10:713,1987.

16. Bonow RO, Henry WL, Kent KM, Ware JW, Glancy DL, Redwood DR, Itscoitz SB, McIntosh CL, Conkle DM, Morrow AG, Epstein SE: Predictors of late death due to congestive heart failure following operation for aortic regurgitation (abstr). Am J Cardiol 41:382,1978.

17. Bonow RO, Picone AL, McIntosh CL, Jones M, Rosing DR, Maron BJ, Lakatos E, Clark RE, Epstein SE: Survival and functional results after valve replacement for aortic regurgitation from 1976 to 1983: impact of preoperative left ventricular function. Circulation 72:1244,1985.

18. Bonow RO, Rosing DR, Maron BJ, McIntosh CL, Jones M, Bacharach SL, Green MV, Clark RE, Epstein SE: Reversal of left ventricular dysfunction after aortic valve replacement for chronic aortic regurgitation: influence of duration of preoperative left ventricular dysfunction. Circulation 70:570,1984.

19. Bonow RO, Rosing DR, McIntosh CL, Jones M, Maron BJ, Lan KKG, Lakatos E, Bacharach SL, Green MV, Epstein SE: The natural history of asymptomatic patients with aortic regurgitation and normal left ventricular function. Circulation 68:509,1983.

20. Borer JS, Bacharach SL, Green MV, Kent KM, Henry WL, Rosing DR, Seides SF, Johnston GS, Epstein SE: Exercise-induced left ventricular dysfunction in symptomatic and asymptomatic patients with aortic regurgitation: assessment with radionuclide cineangiography. Am J Cardiol 42:351,1978.

21. Borer JS, Rosing DR, Kent KM, Bacharach SL, Green MV, McIntosh CJ, Morrow AG, Epstein SE: Exercise-induced left ventricular dysfunction in symptomatic and asymptomatic patients with aortic regurgitation: assessment with radionuclide cineangiography. Am J Cardiol 42:351,1978.

22. Borow KM: Surgical outcome in chronic aortic regurgitation: a physiologic framework for assessing preoperative predictors (editorial). J Am Coll Cardiol 10:1165,1987.

23. Boyd AD, Spencer FC, Isom W, Cunningham JN, Reed GE, Acinapura AJ, Tice DA: Infective endocarditis: an analysis of 54 surgically treated patients. J Thorac Cardiovasc Surg 73:23,1977.

24. Braunwald E, Lambrew CT, Rockoff SD, Ross J Jr, Morrow AG: Idiopathic hypertrophic subaortic stenosis: I. A description of the disease based upon an analysis of 64 patients. Circulation 30:3,1964.

25. Bristow JD, Kremkau EL: Hemodynamic changes after valve replacement with Starr-Edwards prostheses. Am J Cardiol 35:716,1975.

26. Bristow JD, McCord CW, Starr A, Ritzmann LW, Griswold HE: Clinical and hemodynamic results of aortic valvular replacement with a ball valve prosthesis. Circulation 29:36,1964.

27. Bristow JD, Parker BM, Huag WA: Hemopericardium following rupture of a bacterial aortic sinus aneurysm. Am J Cardiol 6:355,1960.

28. Brom AG: Obstruction to the left ventricular outflow tract. In Khonsari S: Cardiac Surgery: Safeguards and Pitfalls in Operative Technique. Rockville, Md, Aspen, 1988, p 276.

29. Buckley MJ, Mundth ED, Daggett WM, Austen WG: Surgical management of the complications of sepsis involving the aortic valve, aortic root, and ascending aorta. Ann Thorac Surg 12:391,1971.

30. Carabello BA: The changing unnatural history of valvular regurgitation. Ann Thorac Surg 53:191,1992.

31. Carabello BA, Green LH, Grossman W, Cohn LH, Koster JK, Collins JJ: Hemodynamic determinants of prognosis of aortic valve replacement in critical aortic stenosis and advanced congestive heart failure. Circulation 62:42,1980.

32. Carabello BA, Usher BW, Hendrix GH, Assey ME, Crawford FA, Leman RG: Predictors of outcome for aortic valve replacement in patients with aortic regurgi-

tation and left ventricular dysfunction: a change in the measuring stick. J Am Coll Cardiol 10:991,1987.

33. Chesler E, Korns ME, Porter GE, Reyes CN, Edwards JE: False aneurysm of the left ventricle secondary to bacterial endocarditis with perforation of the mitral-aortic intervalvular fibrosa. Circulation 37:518,1968.

34. Clark DG, McAnulty JH, Rahimtoola SH: Valve replacement in aortic insufficiency with left ventricular dysfunction. Circulation 61:411,1980.

35. Conkle DM, Jones M, Morrow AG: Treatment of congenital aortic stenosis. Arch Surg 107:649,1973.

36. Cooley DA, Bloodwell RD, Hallman GL, LaSorte AF, Leachman RD, Chapman DW: Surgical treatment of muscular subaortic stenosis: results from septectomy in twenty-six patients. Circulation 35,36(Suppl I):I-124,1967.

37. Cooley DA, Leachman RD, Hallman GL, Gerami S, Hall RJ: Idiopathic hypertrophic subaortic stenosis: surgical treatment including mitral valve replacement. Arch Surg 103:606,1971.

38. Cooley DA, Norman JC, Mullins CE, Grace RR: Left ventricle to abdominal aorta conduits for relief of aortic stenosis. Cardiovasc Dis, Bull Texas Heart Inst 2:376,1975.

39. Copeland JG, Griepp RB, Stinson EB, Shumway NE: Long-term follow-up after isolated aortic valve replacement. J Thorac Cardiovasc Surg 74:875,1977.

40. Cosgrove DM, Rosenkranz ER, Hendren WG, Bartlett JC, Stewart WJ: Valvuloplasty for aortic insufficiency. J Thorac Cardiovasc Surg 102:571,1991.

41. Cribier A, Saoudi N, Berland J, Savin T, Rocha P, Letac B: Percutaneous transluminal valvuloplasty of acquired aortic stenosis in elderly patients: an alternative to valve replacement? Lancet 1:63,1986.

42. Cribier A, Savin T, Berland J, Rocha P, Mechmeche R, Saoudi N, Behar P, Letac B: Percutaneous transluminal balloon valvuloplasty of adult aortic stenosis: report of 92 cases. J Am Coll Cardiol 9:381,1987.

43. Croke RP, Pifarre R, Sullivan H, Gunnar R, Loeb H: Reversal of advanced left ventricular dysfunction following aortic valve replacement for aortic stenosis. Ann Thorac Surg 24:38,1977.

44. Czer LSC, Chaux A, Matloff JM, DeRobertis MA, Nessim SA, Scarlata D, Knan SS, Kass RM, Tsai RP, Blanche C, Gray RJ: Ten-year experience with the St. Jude medical valve for primary valve replacement. J Thorac Cardiovasc Surg 100:44,1990.

45. Czer LSC, Matloff J, Chaux A, DeRobertis M, Yoganathan A, Gray RJ: A 6 year experience with the St. Jude medical valve: hemodynamic performance, surgical results, biocompatibility and follow-up. J Am Coll Cardiol 6:904,1985.

46. Danielson GK, Titus JL, DuShane JW: Successful treatment of aortic valve endocarditis and aortic root abscesses by insertion of prosthetic valve in ascending aorta and placement of bypass grafts to coronary arteries. J Thorac Cardiovasc Surg 67:443,1974.

47. Doty DB, Polanky DB, Jenson CB: Supravalvular aortic stenosis. Repair by extended aortoplasty. J Thorac Cardiovasc Surg 74:362,1971.

48. Duran C, Kumar N, Gometza B, Al Halees Z: Indications and limitations of aortic valve reconstruction. Ann Thorac Surg 52:447,1991.

49. Edmunds LH Jr, Wagner HR, Heymann MA: Aortic valvulotomy in neonates. Circulation 61:421,1980.

50. Elkins RC, Santangelo K, Stelzer P, Randolph JD, Knott-Craig CJ: Pulmonary autograft replacement of the aortic valve: an evolution of technique. J Card Surg 7:108,1992.

51. Fischl SJ, Gorlin R, Herman MV: Cardiac shape and function in aortic valve disease: physiologic and clinical implications. Am J Cardiol 39:170,1977.

52. Frank MJ, Abdulla AM, Canedo MI, Saylors RE: Long-term medical management of hypertrophic obstructive cardiomyopathy. Am J Cardiol 42:993,1978.

53. Frank S, Johnson A, Ross J Jr: Natural history of aortic stenosis. Br Heart J 35:41,1973.

54. Frantz PT, Murray GF, Wilcox BR: Surgical management of left ventricular-aortic discontinuity complicating bacterial endocarditis. Ann Thorac Surg 29:1,1980.

55. Friedman WF, Pappelbaum SJ: Indications for hemodynamic evaluation and surgery in congenital aortic stenosis. Pediatr Clin North Am 18:1207,1971.

56. Frommelt MA, Snider AR, Bove EL, Lupinetti FM: Echocardiographic assess-

ment of subvalvular aortic stenosis before and after operation. J Am Coll Cardiol 19:1018,1992.

57. Gault JH, Covell JW, Braunwald E, Ross J: Left ventricular performance following correction of free aortic regurgitation. Circulation 42:773,1970.

58. Gerosa G, McKay R, Davies J, Ross DN: Comparison of the aortic homograft and the pulmonary autograft for aortic valve or root replacement in children. J Thorac Cardiovasc Surg 102:51,1991.

59. Gerosa G, McKay R, Ross DN: Replacement of the aortic valve or root with a pulmonary autograft in children. Ann Thorac Surg 51:424,1991.

60. Goldschlager N, Pfeifer J, Cohn K, Popper R, Selzer A: The natural history of aortic regurgitation. A clinical and hemodynamic study. Am J Med 54:577,1973.

61. Gonzalez-Lavin L, Scappatura E, Lise M, Ross ND: Mycotic aneurysms of the aortic root: a complication of aortic valve endocarditis. Ann Thorac Surg 9: 551,1970.

62. Greves J, Clark D, Greenberg B, McAnulty J, Starr A, Rahimtoola S: Late survival after valve replacement for severe isolated aortic incompetence (abstr). Am J Cardiol 45:440,1980.

63. Grigg LE, Wigle ED, Williams WG, Daniel LB, Rakowski H: Transesophageal doppler echocardiography in obstructive hypertrophic cardiomyopathy: clarification of pathophysiology and importance in intraoperative decision making. J Am Coll Cardiol 20:42,1992.

64. Grossman W, Jones D, McLaurin LP: Wall stress and patterns of hypertrophy in the human left ventricle. J Clin Invest 56:56,1975.

65. Grunkemeier GL, Starr A, Rahimtoola SH: Prosthetic heart valve performance: long-term follow-up. Curr Probl Cardiol 17:333,1992.

66. Gunther S, Grossman W: Determinants of ventricular function in pressure-overload hypertrophy in man. Circulation 59:679,1979.

67. Henry WL, Bonow RO, Borer JS, Kent KM, Ware JH, Redwood DR, Itscoitz SB, McIntosh CL, Morrow AG, Epstein SE: Evaluation of aortic valve replacement in patients with valvular aortic stenosis. Circulation 61:814,1980.

68. Henry WL, Bonow RO, Borer JS, Ware JH, Kent KM, Redwood DR, McIntosh CL, Morrow AG, Epstein SE: Observations on the optimum time for operative intervention for aortic regurgitation: I. Evaluation of the results of aortic valve replacement in symptomatic patients. Circulation 61:471,1980.

69. Henry WL, Bonow RO, Rosing DR, Epstein SE: Observations on the optimum time for operative intervention for aortic regurgitation: II. Serial echocardiographic evaluation of asymptomatic patients. Circulation 61:484,1980.

70. Henry WL, Clark CE, Epstein SE: Asymmetric septal hypertrophy (ASH): the unifying link in the IHSS disease spectrum. Circulation 47:827,1973.

71. Hirshfield JW, Epstein SE, Roberts AJ, Glancy DL, Morrow AG: Indices predicting long-term survival after valve replacement in patients with aortic regurgitation and patients with aortic stenosis. Circulation 50:1190,1974.

72. Hopkins RA: Cardiac Reconstructions with Allograft Valves. New York, Springer-Verlag, 1989.

73. Horstkotte D, Loogen F: The natural history of aortic valve stenosis. Eur Heart J 9(Suppl E):57,1988.

74. Isom OW, Spencer FC, Glassman E, Teiko P, Boyd AD, Cunningham JN: Long-term results in 1,375 patients undergoing valve replacement with the Starr-Edwards cloth-covered composite-seat prostheses: a six-year appraisal. Ann Surg 186:310,1977.

75. Jack WD II, Kelly DT: Long-term follow-up of valvulotomy for congenital aortic stenosis. Am J Cardiol 38:231,1976.

76. Jamieson WRE, Burr LH, Munro AI, Miyagishima RT, Gerein AN: Cardiac valve replacement in the elderly: clinical performance of biological prostheses. Ann Thorac Surg 48:173,1989.

77. Jones EL, Craver JM, Morris DC, King SB III, Douglas JS Jr, Franch RH, Hatcher CR Jr, Morgan EA: Hemodynamic and clinical evaluation of the Hancock xenograft bioprosthesis for aortic valve replacement (with emphasis on management of the small aortic root). J Thorac Cardiovasc Surg 75:300,1978.

78. Karl TR, Sano S, Brawn WJ, Mee RBB: Critical aortic stenosis in the first month of life: surgical results in 26 infants. Ann Thorac Surg 50:105,1990.

79. Kasten-Sportes CH, Piechaud JF, Sidi D, Kachner J: Percutaneous balloon valvu-

loplasty in neonates with critical aortic stenosis. J Am Coll Cardiol 13:1101,1989.

80. Katz NM, Buckley MJ, Liberthson RR: Discrete membranous subaortic stenosis. Circulation 56:1034,1977.

81. Keane JF, Driscoll DJ, Gersony WM, Hayes CJ, Kidd L, O'Fallon M, Pieroni DR, Wolfe RR, Weidman WH: Second natural history study of congenital heart defects: results of treatment of patients with aortic valvar stenosis. Circulation 87(Suppl I):I-16,1993.

82. Kelly DT, Wulfsberg E, Rowe RD: Discrete subaortic stenosis. Circulation 46: 309,1972.

83. Kelly TA, Rothbart RM, Cooper M, Kaiser DL, Smucker ML, Gibson RS: Comparison of outcome of asymptomatic to symptomatic patients older than 20 years of age with valvular aortic stenosis. Am J Cardiol 61:123,1988.

84. Kennedy JW, Doces J, Stewart DK: Left ventricular function before and following aortic valve replacement. Circulation 56:944,1977.

85. Kennedy KD, Nishimura RA, Holmes DR Jr, Bailey KR: Natural history of moderate aortic stenosis. J Am Coll Cardiol 17:313,1991.

86. Konno S, Imai Y, Iida Y, Nakajima M, Tatsuno K: A new method for prosthetic valve replacement in congenital aortic stenosis associated with hypoplasia of the aortic ring. J Thorac Cardiovasc Surg 70:910,1975.

87. Lababidi Z, Wu J-R, Walls JT: Percutaneous balloon aortic valvuloplasty: results in 23 patients. Am J Cardiol 53:194,1984.

88. Lakier JB, Khaja F, Magilligan DJ Jr, Goldstein S: Porcine xenograft valves: long-term (60–89 month) follow-up. Circulation 62:313,1980.

89. Lakier JB, Lewis AB, Heymann MA, Stanger P, Hoffman JIE, Rudolph AM: Isolated aortic stenosis in the neonate. Natural history and hemodynamic considerations. Circulation 50:801,1974.

90. Lawson RM, Bonchek LI, Menashe V, Starr A: Late results of surgery for left ventricular outflow tract obstruction in children. J Thorac Cardiovasc Surg 71: 334,1976.

91. Leichter DA, Sullivan I, Gersony WM: "Acquired" discrete subvalvular aortic stenosis: natural history and hemodynamics. J Am Coll Cardiol 14:1539,1989.

92. Letac B, Cribier A, Koning R, Lefebvre E: Aortic stenosis in elderly patients aged 80 or older: treatment by percutaneous balloon valvuloplasty in a series of 92 cases. Circulation 80:1514,1989.

93. Leung MP, McKay R, Smith A, Anderson RH, Arnold R: Critical aortic stenosis in early infancy: anatomic and echocardiographic substrates of successful open valvotomy. J Thorac Cardiovasc Surg 101:526,1991.

94. Levinson JR, Akins CW, Buckley MJ, Newell JB, Palacios IF, Block PC, Fifer MA: Octogenarians with aortic stenosis: outcome after aortic valve replacement. Circulation 80(Suppl I):I-49,1989.

95. Linhart JW, Wheat MW: Myocardial dysfunction following aortic valve replacement: the significance of coronary artery disease. J Thorac Cardiovasc Surg 54: 259,1967.

96. Louagie Y, Noirhomme P, Aranguis E, Eucher P, Vanruyssevelt P, Buche M, Dion R, Jaumin P, Schoevaerdts JC: Use of the Carpentier-Edwards porcine bioprosthesis: assessment of a patient selection policy. J Thorac Cardiovasc Surg 104:1013,1992.

97. Lund O, Nielsen TT, Pilegaard HK, Magnussen K, Knudsen MA: The influence of coronary artery disease and bypass grafting of early and late survival after valve replacement for aortic stenosis. J Thorac Cardiovasc Surg 100:327,1990.

98. Lytle BW, Cosgrove DM, Taylor PC, Goormastic M, Stewart RW, Golding LAR, Gill CC, Loop FD: Primary isolated aortic valve replacement: early and late results. J Thorac Cardiovasc Surg 97:675,1989.

99. Macmanus Q, Grunkemeier G, Lambert LE, Teply JF, Harlan BJ, Starr A: Year of operation as a risk factor in the late results of valve replacement. J Thorac Cardiovasc Surg 80:834,1980.

100. Manouguian S, Seybold-Epting W: Patch enlargement of the aortic valve ring by extending the aortic incision into the anterior mitral leaflet. J Thorac Cardiovasc Surg 78:402,1979.

101. Maron BJ, Ferrans VJ, Roberts WC: Myocardial ultrastructure in patients with chronic aortic valve disease. Am J Cardiol 35:725,1975.

102. Maron BJ, Lipson LC, Roberts WC, Savage DD, Epstein SE: "Malignant" hypertrophic cardiomyopathy: identification of a subgroup of families with unusually frequent premature death. Am J Cardiol 41:1133,1978.

103. Maron BJ, Merrill WH, Freier PA, Kent KM, Epstein SE, Morrow AG: Long-term clinical course and symptomatic status of patients after operation for hypertrophic subaortic stenosis. Circulation 57:1205,1978.

104. Matsuki O, Robles A, Gibbs S, Bodnar E, Ross DN: Long-term performance of 555 aortic homografts in the aortic position. Ann Thorac Surg 46:187,1988.

105. McAlpine WA: Heart and Coronary Arteries. Berlin, Heidelberg, New York, Springer-Verlag, 1975.

106. McAnulty JH, Rahimtoola SH: Surgery for infective endocarditis. JAMA 242: 77,1979.

107. McGoon DC, Mankin HT, Vlad P, Kirklin JW: The surgical treatment of supravalvular aortic stenosis. J Thorac Cardiovasc Surg 41:125,1961.

108. Monrad ES, Hess OM, Murakami T, Nonogi H, Corin WJ, Krayenbuehl HP: Time course of regression of left ventricular hypertrophy after aortic valve replacement. Circulation 77:1345,1988.

109. Morrow AG, Reitz BA, Epstein SE, Henry WL, Conkle DM, Itscoitz SB, Redwood DR: Operative treatment in hypertrophic subaortic stenosis: techniques and the results of pre- and postoperative assessment in 83 patients. Circulation 52:88,1975.

110. Mullany CJ, Elveback LR, Frye RL, Pluth JR, Edwards WD, Orszulak TA, Nassef LA, Riner RE, Danielson GK: Coronary artery disease and its management: influence on survival in patients undergoing aortic valve replacement. J Am Coll Cardiol 10:66,1987.

111. Myers JL, Waldhausen JA, Cyran SE, Gleason MM, Weber HS, Baylen BG: Results of surgical repair of congenital supravalvular aortic stenosis. J Thorac Cardiovasc Surg 105:281,1993.

112. Newfeld EA, Muster AJ, Paul MH, Idriss FS, Riker WL: Discrete subvalvular aortic stenosis in childhood. Am J Cardiol 38:53,1976.

113. NHLBI Balloon Valvuloplasty Registry Participants: Percutaneous balloon aortic valvuloplasty: acute and 30-day follow-up results in 674 patients from the NHLBI balloon valvuloplasty registry. Circulation 84:2383,1991.

114. O'Brien MF, Stafford EG, Gardner MAH, Pohlner PG, McGriffin DC, Kirklin JW: A comparison of aortic valve replacement with viable cryopreserved and fresh allograft valves, with a note on chromosomal studies. J Thorac Cardiovasc Surg 94:812,1987.

115. Oyer PE, Stinson EB, Reitz BA, Miller DC, Rossiter SJ, Shumway NE: Long-term evaluation of the porcine xenograft bioprosthesis. J Thorac Cadiovasc Surg 78: 343,1979.

116. Pantely G, Morton M, Rahimtoola SH: Effects of successful, uncomplicated valve replacement on ventricular hypertrophy, volume, and performance in aortic stenosis and in aortic incompetence. J Thorac Cardiovasc Surg 75:383,1978.

117. Parker FB, Thomas FD, Poirier RA, Markowitz AHM, Eich RH: Left ventricular function following aortic valve replacement. J Thorac Cardiovasc Surg 79: 121,1980.

118. Peterson CR, Herr R, Crisera RV, Starr A, Bristow JD, Griswold HE: The failure of hemodynamic improvement after valve replacement surgery: etiology, diagnosis, and treatment. Ann Intern Med 66:1,1967.

119. Pupello DF, Blank RH, Bessone LN, Harrison E, Sbar S: Surgical management of the small aortic annulus: hemodynamic evaluation. Chest 74:163,1978.

120. Rahimtoola SH: Early valve replacement for preservation of ventricular function? Am J Cardiol 40:472,1977.

121. Rahimtoola SH: Perspective on valvular heart disease: an update. J Am Coll Cardiol 14:1,1989.

122. Rapaport E: Natural history of aortic and mitral valve disease. Am J Cardiol 35: 221,1975.

123. Rastan H, Koncz J: Aortoventriculoplasty. J Thorac Cardiovasc Surg 71:920,1976.

124. Rastelli GB, McGoon DC, Ongley PA, Mankin GT, Kirklin JW: Surgical treatment of supravalvular aortic stenosis. Report of 16 cases and review of the literature. J Thorac Cardiovasc Surg 51:873,1966.

125. Rhodes LA, Colan SD, Perry SB, Jonas RA, Sanders SP: Predictors of survival in neonates with critical aortic stenosis. Circulation 84:2325,1991.

126. Richardson JV, Karp RB, Kirklin JW, Dismukes WE: Treatment of infective endocarditis: a 10-year comparative analysis. Circulation 58:589,1978.

127. Richardson JV, Kouchoukos NT, Wright JO III, Karp RB: Combined aortic valve replacement and myocardial revascularization: results in 220 patients. Circulation 59:75,1979.

128. Rittenhouse EA, Sauvage LR, Stamm SJ, Mansfield PB, Hall DG, Herndon PS: Radical enlargement of the aortic root and outflow tract to allow valve replacement. Ann Thorac Surg 27:367,1979.

129. Ross DN: Homograft replacement of the aortic valve. Lancet 2:487,1962.

130. Ross DN: Replacement of the aortic and mitral valves with a pulmonary autograft. Lancet 2:956,1967.

131. Ross DN: Technique of aortic valve replacement with a homograft orthotopic replacement. Ann Thorac Surg 52:154,1991.

132. Ross J Jr, Braunwald E: Aortic stenosis. Circulation 38(Suppl V):V-61,255,1976.

133. Ross J Jr, Sonnenblick EH, Taylor RR, Spotnitz HM, Covell JW: Diastolic geometry and sarcomere lengths in the chronically dilated canine left ventricle. Circ Res 28:49,1971.

134. Ross J Jr: Afterload mismatch and preload reserve: a conceptual framework for the analysis of ventricular function. Prog Cardiovasc Dis 18:255,1976.

135. Ross J Jr: Afterload mismatch in aortic and mitral valve disease: implications for surgical therapy. J Am Coll Cardiol 5:811,1985.

136. Russell RO: Timing of aortic valve replacement in chronic aortic regurgitation (editorial). J Am Coll Cardiol 11:930,1988.

137. Safian RD, Berman AD, Diver DJ, McKay LL, Come PC, Riley MF, Warren SE, Cunningham MJ, Wyman RM, Weinstein JS, Grossman W, McKay RG: Balloon aortic valvuloplasty in 170 consecutive patients. N Engl J Med 319:125,1988.

138. Samuels DA, Cureman GD, Friedlich AL, Buckley MU, Austen WG: Valve replacement for aortic regurgitation: long-term follow-up with factors influencing the results. Circulation 60:647,1979.

139. Sandor GGS, Olley PM, Trusler GA, Williams WG, Rowe RD, Morch JE: Long-term follow-up of patients after valvotomy for congenital valvular aortic stenosis in children: a clinical and actuarial follow-up. J Thorac Cardiovasc Surg 80:171,1980.

140. Sanfilippo AJ, Picard MH, Newell JB, Rosas E, Davidoff R, Thomas JD, Weyman AE: Echocardiographic assessment of patients with infectious endocarditis: prediction of risk for complications. J Am Coll Cardiol 18:1191,1991.

141. Sapsford RN, Blackstone EH, Kirklin JW, Karp RB, Kouchoukos NT, Pacifico AD, Roe CR, Bradley EL: Coronary perfusion versus cold ischemic arrest during aortic valve surgery: a randomized study. Circulation 49:1190,1974.

142. Shumacker HB Jr: Aneurysms of the aortic sinuses of Valsalva due to bacterial endocarditis, with special reference to their operative management. J Thorac Cardiovasc Surg 63:896,1972.

143. Slaughter L, Morris JE, Starr A: Prosthetic valvular endocarditis: a 12-year review. Circulation 47:1319,1973.

144. Smith N, McAnulty JH, Rahimtoola SH: Severe aortic stenosis with impaired left ventricular function and clinical heart failure: results of valve replacement. Circulation 58:255,1978.

145. Starr A, Dotter C, Griswold HE: Supravalvular aortic stenosis: diagnosis and treatment. J Thorac Cardiovasc Surg 81:134,1961.

146. Starr A, Grunkemeier G, Lambert LE, Thomas DR, Sugimura S, Lefrak EA: Aortic valve replacement: a ten-year follow-up of noncloth-covered vs cloth-covered caged ball prostheses. Circulation 56(Suppl II):II-133,1977.

147. Stewart JR, Merrill WH, Hammon JW Jr, Graham TP, Bender HW: Reappraisal of localized resection for subvalvar aortic stenosis. Ann Thorac Surg 50:197,1990.

148. Strom J, Becker R, Davis R, Matsumoto M, Frishman W, Sonnenblick EH, Frater RWM: Echocardiographic and surgical correlations in bacterial endocarditis. Circulation 62(Suppl I):I-164,1980.

149. Syracuse DC, Gaudiani VA, Kastl DG, Henry WL, Morrow AG: Intraoperative, intracardiac echocardiography during left ventriculotomy and myectomy for hypertrophic subaortic stenosis. Circulation 58(Suppl I):I-23,1978.

150. Thompson R, Yacoub M, Ahmed M, Seabra-Gomes R, Rickards A, Towers M: Influence of preoperative left ventricular function on results of homograft replacement of the aortic valve for aortic stenosis. Am J Cardiol 43:929,1979.
151. Tompsett R, Lubash GD: Aortic valve perforation in bacterial endocarditis. Circulation 23:662,1961.
152. Tsai TP, Matloff JM, Gray RJ, Chaux A, Kass RM, Lee ME, Czer LSC: Cardiac sugery in the octogenarian. J Thorac Cardiovasc Surg 91:924,1986.
153. Turley K, Bove EL, Amato JJ, Iannettoni M, Yeh J, Cotroneo JV, Galdieri RJ: Neonatal aortic stenosis. J Thorac Cardiovasc Surg 99:679,1990.
154. Utley JR: Annular erosion and pericarditis: complications of endocarditis of the aortic root. J Thorac Cardiovasc Surg 64:76,1972.
155. Wheller JJ, Hosier DM, Teske DW, Craenen JM, Kilman JW: Results of operation for aortic valve stenosis in infants, children, and adolescents. J Thorac Cardiovasc Surg 96:474,1988.
156. Wigle ED, Labrosse CJ: Sudden, severe aortic insufficiency. Circulation 32:708,1965.
157. Wong JB, Salem DN, Pauker SG: You're never too old (editorial). N Engl J Med 328:971,1993.
158. Zeevi B, Keane JF, Castaneda AR, Perry SB, Lock JE: Neonatal critical valvar aortic stenosis: a comparison of surgical and balloon dilatation therapy. Circulation 80:831,1989.

14

Tricuspid Valve Surgery

The evolution over the last several decades of surgery for acquired disease of the tricuspid valve is characterized by steady movement away from replacement and toward techniques that conserve the valve. Replacement of the valve has become uncommon, occurring in less than 5% of patients undergoing tricuspid valve surgery. Conservative surgery of the valve—anuloplasty, occasionally in association with commissurotomy—remains an area of some controversy, involving indications for surgery, choice of anuloplasty technique, and details of technique. In this chapter, we will illustrate two common methods of anuloplasty, the Carpentier and the DeVega, illustrate commissurotomy, and discuss valve replacement.

Anuloplasty

Indications for Surgery

Surgery of the tricuspid valve has long been a challenge.[11,12] Methods of evaluating the severity of tricuspid insuffficiency—whether clinical, hemodynamic, or operative—all involve a degree of subjectivity. The variable early results of valve repair or valve replacement led to differing recommendations regarding management of the tricuspid valve during mitral or mitral and aortic surgery, from doing nothing[3] to reparative operations[6,24] to tricuspid replacement in the majority of cases.[2,4,23,28,29] As the poor late results from tricuspid valve replacement[17] have become more apparent and the results of anuloplasty have become more predictable and reproducible, anuloplasty has become the method of choice for management of most cases of moderate to severe tricuspid insufficiency.

Tricuspid insufficiency is usually caused by right ventricular hypertension, right ventricular enlargement, and anular dilatation, secondary to mitral and/ or aortic valvular disease, commonly referred to as "functional" regurgitation. It may also be caused by rheumatic disease of the anulus, valve leaflets, and subvalvular mechanism—"organic" regurgitation. Tricuspid regurgitation can also be caused by trauma. In rare instances, tricuspid regurgitation can be caused by myxomatous degeneration.

The degree of regurgitation can vary from very mild, with only a soft murmur and normal right atrial pressure, to severe, with pulsating neck veins, an enlarged and pulsating liver, and right atrial hypertension. Severe regurgitation requires operative management, whereas mild regurgitation does not. The difficult decision occurs in moderate regurgitation, where clinical signs are minimal or absent, and only a slight degree of right atrial hypertension is present. Operative assessment of severity of tricuspid regurgitation is helpful in this situation.

Digital exploration of the right atrium is performed through the appendage prior to insertion of the caval cannula. The extent, width, and strength of the regurgitant jet is determined, and the valve is palpated. Operative findings can be influenced by changes in right ventricular pressure and cardiac output secondary to anesthesia and opening the chest, and must be balanced with preoperative clinical and hemodynamic assessment.

Surgical Strategy

Myocardial Preservation
The usual method of myocardial preservation is cold blood potassium cardioplegia (Chapter 6). This provides a still, dry field for anuloplasty.

Associated Procedures
Any surgery on the mitral or aortic valve is performed prior to the tricuspid procedure.

Choice of Anuloplasty Technique
There are several anuloplasty techniques from which to choose[33]: (1) lateral anuloplasty with obliteration of the posterior leaflet, resulting in a bicuspid valve[18,19]; (2) semicircular ring anuloplasty by the method of DeVega[9] and its modifications[1]; and (3) Carpentier ring anuloplasty[6,7] and its modifications.[10,15] Our preference is for the DeVega or Carpentier technique.

Surgical Anatomy

The three leaflets of the tricuspid valve are the anterior, posterior, and septal (Fig. 14-1). There are two main papillary muscles supporting the valve: the *anterolateral*, with chordae tendineae inserting on the anterior and posterior leaflets, and the *posteromedial*, with chordae inserting on the septal leaflet.[27]

The atrioventricular (AV) node is located just medial to the orifice of the coronary sinus. The bundle of His begins as a continuation of the AV node at the right fibrous trigone, also called the central fibrous body: the confluence of the AV valves, atrial septum, membranous ventricular septum, and aortic

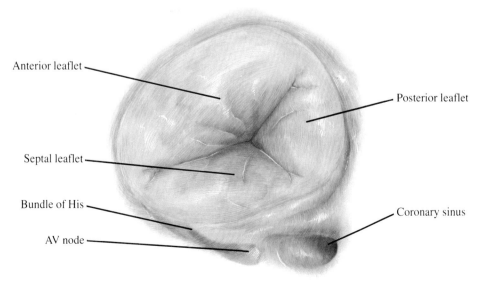

Anterior leaflet

Posterior leaflet

Septal leaflet

Bundle of His

Coronary sinus

AV node

14-1

valve ring. The His bundle pierces the membranous ventricular septum or skirts the septum posteriorly to enter the summit of the muscular ventricular septum, where it gives off multiple branches to the left ventricle.[16,31]

Surgical Technique

Carpentier Ring Anuloplasty

Coauthored by Alain Carpentier

The basis of the Carpentier ring anuloplasty is anulus remodeling: both dilatation and deformation are corrected. Right ventricular volume and pressure overload cause a change in shape of the tricuspid anulus as well as in size: the anulus becomes circular, losing its normal ovoid shape.[5-7,14] This change in shape moves the anterior and posterior leaflets out of apposition with each other and with the septal leaflet. Implantation of the Carpentier ring brings the anular shape back to normal. The aim is to correct the tricuspid insufficiency by creating a valve orifice with normal morphology without any appreciable narrowing of the orifice.

Use of the ring allows plication of the anulus where the dilatation is most prominent—at the commissures. The ring is flexible, with a large opening at the anteroseptal commissure and septal leaflet, preventing injury to the bundle of His.

The size of the ring is chosen either by measurement at the base of the septal leaflet, which is not affected by anular dilatation, or by fitting the ring to the size of the anterior leaflet (Fig. 14–2). Horizontal mattress sutures are then placed in the anulus and through the fabric of the ring (Fig. 14–3). Plication takes place at the commissures. The ring is seated and tied (Fig. 14–4). Competence of the valve is checked by injecting saline into the right ventricle with a large bulb syringe.

DeVega Anuloplasty

A suture of 2–0 polypropylene is passed through a pledget of Teflon, and the suture line is begun near the commissure between the anterior and septal leaflets (Fig. 14–5). Bites are taken just into or near the anulus as the suture line proceeds laterally around the anterior leaflet.

Near the commissure between the posterior and septal leaflets the suture is

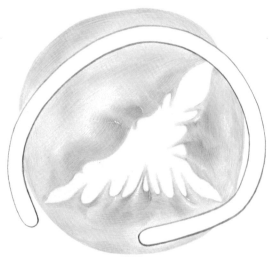

14–2

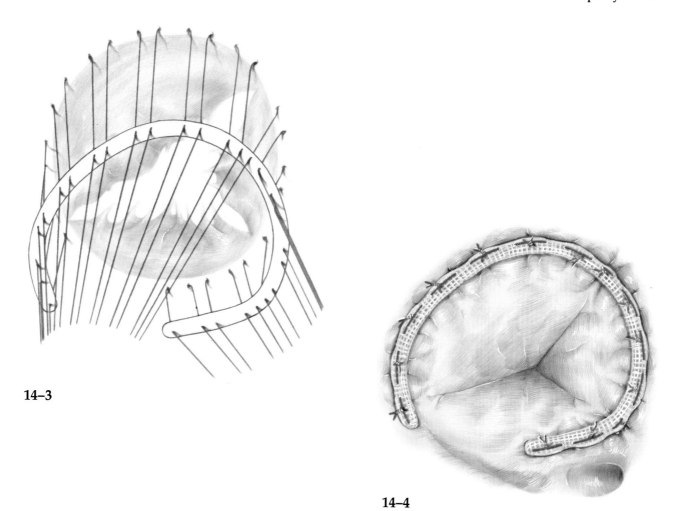

14–3

14–4

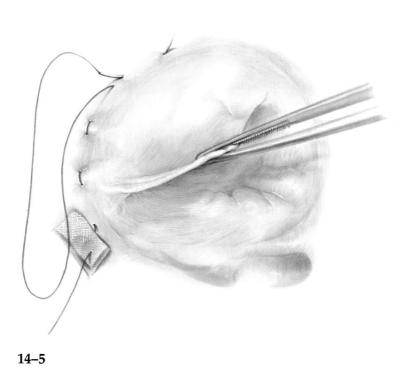

14–5

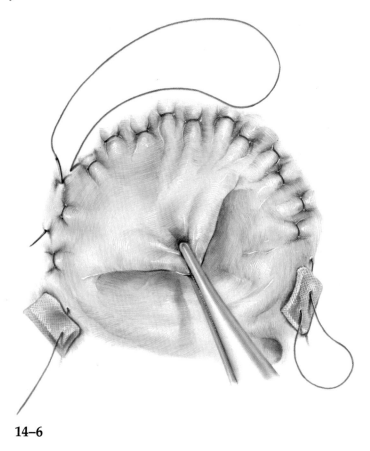

14–6

passed through another Teflon pledget and is carried back to its origin, taking bites just outside the inner suture line (Fig. 14–6).

A valve sizer appropriate to the patient's size is placed in the anulus for calibration. The suture is then tied over the medial pledget as the suture is gathered and the anulus is brought against the sizer. The competence of the valve is assessed by injecting cold saline into the right ventricle with a large bulb syringe.

Results

Operative mortality is in the range of 5%–15%.[9,19] Good functional and hemodynamic results have been reported with a number of techniques.[6,8,9,10,12,15,18,19,32] Grondin and colleagues[12] reported 17 patients studied after a DeVega anuloplasty and 32 studied after Carpentier ring anuloplasty. Tricuspid insufficiency was absent or trivial in 75%, even in the presence of elevated right ventricular pressures. The DeVega technique may be less predictable than the ring technique and can create tricuspid stenosis.[13,22]

Commissurotomy

Indications for Surgery

Organic tricuspid valve disease is becoming rare in the United States and many European countries. In other areas of the world, however, it is quite common.

Organic involvement of the valve can create stenosis by fusion of the commissures. Stenosis is usually part of a mixed lesion including regurgitation. Most valves with stenosis can be repaired with commissurotomy and anuloplasty. Any valve with more than a 5 mm Hg gradient should be explored.

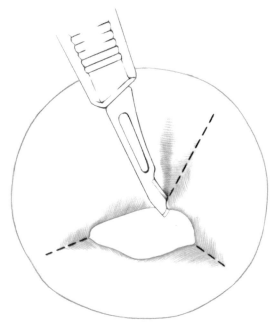

14–7

Surgical Technique

The commissures are incised with a knife to within about 3 mm of the anulus (Fig. 14–7). Usually nothing needs to be done to the chordae. An anuloplasty should be performed to correct the insufficiency. The use of a prosthetic ring in this situation is important to avoid narrowing of the orifice.

Replacement

Indications for Surgery

Traumatic injury of the tricuspid valve is usually an indication for replacement.[30] Leaflet tears and ruptured chordae may be repaired. Symptoms may not occur until many years following injury. Tricuspid valve replacement is also indicated in some symptomatic patients with Ebstein's disease.[21] Replacement may be indicated in symptomatic patients late after tricuspid valve excision for endocarditis.

Replacement for organic or functional tricuspid disease is rarely indicated. A less than perfect repair is preferable to replacement. An insufficient valve should be replaced only if there is rupture of multiple chordae or other irreparable damage. A valve with mixed stenosis and insufficiency should be replaced only if the chronic inflammation and scarring are so extensive that the leaflets are shrunken and curled and the chordae are thickened and shortened.

Surgical Strategy

Choice of Prosthesis
Mechanical prostheses in the tricuspid position are prone to thrombotic obstruction.[17,25,26] The struts of caged-ball valves frequently penetrate the right ventricular endocardium, resulting in restriction of ball excursion. This is usually a gradual process. Tilting-disc valves may have restriction on disc movement due to thrombus formation; this can cause catastrophic malfunction. The wedge-shaped right ventricular cavity conforms poorly to both types of mechanical prosthesis.

Our preference is for a bioprosthesis. The bioprostheses, with central flow and absence of areas prone to thrombus formation and propagation, are likely to provide superior performance in the tricuspid position, at least over the short term (3–8 years).

Surgical Technique

The valve is excised, leaving about 4 mm of the base of the septal leaflet. Horizontal mattress sutures with pledgets on the atrial side are placed in the anulus of the anterior and posterior leaflets. The sutures are placed through leaflet tissue of the septal leaflet, in order to avoid injury to the His bundle.

Results

Replacement of the tricuspid valve, in association with replacement of the mitral and/or aortic valves, can be performed with operative mortality as low as 10%–15%.[4,29] Functional improvement occurs in 85%–95%.[17,25] McGrath and colleagues[20] reported that 70% of patients were free of reoperation for valve failure 10 years following tricuspid valve replacement with a Carpentier-Edwards bioprosthesis. Late survival is variable, but can be as high as 70% at 3 years.[25]

References

1. Alonso-Lej F: Discussion of Duran et al: Clinical and hemodynamic performance of a totally flexible prosthetic ring for atrioventricular valve reconstruction. Ann Thorac Surg 22:463,1976.
2. Boyd AD, Engelman RM, Isom OW, Reed GE, Spencer FC: Tricuspid annuloplasty: five and one-half years' experience with 78 patients. J Thorac Cardiovasc Surg 68:344,1974.
3. Braunwald NS, Ross J Jr, Morrow AG: Conservative management of tricuspid regurgitation in patients undergoing mitral valve replacement. Circulation 35(Suppl I):I-63,1967.
4. Breyer RH, McClenathan JH, Michaelis LL, McIntosh CL, Morrow AG: Tricuspid regurgitation: a comparison of nonoperative management, tricuspid annuloplasty, and tricuspid valve replacement. J Thorac Cardiovasc Surg 72:867,1976.
5. Carpentier A: Cardiac valve surgery—the "French correction." J Thorac Cardiovasc Surg 86:323,1983.
6. Carpentier A, Deloche A, Hanania G, Forman J, Sellier P, Piwnica A, Dubost C: Surgical management of acquired tricuspid valve disease. J Thorac Cardiovasc Surg 67:53,1974.
7. Carpentier A, Relland J: Carpentier rings and tricuspid insufficiency (letter). Ann Thorac Surg 27:95,1979.
8. Deloche A, Guerinon J, Fariani JM, Morillo F, Caramanian M, Carpentier A, Maurice P, Dubost C: Etude anatomique des valvuloplasties rhumatismales tricuspidiennes. Arch Mal Coeur 67:5,1974.
9. DeVega NG: La anuloplastia selectiva, reguable y permanente. Rev Esp Cardiol 25:6,1972.
10. Duran CG, Ubago JLM: Clinical and hemodynamic performance of a totally flexible prosthetic ring for atrioventricular valve reconstruction. Ann Thorac Surg 22:458,1976.
11. Grondin P, Lepage G, Castongnay Y, Meere C: The tricuspid valve: a surgical challenge. J Thorac Cardiovasc Surg 53:7,1967.
12. Grondin P, Meere C, Limet R, Lopez-Bescos L, Delcan JL, Rivera R: Carpentier's annulus and DeVega's annuloplasty: the end of the tricuspid challenge. J Thorac Cardiovasc Surg 70:852,1975.
13. Haerten K, Seipel L, Loogen F, Herzer J: Hemodynamic studies after DeVega's tricuspid anuloplasty. Circulation 58(Suppl I):I-28,1978.
14. Hansing CE, Rowe GG: Tricuspid insufficiency: a study of hemodynamics and pathogenesis. Circulation 45:793,1972.

15. Hecart J, Blaise C, Bex JP, Bajolet A: Technique for tricuspid annuloplasty with a flexible linear reducer. J Thorac Cardiovasc Surg 79:689,1980.

16. James TN: Morphology of the human atrioventricular node, with remarks pertinent to its electrophysiology. Am Heart J 62:756,1961.

17. Jugdutt BI, Fraser RS, Lee SJK, Rossall RE, Callaghan JC: Long-term survival after tricuspid valve replacement. J Thorac Cardiovasc Surg 74:20,1977.

18. Kay JH, Masselli-Campagna G, Tusju HK: Surgical treatment of tricuspid insufficiency. Ann Surg 162:53,1965.

19. Kay JH, Mendez AM, Zubiate P: A further look at tricuspid annuloplasty. Ann Thorac Surg 22:498,1976.

20. McGrath LB, Chen C, Bailey BM, Fernandez J, Laub GW, Adkins MS: Early and late phase events following bioprosthetic tricuspid valve replacement. J Card Surg 7:245,1992.

21. Melo J, Saylam A, Knight R, Starr A: Long-term results after surgical correction of Ebstein's anomaly. J Thorac Cardiovasc Surg 78:233,1979.

22. Meyer J, Bircks W: Predictable correction of tricuspid insufficiency by semicircular annuloplasty. Ann Thorac Surg 23:574,1977.

23. Pluth JR, Ellis FH Jr: Tricuspid insufficiency in patients undergoing mitral valve replacement: conservative management, annuloplasty, or replacement. J Thorac Cardiovasc Surg 58:484,1969.

24. Reed GE, Boyd AD, Spencer FC, Engelman RM, Isom OW, Cunningham JN: Operative management of tricuspid regurgitation. Circulation 54(Suppl III):III-96,1976.

25. Sanfelippo PM, Giuliani ER, Danielson GK, Wallace RB, Pluth JR, McGoon DC: Tricuspid valve prosthetic replacement: early and late results with the Starr-Edwards prosthesis. J Thorac Cardiovasc Surg 71:441,1976.

26. Schoevaerdts JC, Jaumin P, Piret L, Kremer R, Ponlot R, Chalant CH: Tricuspid valve surgery. J Cardiovasc Surg 18:397,1977.

27. Silver MD, Lam JHC, Ranganathan N, Wigle ED: Morphology of the human tricuspid valve. Circulation 43:333,1971.

28. Starr A: Acquired disease of the tricuspid valve. *In* Sabiston DC Jr, Spencer FC (eds): Gibbon's Surgery of the Chest. Philadelphia, WB Saunders Co, 1976, p 1176.

29. Starr A, Herr RH, Wood JA: Tricuspid replacement for acquired valve disease. Surg Gynecol Obstet 122:1295,1966.

30. Tachovsky TJ, Giuliani ER, Ellis FH Jr: Prosthetic valve replacement for traumatic tricuspid insufficiency. Am J Cardiol 26:196,1970.

31. Titus JL: Normal anatomy of the human cardiac conductive system. Mayo Clin Proc 48:23,1973.

32. Wei J, Chang C, Lee F, Lai W: DeVega's semicircular annuloplasty for tricuspid valve regurgitation. Ann Thorac Surg 55:482,1993.

33. West PN, Weldon CS: Reconstructive valve surgery. Ann Thorac Surg 25:167,1978.

15

Patent Ductus Arteriosus

Robert Gross stated that his first ligation of a patent ductus arteriosus in 1938 "formed the opening wedge in the surgical attack on congenital cardiovascular anomalies."[9] Ligation or division of the ductus has become a simple procedure associated with almost no morbidity or mortality. However, the complication of operative hemorrhage from a torn or insufficiently sutured ductus is so serious that the operation should always be approached with respect, proper planning, and meticulous technique.

Indications for Surgery

The Infant

Patent ductus arteriosus is common in the premature infant. Almost all infants with birth weights of less than 1000 g and nearly two-thirds of all infants with birth weights of less than 1750 g have clinical evidence of a persistently patent ductus.[24] Closure of the ductus in these infants usually occurs during the first weeks of life.

Closure of the ductus may not occur, however, which may lead to the development of congestive heart failure that does not respond to medical therapy. Large left-to-right shunts can be documented in this group of infants. Echocardiographic assessment of left-to-right shunting is an accurate means of noninvasive diagnosis for these infants.[2,18,25,26]

Pharmacologic closure of the ductus using indomethacin,[7] a drug that counteracts prostaglandin activity, is effective in premature infants.[30] Gersony and co-workers[8] reported a randomized trial to evaluate the role of indomethacin in premature infants weighing less than 1750 g. They found that indomethacin given concurrently with usual medical therapy at the time of diagnosis resulted in ductal closure in 79% of patients compared to 35% with placebo. They also found that the patients in the indomethacin group who required surgery did not have any higher risk because of the use of indomethacin. Even in these ill infants, surgery is a safe approach, several series reporting no operative mortality.[5,17,29]

The Child

Surgical treatment of a patent ductus arteriosus in the child is indicated in spite of absence of symptoms. Several studies have shown that a patent ductus arteriosus is associated with a shortened life span. In Abbott's 1936 series[1] of autopsies of 92 patients with patent ductus arteriosus, the average

age at death was 24 years. A similar study by Keys[13] in 1943 showed an average age at death of 35 years. Campbell's[4] study of the natural history of patent ductus arteriosus indicated that one-third of patients die within the first 40 years of life. Heart failure or endarteritis is the usual cause of death. The risk of endarteritis is probably from 0.5% to 1%/year.

The unfavorable natural history of the defect and the extremely low risk of surgery in the child justify surgical intervention even in the absence of symptoms. If a left-to-right shunt persists, surgical treatment is indicated even in the presence of pulmonary hypertension. The operative mortality in the child approaches zero.

The Adult

Surgical treatment is indicated in the adult if there is persistence of a left-to-right shunt. Pulmonary hypertension does not contraindicate surgery in the presence of a left-to-right shunt.[3] A balanced shunt is a contraindication to operation.

Surgical Strategy

Ligation Versus Division

The objective of surgical treatment of patent ductus arteriosus is a complete and permanent interruption of the blood flow from the aorta into the pulmonary artery. This can be accomplished by either ligation or division.

During the early years of ductal surgery, ligation fell from favor because it was associated with an unacceptable incidence of persistence or recurrence of ductal flow. Gross[9] reported that 10% of a series of 43 cases showed persistence of flow and another 10% showed later recurrence. Persistence of flow was due to inadequate ligation, most likely caused by the timidity of surgeons who feared cutting through the ductus with the thin silk sutures in use at that time. Recurrence was probably caused by the thin silk sutures gradually cutting through the tissue, with eventual formation of a fistula between the aorta and the pulmonary artery. The use of either cotton or silk tape for ligation has solved these problems. In our experience, as well as that of others,[21] ligation is as effective and permanent as division and is usually a simpler and safer procedure. Ligation should not be performed in the calcified ductus, for which special techniques are usually necessary.

In the usual ductus we use ligation (Children's Cardiac Center of Oregon/Portland) or division (Sutter/Sacramento). When properly performed, either gives excellent results.

The Difficult Ductus

The ductus associated with calcification and the recurrent ductus can provide additional challenge. Safe division can be accomplished by control of the pulmonary artery end of the ductus and occlusion of the aorta above and below the ductus, removal of an ellipse of aorta, and Dacron patch repair of the aortic defect.[6] The ductal orifice may also be closed with a patch through an opening in the lateral aorta.[19,22] The complicated patent ductus may also be closed through the pulmonary artery using cardiopulmonary bypass and profound hypothermia with low flow or circulatory arrest.[15,20] Hypotension during clamping can be used for a potentially friable ductus. Groin cannulation can also be performed in the case of a large, thin ductus so that femoral-femoral bypass and aortic clamping above and below the ductus can be rapidly instituted if difficulties are encountered.

Intrapericardial Ligation

Retraction of the pulmonary artery inferiorly exposes the ductus for dissection and ligation.[14] We usually perform ligation after institution of cardiopulmonary bypass during the period of systemic cooling. The ductus should be ligated if there is any suspicion of patency when circulatory arrest is used and the right heart or pulmonary artery is opened. A small open ductus can provide an opening for entrance of air into the aorta during the period of arrest.

Transcatheter Closure

Rashkind[23] performed the first successful transcatheter closure of a patent ductus arteriosus in 1977. The equipment and technique have undergone modification since that time and transcatheter closure can now be accomplished with a low morbidity and no mortality.[16,28] However, recurrent shunting found by color-flow doppler can be as high as 38% at one year, although this decreases with the passage of time.[11] This small degree of shunting, which is usually not detectable clinically, may be entirely benign.[16] More studies will be necessary to determine whether transcatheter closure is as predictable and reliable as surgery in eliminating ductal flow. As of mid-1993, the United States Food and Drug Administration had not approved the catheter device.[27]

Surgical Anatomy

Important anatomic relations must be understood in order to interrupt the ductus without injury to the ductus, surrounding vessels, or adjacent nerves (Fig. 15–1). The superior border of the ductus often forms an acute angle with the distal aortic arch, and a narrow plane is present between the superior border of the ductus and the inferior aspect of the aortic arch. The most common mistake in surgery on infants is mistaking the ductus for the aortic arch.

The pericardium is attached as a fold over the anterior portion of the ductus, and in this region proper dissection is necessary to open the correct tissue plane. The vagus nerve descends beneath the pleura overlying the ductus and gives off the recurrent laryngeal nerve, which sweeps around the ductus in close proximity and then passes behind the aortic arch to ascend to the larynx. Connective tissue adherent to the posterior ductus is best dissected sharply prior to passing a clamp behind the ductus. Excessive blunt dissection behind the ductus can cause laceration of the posterior wall and life-threatening hemorrhage.

The intrapericardial location of the normally positioned ductus is just above the bifurcation of the main pulmonary artery. Its direction is superior and slightly to the left. When the great arteries are transposed, relations are somewhat different: the ductus is located more medially under the inferior portion of the aortic arch. This can make encircling the ductus in transposition more difficult than in normally related great arteries.

Surgical Technique

Thoracic Incision

Although the ductus can be approached anteriorly, as in the original operation by Gross,[10] our preference is a posterolateral thoracotomy through the

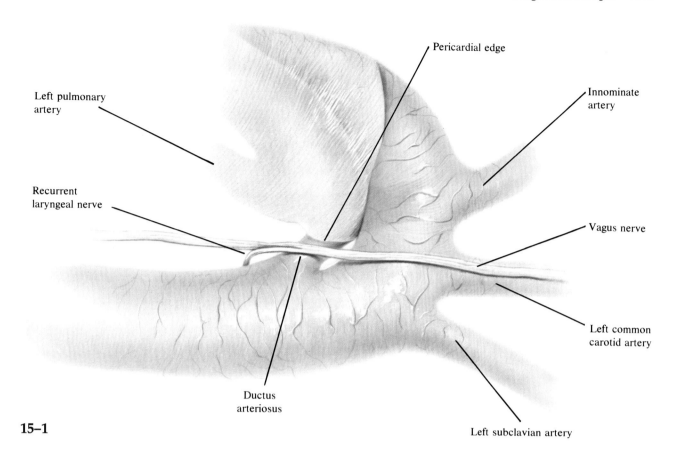

Left pulmonary
artery

Recurrent
laryngeal nerve

Pericardial edge

Innominate
artery

Vagus nerve

Left common
carotid artery

Ductus
arteriosus

Left subclavian artery

15–1

fourth or third interspace, as described by Jones.[12] Little, if any, of the serratus anterior need be divided.

Dissection

Pleural incision is made over the aorta posterior to the vagus nerve and carried up to the subclavian artery in order to adequately expose the distal arch (Fig. 15-2). The vagus and recurrent nerves are reflected anteriorly, avoiding division of the pulmonary branches. The pleural edges are suspended to wound towels.

Sharp dissection is used to open the planes above (Fig. 15-3) and below (Fig. 15-4) the ductus and behind the aorta (Fig. 15-5) above and below the ductus. Tissue around the ductus is gripped for retraction; it is best to avoid gripping the ductus, particularly in the infant. Tapes are then passed around the aorta above (Fig. 15-6) and below the ductus. The tapes are used to retract the aorta for posterior dissection of the ductus, and they provide easy control of the aorta should the ductus be injured at any subsequent step in the procedure.

Ligation

Following complete dissection of the ductus, a cotton tape and heavy silk are passed around it (Fig. 15-7). The ductus is then doubly ligated (Figs. 15-8, 15-9).

Division

Following complete dissection of the ductus, as illustrated previously, clamps are placed on the aortic end and the pulmonary artery end, and the ductus is

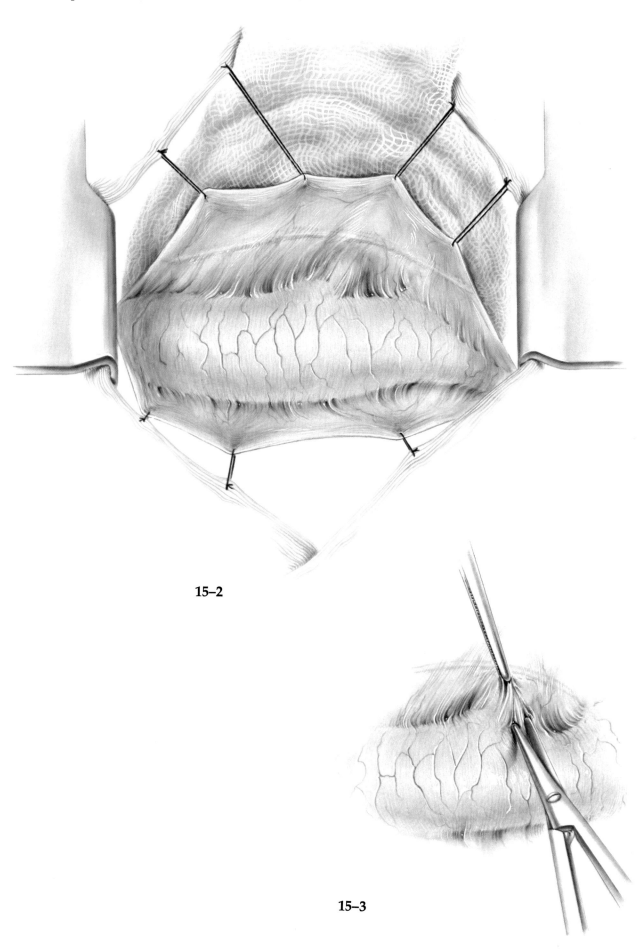

15–2

15–3

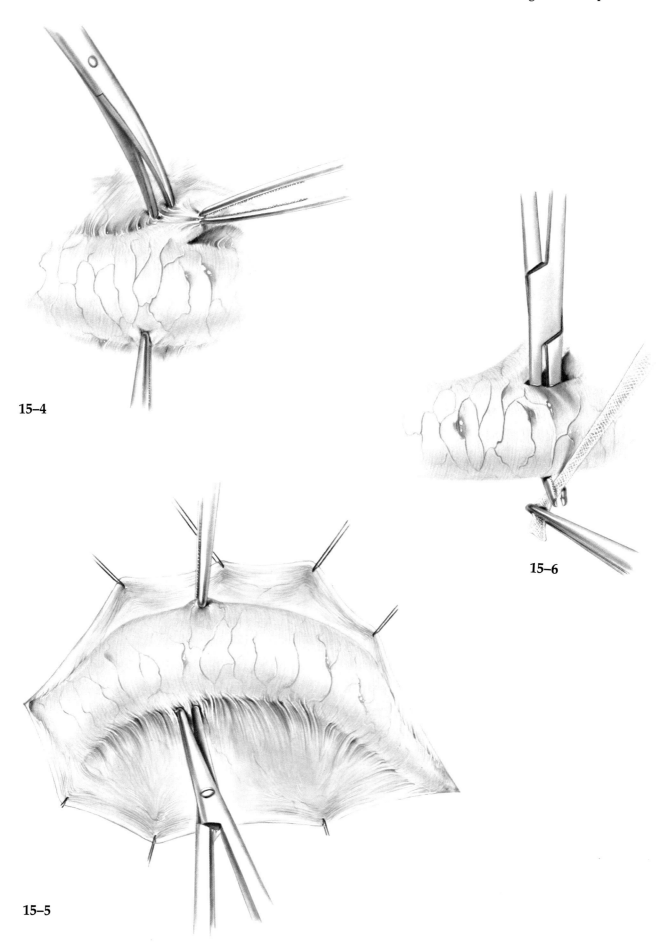

15–4

15–6

15–5

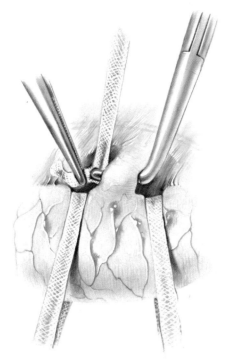

15–7

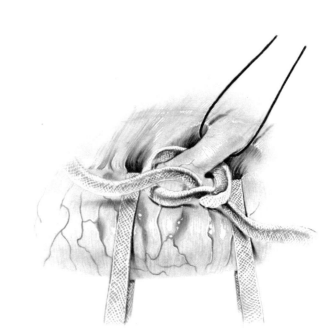

15–8

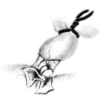

15–9

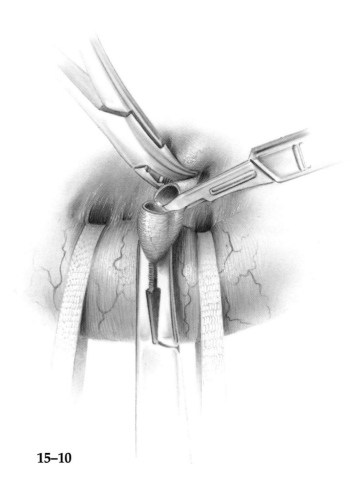

15–10

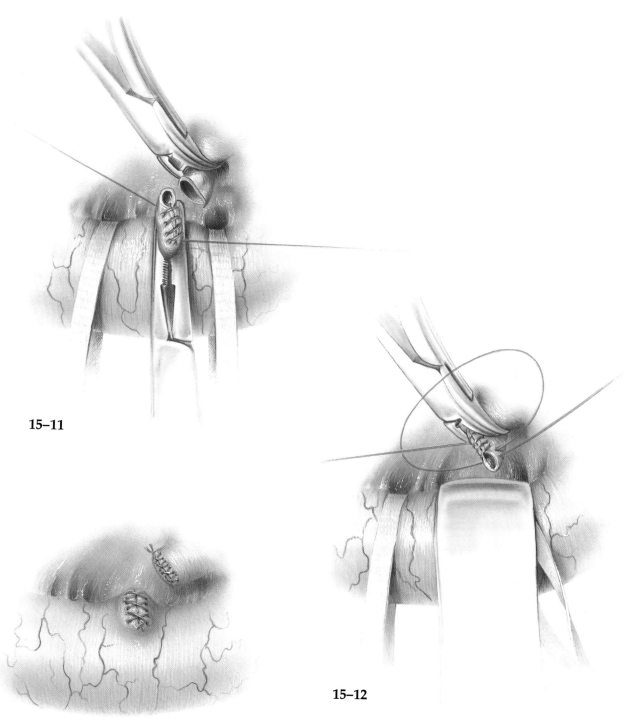

15–11

15–12

15–13

divided (Fig. 15–10). A polypropylene suture (usually 5–0) is then run down
and back the aortic end (Fig. 15–11). The clamp is then usually removed from
the aortic end and the aorta is retracted laterally with the tapes or a small
malleable retractor, for better exposure of the pulmonary end. The pulmonary artery end is then sutured (Fig. 15–12), completing the division (Fig. 15–
13).

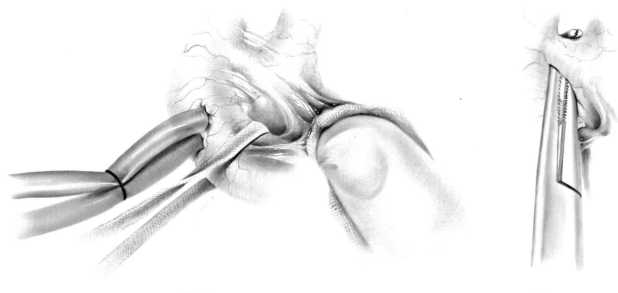

15–14   15–15

Intrapericardial Ligation

An assistant retracts the pulmonary infundibulum inferiorly, placing the pulmonary artery on stretch. Dissection begins at the base of the left pulmonary artery and is continued on both sides of the ductus (Fig. 15–14). It is important to clearly identify the left and right pulmonary arteries to assure proper identification of the ductus. If the structures are not carefully identified and if excessive traction is placed on the pulmonary artery, the descending aorta can be mistaken for the ductus. A clamp is then placed around the ductus (Fig. 15–15) and a ligature passed and tied while the pump flow is momentarily lowered to lower the systemic pressure.

References

1. Abbott ME: Atlas of Congenital Cardiac Disease. New York, American Heart Association, 1936, p 61.
2. Allen HD, Sahn DJ, Goldberg SJ: New serial contrast technique for assessment of the left to right shunting patent ductus arteriosus in the neonate. Am J Cardiol 41: 288,1978.
3. Black LL, Goldman BS: Surgical treatment of the patent ductus arteriosus in the adult. Ann Surg 175:290,1972.
4. Campbell N: Natural history of persistent ductus arteriosus. Br Heart J 30:4,1968.
5. Clark DR, Paton BC, Way GL, Stewart JR: Patent ductus arteriosus ligation and respiratory distress syndrome in premature infants. Ann Thorac Surg 22:138,1976.
6. Cooley DA: Techniques in Cardiac Surgery, 2nd ed. Philadelphia, WB Saunders Co, 1984, p 31.
7. Friedman WF, Hirschklau MJ, Printz MP, Pitlick PT, Kirkpatrick SE: Pharmacologic closure of patent ductus arteriosus in the premature infant. N Engl J Med 295:526,1976.
8. Gersony WM, Peckham GJ, Ellison RC, Miettinen OS, Nadas AS: Effects of indomethacin in premature infants with patent ductus arteriosus: results of a national collaborative study. J Pediatr 102:895,1983.
9. Gross RE: The patent ductus arteriosus: observation on diagnosis and therapy in 525 surgically treated cases. Am J Med 12:472,1952.
10. Gross RE, Hubbard JP: Surgical ligation of a patent ductus arteriosus. Report of the first successful case. JAMA 112:729,1939.

11. Hosking MCK, Benson LN, Musewe N, Dyck JD, Freedom RM: Transcatheter occlusion of the persistently patent ductus arteriosus: forty-month follow-up and prevalence of residual shunting. Circulation 84:2313,1991.

12. Jones JC: Twenty-five years' experience with surgery of patent ductus arteriosus. J Thorac Cardiovasc Surg 50:149,1965.

13. Keys A, Shapiro MJ: Patency of the ductus arteriosus in adults. Am Heart J 25: 158,1943.

14. Kirklin JW, Silver AW: Technique of exposing the ductus arteriosus prior to establishing extracorporeal circulation. Mayo Clin Proc 33:423,1958.

15. Lam CR: A safe technique for closure of the recurrent patent ductus arteriosus. J Thorac Cardiovasc Surg 72:232,1976.

16. Latson LA: Residual shunts after transcatheter closure of patent ductus arteriosus: a major concern or benign "techno-malady"? (editorial) Circulation 84:2591,1991.

17. Levitsky S, Fisher E, Vidyasagar D, Hastreiter AR, Bennett EJ, Raju TNK, Roger K: Interruption of patent ductus arteriosus in premature infants with respiratory distress syndrome. Ann Thorac Surg 22:131,1976.

18. Liao PK, Su WJ, Hung JS: Doppler echocardiographic flow characteristics of isolated patent ductus arteriosus: better delineation by doppler color flow mapping. J Am Coll Cardiol 12:1285,1988.

19. Morrow AG, Clark WD: Closure of calcified patent ductus arteriosus: a new operative method utilizing cardiopulmonary bypass. J Thorac Cardiovasc Surg 51: 534,1964.

20. O'Donovan TG, Beck W: Closure of the complicated patent ductus arteriosus. Ann Thorac Surg 25:464,1978.

21. Panagopoulos PG, Tatooles CJ, Aberdeen E, et al: Patent ductus arteriosus in infants and children. A review of 936 operations. Thorax 26:137,1971.

22. Pifarre R, Rice PL, Nemickas R: Surgical treatment of calcified patent ductus arteriosus. J Thorac Cardiovasc Surg 65:625,1973.

23. Rashkind WJ, Mullins CE, Hellenbrand WE, Tait MA: Nonsurgical closure of patent ductus arteriosus: clinical application of the Rashkind PDA Occluder System. Circulation 75:583,1987.

24. Rudolph AM: Congenital Diseases of the Heart. Chicago, Year Book, 1974.

25. Silverman NH, Lewis AB, Heymann MA, et al: Echocardiographic assessment of ductus arteriosus shunt in premature infants. Circulation 50:821,1974.

26. Swensson RE, Valdes-Cruz LM, Sahn DJ, Sherman FS, Chung KJ, Scagnelli S, Hagen-Ansert S: Real-time doppler color flow mapping for detection of patent ductus arteriosus. J Am Coll Cardiol 8:1105,1986.

27. USCI/Bard: Personal communication. 1993.

28. Wessel DL, Keane JF, Parness I, Lock JE: Outpatient closure of the patent ductus arteriosus. Circulation 77:1068,1988.

29. Williams WH, Gelband H, Boncalari E, Bauer C, Garcia O, Tamer D, Kaiser GA: The ductus debate: ligation in prematurity? Ann Thorac Surg 22:151,1976.

30. Yeh TF, Luken JA, Thalji A, Raval D, Carr I, Pildes RS: Intravenous indomethacin therapy in premature infants with persistent ductus arteriosus—a double-blind controlled study. J Pediat 98:137,1981.

16

Coarctation of the Aorta

Coarctation of the thoracic aorta was first resected successfully in 1944.[20] Although resection has remained the most common method of repair, additional operations have been developed to encompass the anatomic variations of coarctation. The objective of all procedures is permanent relief of any gradient across the coarctation and establishment of normal, pulsatile flow to the lower body.

Hemorrhage, the most common operative complication, can be avoided by knowledge of anatomic variations, delicate dissection and suturing, proper choice of operation, and proper anesthetic management. The rare but dreaded complication of paraplegia can almost be eliminated by proper choice of surgical approach based on preoperative and operative assessment of adequacy of collateral circulation.

Percutaneous Balloon Angioplasty

The development of percutaneous balloon angioplasty in the early 1980s[37,41,42,67] has added another option in the treatment of coarctation and has stimulated considerable controversy.[54,55,74,75] The results of balloon angioplasty are different in the three groups of patients: neonates and infants, children with unoperated coarctation, and children with recurrent coarctation.

Balloon angioplasty in neonates and infants is associated with a high incidence of recoarctation.[56] The average rate of recoarctation in a compiled series of eight reports comprising 57 patients was 57%.[34]

Balloon angioplasty in the unoperated child results in a transmural tear of the vessel wall through the intima and media, depending on the adventitia to maintain vascular integrity.[9,75] Balloon angioplasty can be performed in children with unoperated coarctation with an absence of mortality and a low incidence of morbidity,[63] but is associated with a troubling incidence of aneurysms, with incidences as high as 20%–40%,[18,63] and a high incidence of residual or recurrent gradients.[7] Shaddy and colleagues[63] found an incidence of restenosis of 25% following angioplasty. Although aneurysms following angioplasty have not been shown to lead to rupture on early follow-up,[75] the eventual fate of these aneurysms is yet to be determined.

Balloon angioplasty for recurrent coarctation has given the most favorable results and seems equally successful regardless of whether the prior procedure was resection and end-to-end anastomosis, subclavian flap angioplasty, or synthetic patch angioplasty. Balloon angioplasty can be performed with absence of mortality, low morbidity, effective reduction of the gradient, restenosis of only 10%–15%, and aneurysm formation of only 2%–4%.[3,19,31,55]

Balloon angioplasty does not seem appropriate for neonates and infants, remains questionable for children with unoperated coarctation, and is a reasonable option for children with recurrent coarctation.

Indications for Surgery

The Infant

The usual presentation of coarctation in infancy is congestive heart failure. A small percentage of these infants will respond to vigorous medical therapy, and surgery can be postponed months or years. However, most infants with coarctation and congestive heart failure have associated extracardiac and intracardiac defects (patent ductus arteriosus, ventricular septal defect, aortic valve abnormalities) and respond poorly to medical therapy.[65] In these infants continued medical therapy in the face of unresponsive congestive heart failure is associated with a mortality approaching 100%. Urgent surgery is necessary for survival. The clinical condition of neonates can often be improved preoperatively by administration of prostaglandin E_1 and inotropes.[26]

Optimum management of intracardiac defects at the time of coarctation repair remains somewhat controversial.[26,38,53] Ventricular septal defect, the most common intracardiac defect, has been palliated in the past by pulmonary artery banding. However, pulmonary artery banding can be associated with high mortality in these infants.[28,43] Park and colleagues[53] have reported a series of 39 infants with coarctation of the aorta and ventricular septal defect, most of whom were managed by initial coarctation repair alone. Of the 39 infants, 41% never required a second operation for ventricular septal defect closure. We presently repair the coarctation and ligate the ductus arteriosus. Persistence of congestive heart failure in the postoperative period is the indication for closure of the ventricular septal defect.

The Child and the Adult

Coarctation of the thoracic aorta usually presents as upper extremity hypertension in the child and the adult. Surgical repair is indicated because the natural history of the defect results in premature death. A review by Reifenstein[57] in 1947 of 104 autopsied cases of "adult type" of coarctation found an average age at death of 35 years. The majority of deaths were caused by rupture of the aorta or intracranial arteries, congestive heart failure, and bacterial endocarditis.

Surgical Strategy

Choice of Operation: Neonate and Infant

The anatomy of the coarctation and the age of the patient determine our choice of operation for coarctation. Beginning in the mid-1970s, we began performing the subclavian artery patch angioplasty in the neonate and infant, using the left subclavian artery as a living patch over the coarctation, as described by Waldhausen.[73] We were disappointed by the high incidence (30%–60%)[16] of recurrent coarctation that occurred following resection and end-to-end anastomosis, using the surgical techniques of that time. We have since become disappointed with the incidence of recurrent coarctation following subclavian flap angioplasty, particularly in infants below the age of 2 months,[47] and presently perform either resection and extended end-to-end anastomosis or resection and subclavian flap repair, with a preference for the resection and extended end-to-end anastomosis.

The conclusions of the studies comparing resection to subclavian flap repair are conflicting. Some studies conclude that subclavian flap repair is better,[36,52,60] some conclude that resection and end-to-end anastomosis is better,[24,70] and others conclude that there is no difference between the two techniques.[6,69,79] The differing conclusions are probably explained by the facts that none of the studies was a randomized study; there were differences in time frames, personnel, and surgical technique; and there were probably differences in patient mix.

Variables in surgical technique can affect the outcome of both resection and end-to-end anastomosis and subclavian flap repair. The outcome of resection can be affected by the extent of resection, the circumference of the anastomosis, the suture technique, the suture material (absorbable or nonabsorbable), and the tension on the suture line. The outcome of subclavian flap repair can be affected by multiple factors, including suture technique, suture material (absorbable or nonabsorbable), tension on the suture line, incomplete excision of coarctation ridge, and the length of the flap beyond the coarctation.

The usual cause of recurrent coarctation following subclavian flap repair is lumen stenosis caused by proliferation of coarctation ridge tissue of the posterior wall.[47,59] This stimulated the modification of the subclavian flap procedure to resection and subclavian flap, as described by Dietl.[21,22] At Sutter/Sacramento, we independently began doing resection and subclavian flap repair in 1985, for the same reason. Dietl and co-workers[22] have found resection and subclavian flap to be superior to subclavian flap alone in a series of their patients. They now prefer to detach the subclavian artery and use its base for augmenting the circumferential suture line, thereby preserving normal subclavian artery blood flow.[22]

It is becoming clear that it is possible to obtain low recurrence rates following repair of coarctation with resection and end-to-end anastomosis, often with an extension of the incision under the subclavian artery and with an oblique incision of the aorta beyond the coarctation: resection and extended end-to-end anastomosis.[38,39,72] The long-term effects of subclavian flap repair on forearm vascular function and growth are minimal, with Shenberger and colleagues[64] showing normal forearm blood flow and only minor differences in anthropometric measurements. If all other things are equal, however, preservation of normal subclavian blood flow would favor resection and extended end-to-end anastomosis.

Choice of Operation: Child

Our usual operation for discrete coarctation in the child is resection and primary anastomosis. If mobility of the proximal and distal aorta is decreased, as can occur in the older child or the adult, tube graft interposition can be used. Bypass grafts from the left subclavian artery or ascending aorta to the descending aorta can be used to treat long-segment coarctation, recoarctation, or coarctation occurring in the aortic arch.[23,32,77] Left thoracotomy can be avoided in recoarctation or unusual forms by performing a bypass graft from the ascending aorta to the abdominal aorta through a midline sternotomy extended into a midline laparotomy.[17]

Assessment of Spinal Cord Blood Supply During Aortic Clamping

Assessment of collaterals is important in maximizing the adequacy of spinal cord blood supply during aortic clamping and decreasing or eliminating the occurrence of postoperative paraplegia.[10] The anterior spinal artery is not always a continuous channel, but may divide into end arteries at several different levels. If the anterior spinal artery is divided into end arteries below the coarctation, spinal cord blood supply depends on collateral flow during the period of aortic cross-clamping. If collateral flow is adequate, spinal cord ischemia is extremely rare, regardless of the number of intercostals divided or the duration of aortic occlusion.[10]

Lack of satisfactory collateral flow is suggested preoperatively by pulses in the lower extremities, lack of hypertension in the arms, and lack of collateral vessels on angiography. Deficient collateral flow should be strongly suspected in the case of recurrent coarctation.

Most children with coarctation will have adequate collaterals, as indicated by angiography and clinical examination and can undergo simple clamping and an expeditious resection and anastomosis with a very low risk of spinal cord injury. In special situations where collateral flow is questionable, it has been suggested that collateral flow can be assessed operatively by clamping the aorta above the coarctation and checking distal aortic pressure. A distal aortic pressure of 50 mm Hg or more has been suggested to indicate adequate collateral flow.[10,30,76] If collateral flow is inadequate, resection can be performed using partial cardiopulmonary bypass or a shunt, or a bypass graft can be performed from above the coarctation to below,[23] with partial occluding clamps placed so as not to interfere with flow through the area of coarctation.

Surgical Anatomy

Usual Anatomy

Coarctation of the thoracic aorta is a congenital narrowing or stricture usually located just distal to the origin of the left subclavian artery (Fig. 16–1). Coarc-

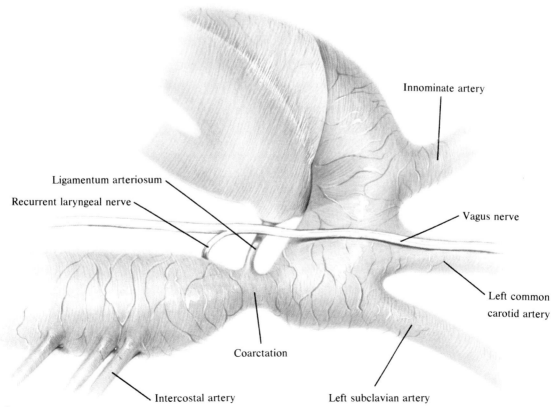

Innominate artery

Ligamentum arteriosum

Recurrent laryngeal nerve

Vagus nerve

Left common carotid artery

Coarctation

Intercostal artery

Left subclavian artery

16–1

tation may also occur between the left carotid artery and the subclavian artery or at the level of the subclavian artery involving its origin. These locations occur in less than 5% of cases.[13,68]

Keith[35] has classified coarctation in terms of location as being "preductal" or "postductal." The anatomy of the coarctation and surrounding structures is usually different in these two types, and preductal coarctation is associated with a high incidence of intracardiac defects.

Preductal coarctation is often associated with a hypoplastic aortic arch and hypoplastic isthmus narrowing proximal to the membranous portion of coarctation narrowing. There is evidence that a diminished flow in utero through the aortic arch is responsible for aortic arch abnormalities and coarctation.[48,49] Such reduced aortic arch flow could result from subtle obstruction at the aortic valve, mitral valve, or foramen ovale.[48] The coarctation is usually just above the junction of the ductus arteriosus and the aorta. The ductus arteriosus is sometimes larger than the aortic arch in this malformation. Intercostal arteries are normal. Preductal coarctation usually presents in infancy, is associated with a high incidence of intracardiac defects, and often requires urgent surgical treatment.

Postductal or juxtaductal coarctation is the most common form presenting in childhood or adulthood, although it may present in the neonatal period of infancy. The narrowing is at or just distal to the ductus arteriosus or ligamentum arteriosum. In the child or young adult this is usually 1–2 cm distal to the subclavian artery. The external diameter of the aorta, although narrow, is considerably wider than the diameter of the lumen. The aortic wall at the site of the coarctation has a thickening and infolding of the media, forming a diaphragm that may have either a lumen as small as 1 mm or no lumen at all.

The aorta just distal to the coarctation is often dilated, which increases with age. The intercostal arteries arise at a variable distance from the coarctation, usually within 1–2 cm. These arteries form part of the network of collateral circulation and are often greatly enlarged, attaining sizes several times normal. They are often tortuous, thin-walled, and extremely friable. Bronchial arteries also arise in the area of the intercostals.

Unusual Anatomy

Immobile Aorta or Long-Segment Coarctation
Resection and graft interposition is used for these conditions.

Coarctation Involving the Left Subclavian
Occurring in less than 5% of cases,[13,68] this condition is indicated clinically by absence of pulses in the left arm and left chest wall. Angiography provides confirmation. The coarctation can be resected and the subclavian artery reimplanted by using its base as an onlay patch (Fig. 16–18).

Coarctation Between Left Carotid and Left Subclavian
This lesion is difficult to resect. We have chosen to perform bypass from the ascending aorta to the descending aorta in this unusual form of coarctation. The distal anastomosis is performed through a left thoracotomy; the proximal anastomosis is performed through a median sternotomy.

Right Subclavian Artery Arising Distal to Coarctation
This rare anatomic variation is suggested clinically by absence of pulses in the right arm and right chest wall. Preoperative knowledge of its presence does not change the basic approach to the coarctation, but adjustments in dissection and clamp placement may be called for, depending on the proximity between the coarctation and the right subclavian artery.

Recurrent Coarctation
Reoperation for recurrent coarctation is associated with increased morbidity and mortality, particularly when re-resection is performed. The area of the

recoarctation is difficult to dissect. If the aorta around the previous anastomosis is friable, stitches may hold poorly and the jaws of the clamp may injure the aorta. Partial correction of the coarctation may have caused decreased or absent collaterals, thereby increasing the possibility of ischemic spinal cord injury if the aorta is cross-clamped.

Because of these factors we prefer bypass grafting for many cases of recurrent coarctation.[32] This avoids extensive dissection in the area of previous repair and avoids jeopardizing the spinal cord blood flow by cross-clamping the aorta. Bypass can be performed from the proximal segment to the descending aorta or from the ascending aorta to the descending aorta.[17,23,77]

Surgical Technique

Resection and Subclavian Artery Patch Angioplasty

A left posterolateral thoracotomy is made through the fourth intercostal space. The pleura is incised over the aorta, and the incision is carried up the subclavian artery. Retraction of the medial pleural flap carries the vagus and recurrent laryngeal nerve medially. The ductus, distal aorta, area of coarctation, left subclavian artery, and arch up to the left carotid artery are dissected (Fig. 16–2). A heavy silk tie is passed around the ductus. The branches of the subclavian artery are tied, with tying of the vertebral artery to prevent subsequent development of a subclavian steal syndrome. The ductus is ligated. A vascular clamp is placed across the aortic arch between the left carotid artery and the left subclavian artery. Another clamp is placed distal to the coarctation. Heparin is not routinely used. The distal subclavian artery is ligated and divided. A lateral incision is made in the aorta below the coarcta-

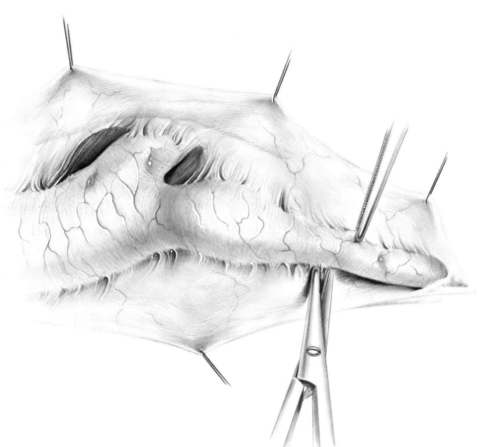

16–2

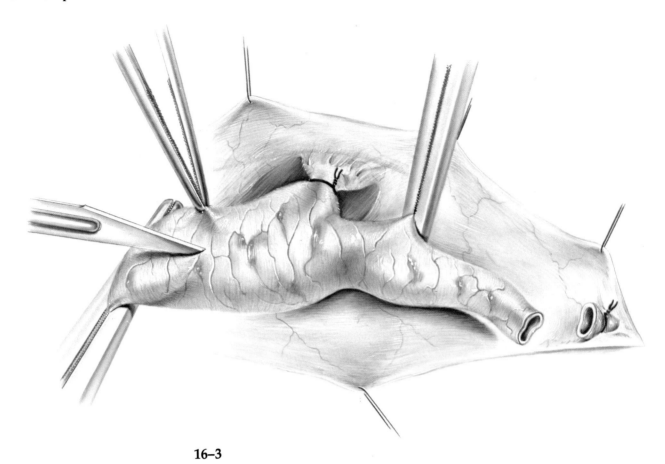

16–3

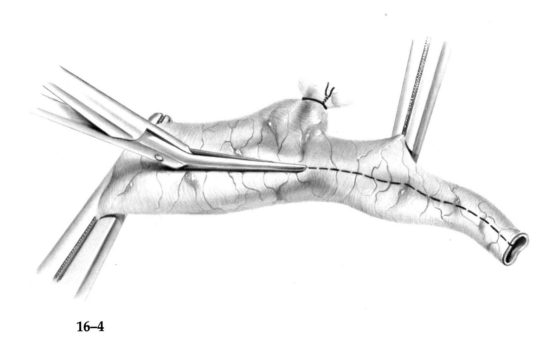

16–4

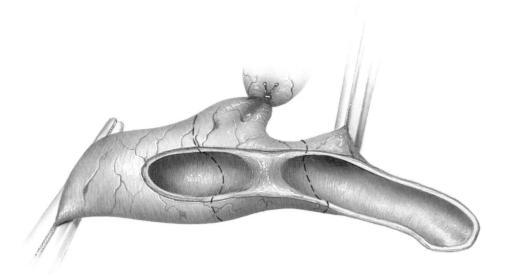

16-5

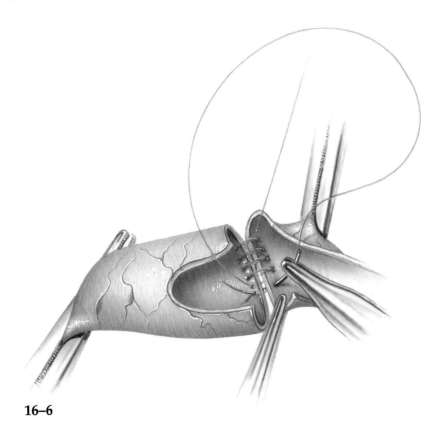

16-6

tion (Fig. 16-3) and carried through the area of coarctation into the subclavian artery (Fig. 16-4). The aorta is transected above and below the coarctation (Fig. 16-5). The posterior anastomosis is completed (Fig. 16-6). The sutures used are 6-0 absorbable polydioxanone (Sutter/Sacramento) or 6-0 prolene (Children's Cardiac Center of Oregon/Portland). Polydioxanone suture has been shown experimentally[51] and clinically[4,50] to provide a secure suture line and allow for growth. The subclavian artery flap is then brought down and sutured, with the posterior suture line suture tied to the flap suture when it is reached (Figs. 16-7, 16-8).

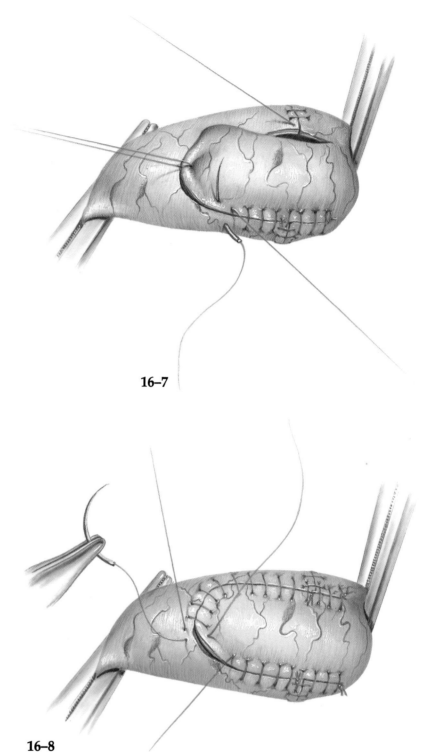

16–7

16–8

Resection with Extended End-to-End Anastomosis

A left posterolateral thoracotomy is made and the area of coarctation, ductus, left subclavian, and arch between the left carotid artery and left subclavian artery are dissected. A clamp is placed across the subclavian and distal arch and another clamp on the distal aorta, and the aorta is transected above and below the coarctation (Fig. 16-9). The underside of the distal aortic arch is incised past the base of the left subclavian artery (Fig. 16-10). The anastomosis is then performed with running 6-0 suture (Figs. 16-11, 16-12).

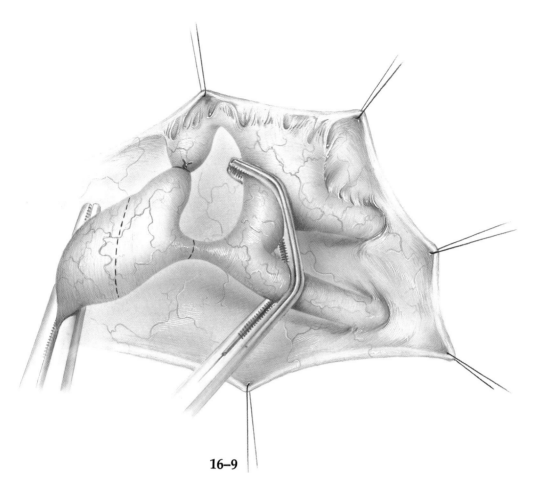

16–9

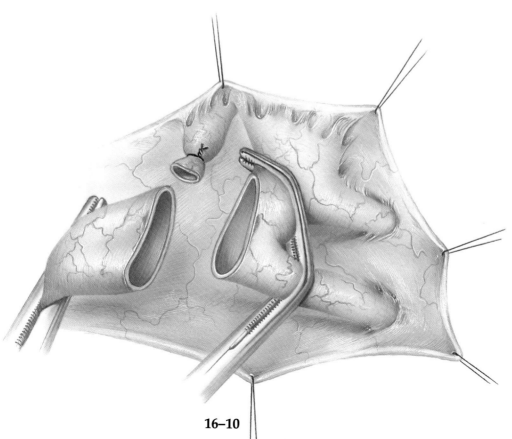

16–10

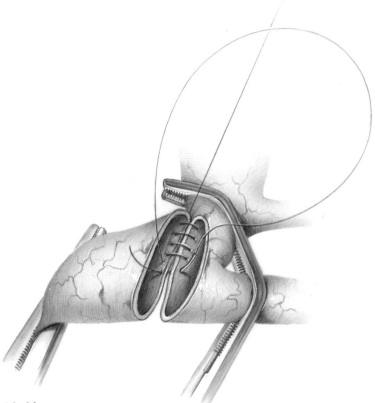

16–11

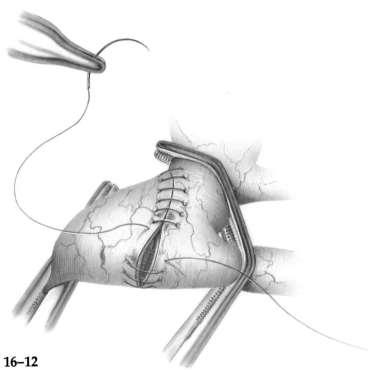

16–12

Resection with Primary Anastomosis

A left posterolateral thoracotomy is made through the fourth intercostal space. Careful incision of the latissimus and trapezius is necessary to identify and control the numerous large collateral arteries. These arteries are divided and ligated, since electrocoagulation is often ineffective or can result in delayed hemorrhage.

Pleural incision is as described previously. Dissection includes the proximal left subclavian artery, distal aortic arch, coarctation, ligamentum arteriosum, distal aorta, and intercostal arteries (Fig. 16–13). An artery may arise posteriorly around the origin of the left subclavian artery. This artery, not found in normal subjects, is called Abbott's artery, after its first description in 1928 by Maude Abbott.[1]

Intercostal arteries must be dissected with utmost care, since hemorrhage arising from them can be a major operative complication. The lateral intercostals are usually seen easily. The medial intercostals are often hidden under the aorta and can be injured by blind dissection behind the aorta or excessive retraction of the aorta.

Dissection well up onto the aortic arch and well onto the aorta distal to the coarctation provides mobile aorta for reapproximation after resection and usually permits an anastomosis without tension. Adequate dissection can provide for 2 cm of resection in the child.

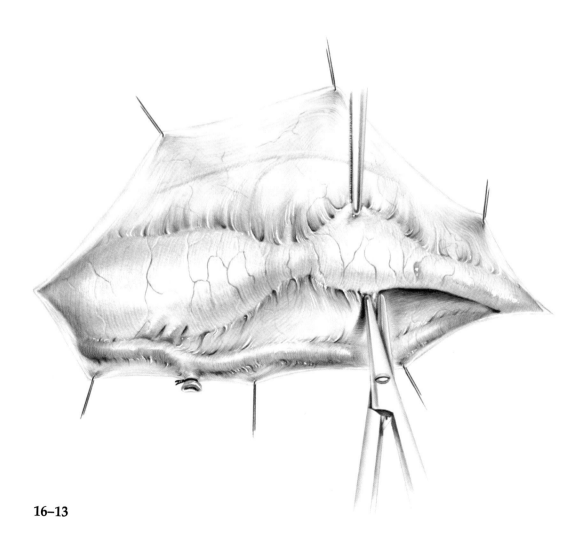

16–13

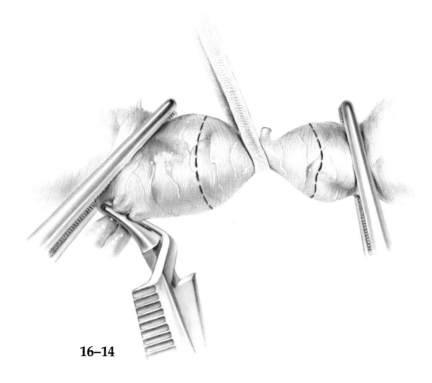

16–14

Proximal clamp placement is dictated by the distance between the subclavian artery and the coarctation (Fig. 16-14). If the length of aorta is not sufficient with the clamp placed below the left subclavian, the clamp may be placed across the base of the subclavian artery and across the arch just distal to the left carotid.

The distal clamp should be placed so as to provide 1 cm or more of aortic cuff for suturing after resection of the coarctation. This may require placement of the clamp below one or more sets of intercostals. In this situation we prefer to clamp the intercostals with small bulldog clamps. They may be divided, but during tying troublesome bleeding can occur from tearing of the friable walls.

The aorta above the coarctation should be resected at the level where its diameter equals that of the distal arch or the segment just below the subclavian. A 14-mm diameter is adequate in the adult.[11] Often, only 1-2 cm needs to be resected. A lumen equal to the distal arch at the end of repair will not have a gradient. Resecting into the dilated distal aorta or excessive tailoring of the proximal segment will not provide any hemodynamic advantage and can introduce severe technical disadvantages, such as excessive tension of the anastomosis.

The primary anastomosis is made with 5-0 polydioxanone or 5-0 polypropylene. A running suture is used for the posterior row (Fig. 16-15) and interrupted sutures for the anterior (Fig. 16-16). If absorbable polydioxanone is used, a running suture is used for the entire suture line.

Additional Procedures

Subclavian Aortoplasty
Meier and colleagues[46] have described the technique of detaching the subclavian, opening it longitudinally on its posterior aspect, incising the anterior wall of the aorta through the coarctation, excising the coarctation membrane, and suturing the subclavian flap over the aorta (Fig. 16-17). This technique can also be combined with resection of the coarctation (Fig. 16-18).

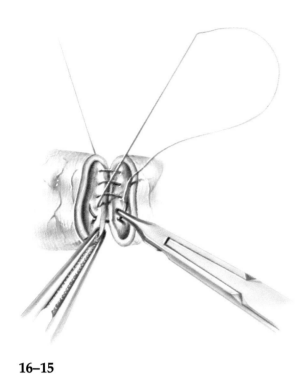

16–15

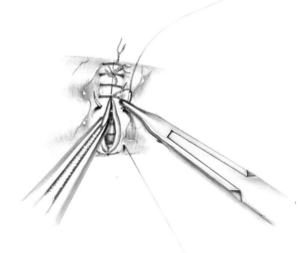

16–16

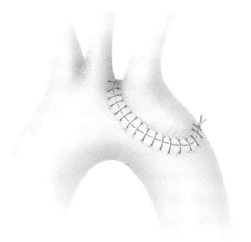

16–17

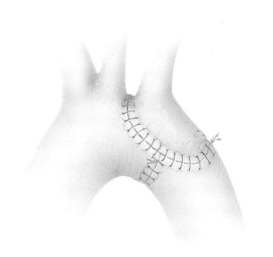

16–18

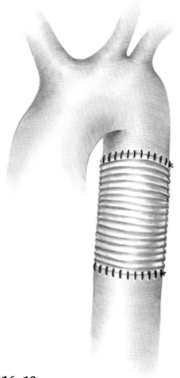

16–19

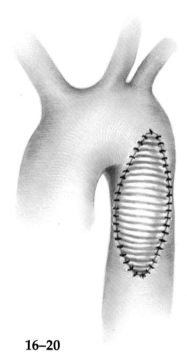

16–20

Graft Interposition

Long-segment coarctation may be repaired by resection and interposition of a segment of Dacron graft (Fig. 16–19).

Patch Aortoplasty

A lateral incision is made from the proximal aorta down through the coarctation onto the distal aorta. The inner membrane of the coarctation is excised, and a diamond-shaped patch is sutured in place, with the widest area of the patch at the area of coarctation. A patch that is cut out of a knitted Dacron tube graft of appropriate size and preclotted has a better contour than one cut from a flat Dacron patch (Fig. 16–20).

Late development of aneurysm at the site of repair is a disadvantage of prosthetic patch aortoplasty.[2,12,14] Aert and colleagues[2] found that 20% of their patients required reoperation a mean of 9 years following patch aortoplasty. Clarkson and co-workers[14] found an actuarial incidence of aneurysm formation of 38% at 14 years following patch aortoplasty.

Bypass Grafts

Long-segment coarctation or recurrent coarctation may be treated with a bypass graft from the aorta and base of the subclavian to below the coarctation (Fig. 16–21).

A bypass graft can also be placed from the ascending aorta to the descending aorta (Fig. 16–22). Our technique for this procedure is to perform the descending aorta anastomosis through a posterolateral thoracotomy after the administration of heparin. The graft is then filled with blood and placed in the upper part of the pleural cavity medial to the lung. The thoracotomy is closed. The patient is then placed supine and a sternotomy incision made, the left pleura is opened, and the graft is located. The pericardium is opened and the graft is anastomosed to the ascending aorta.

An additional possible bypass graft is from the ascending aorta to the abdominal aorta (Fig. 16–23).

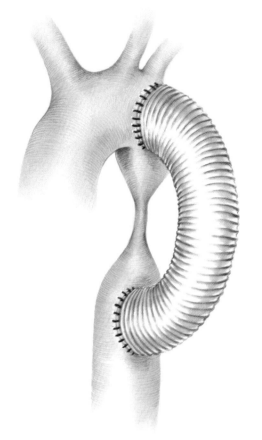

16–21

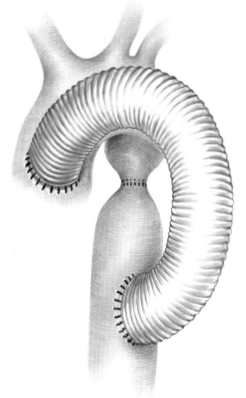

16–22

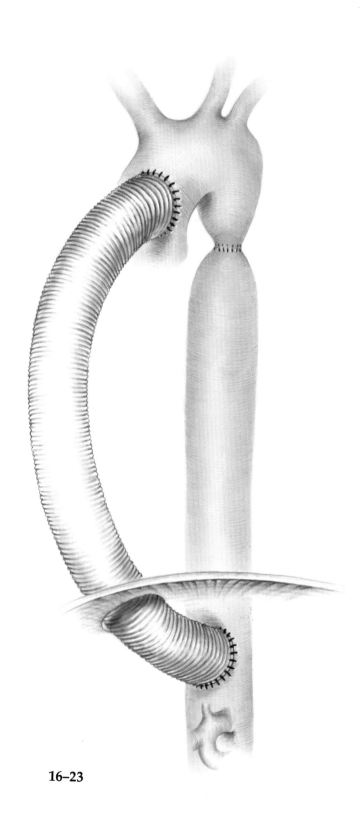

16–23

Postoperative Paradoxical Hypertension

Incidence

Hypertension is common following repair of coarctation of the aorta. The incidence in the literature varies, depending upon the definition of hypertension and the frequency of blood pressure measurement. An incidence as high as 100% has been reported.[58] There are two phases of the hypertension—an early phase occurring immediately or several hours after repair and a second phase occurring on the second or third postoperative day.[61] Hypertension in the postoperative period can cause mesenteric arteritis and bowel infarction as well as bleeding from the surgical repair.

Physiology

The mechanisms invoked to explain the postoperative hypertension in patients with coarctation include increased catecholamine secretion, carotid baroreceptor resetting, and increased renin production. The sympathetic nervous system is responsible for the initial phase of hypertension after coarctation resection, and the renin-angiotensin system may play a major role in the second phase of hypertension and in the pathogenesis of mesenteric arteritis.[58,62]

Mild abdominal pain may occur in the absence of hypertension in the postoperative period, but mesenteric arteritis is almost always associated with severe, persistent hypertension. Mesenteric arteritis is characterized by abdominal pain and tenderness, ileus, vomiting, intestinal bleeding, fever, and leukocytosis.[29] The pathologic finding is a necrotizing arteritis in vessels below the site of the coarctation, especially the branches of the superior mesenteric artery.[45] Mesenteric arteritis can progress to bowel infarction, requiring laparotomy.

Treatment

Preoperative administration of propranolol for 2 weeks before surgery can reduce the incidence and severity of postoperative hypertension.[25]

Postoperative hypertension should be vigorously treated. Treatment of hypertension appears to eliminate the occurrence of mesenteric arteritis. Although reserpine and trimethaphan have been used in the past, our present drug of choice is nitroprusside. Its rapid onset and rapid reversibility make it effective and safe. Esmolol is also an effective treatment of postoperative hypertension.[66,71] It has the advantage that it can be administered as a continuous infusion and, since it has a very short half-life, is easily titrated. Esmolol may come to supplant nitroprusside as the main drug for the treatment of postoperative hypertension. The hypertension is usually of short duration, abating before the sixth postoperative day.[58] In some patients longer-term oral treatment is necessary, and propranolol is an effective drug in this group.[78]

Results

Neonates and Infants

Mortality of coarctation repair in neonates and infants depends on the presence and severity of associated conditions. The operative mortality reported between 1984 and 1991 in neonates and infants undergoing subclavian flap repair or resection and end-to-end anastomosis has ranged from 0% to 24%, with an average mortality of a collected series totaling 1189 patients being 12%.[34] The recoarctation rate in the same series of patients ranged from 2% to 25% with an average of 14%.[34] Vouhe and colleagues[72] reported operative mortality of 0% in pure coarctation or coarctation with patent ductus arteriosus, 4% in coarctation with ventricular septal defect, and 36% in coarctation with complex intracardiac anomalies.

The severe congestive heart failure present in these ill infants is usually reversible. Severe depressions of left ventricular ejection fraction and cardiac output usually return postoperatively to normal.[27]

Children and Adults

Operative mortality is extremely low following coarctation repair in children. We have had no mortality in patients 1–30 years of age during the past 3 decades. Operative mortality is higher in patients over 40 years of age.[8]

The completeness and permanence of the reversibility of hypertension are related to age at repair. Stansel and colleagues[68] report cure of hypertension in almost all patients repaired before the age of 10 years. Maron and colleagues[44] carefully evaluated 59 patients who underwent coarctation repair at a mean age of 22 years; of these, 31% had systemic hypertension in the absence of clinical evidence of persistent or recurrent coarctation. The increasing incidence of irreversible hypertension with increasing age strongly supports repair of coarctation at an early age, preferably before 10 years.

Most patients have normal blood pressure at rest and during exercise following repair of coarctation,[5,40] although systolic hypertension may develop during exercise in patients without residual resting gradients across the area of coarctation.[33] Balderston and colleagues[5] studied 31 children during exercise following repair of coarctation. The mean age at operation was 41 months and the mean age at study was 134 months. They found above-average work capacity and normal exercise systolic blood pressure.

The long-term clinical course following repair of coarctation of the aorta is determined by the age at the time of repair. Cohen and co-workers[15] studied 646 patients who underwent coarctation repair at the Mayo Clinic from 1946 to 1981. They found that patients less than 14 years of age at the time of repair had a survival at 20 years of 91%, whereas patients older than 14 years at the time of repair had a 20-year survival of 79%. The best survivorship was observed in patients operated on at 9 years of age or less. Coronary artery disease was the most common cause of late death.

References

1. Abbott ME: Coarctation of the aorta of the adult type. Am Heart J 3:574,1928.
2. Aert H, Laas J, Bednarski P, Koch U, Prokop M, Borst HG: High incidence of aneurysm formation following patch plasty repair of coarctation. Eur J Cardiothorac Surg 7:200,1993.
3. Allen HD, Marx GR, Ovitt TW, Goldberg SJ: Balloon dilatation angioplasty for coarctation of the aorta. Am J Cardiol 57:828,1986.
4. Arenas JD, Myers JL, Gleason MM, Vennos A, Baylen BG, Waldhausen JA: End-to-end repair of aortic coarctation using absorbable polydioxanone suture. Ann Thorac Surg 51:413,1991.
5. Balderston SM, Daberkow E, Clarke DR, Wolfe RR: Maximal voluntary exercise variables in children with postoperative coarctation of the aorta. J Am Coll Cardiol 19:154,1992.
6. Beekman RH, Rocchini AP, Behrendt DM, Bove EL, Dick M II, Crowley DC, Snider AR, Rosenthal A: Long-term outcome after repair of coarctation in infancy: subclavian angioplasty does not reduce the need for reoperation. J Am Coll Cardiol 8:1406,1986.
7. Beekman RH, Rocchini AP, Dick M II, Snider AR, Crowley DC, Serwer GA, Spicer RL, Rosenthal A: Percutaneous balloon angioplasty for native coarctation of the aorta. J Am Coll Cardiol 10:1078,1987.
8. Braimbridge MV, Yen A: Coarctation in the elderly. Circulation 31:209,1965.

9. Brandt B, Marvin WJ, Rose EF, Mahoney LT: Surgical treatment of coarctation of the aorta after balloon angioplasty. J Thorac Cardovasc Surg 94:715,1987.

10. Brewer LA, Fosburg RG, Mulder GA, Verska JJ: Spinal cord complications following surgery for coarctation of the aorta. J Thorac Cardiovasc Surg 64:368,1972.

11. Brom AG: Narrowing of the aortic isthmus and enlargement of the mind. J Thorac Cardiovasc Surg 50:166,1965.

12. Bromberg BI, Beekman RH, Rocchini AP, Snider RA, Bank ER, Heidelberger K, Rosenthal A: Aortic aneurysm after patch aortoplasty repair of coarctation: a prospective analysis of prevalence, screening tests and risks. J Am Coll Cardiol 14:734,1989.

13. Clagett OT, Kirklin JW, Edwards JE: Anatomic variations and pathologic changes in coarctation of the aorta: a study of 124 cases. Surg Gynecol Obstet 98:103,1954.

14. Clarkson PM, Brandt PWT, Barratt-Boyes BG, Rutherford JD, Kerr AR, Neutze JM: Prosthetic repair of coarctation of the aorta with particular reference to Dacron onlay patch grafts and late aneurysm formation. Am J Cardiol 56:342,1985.

15. Cohen M, Fuster V, Steele PM, Driscoll D, McGoon DC: Coarctation of the aorta: long-term follow-up and prediction of outcome after surgical correction. Circulation 80:840,1989.

16. Connors JP, Hartmann AF, Weldon CS: Considerations in the surgical management of infantile coarctation of the aorta. Am J Cardiol 36:489,1975.

17. Cooley DA: Techniques in Cardiac Surgery, 2nd ed. Philadelphia, WB Saunders Co, 1984, p 49.

18. Cooper RS, Ritter SB, Rothe WB, Chen CK, Griepp R, Golinko RJ: Angioplasty for coarctation of the aorta: long-term results. Circulation 75:600,1987.

19. Cooper SG, Sullivan ID, Wren C: Treatment of recoarctation: balloon dilation angioplasty. J Am Coll Cardiol 14:413,1989.

20. Crafoord C, Nylin G: Congenital coarctation of the aorta and its surgical treatment. J Thorac Surg 14:347,1945.

21. Dietl CA, Torres AR: Coarctation of the aorta: anastomotic enlargement with subclavian artery: two new surgical options. Ann Thorac Surg 43:224,1987.

22. Dietl CA, Torres AR, Favaloro RG, Fessler CL, Grunkemeier GL: Risk of recoarctation in neonates and infants after repair with patch aortoplasty, subclavian flap, and the combined resection-flap procedure. J Thorac Cardiovasc Surg 103:724,1992.

23. Edie RN, Janani J, Attai LA, Malm JR, Robinson G: Bypass grafts for recurrent or complex coarctations of the aorta. Ann Thorac Surg 20:558,1975.

24. Fenchel G, Steil E, Seybold-Epting W, Seboldt H, Apitz J, Hoffmeister H-E: Repair of symptomatic aortic coarctation in the first three months of life: early and late results after resection and end-to-end anastomosis and subclavian flap angioplasty. J Cardiovasc Surg 29:257,1988.

25. Gidding SS, Rocchini AP, Beekman R, Szpunar CA, Moorehead C, Behrendt D, Rosenthal A: Therapeutic effect of propranolol on paradoxical hypertension after repair of coarctation of the aorta. N Engl J Med 312:1224,1985.

26. Goldman S, Hernandez J, Pappas G: Results of surgical treatment of coarctation of the aorta in the critically ill neonate: including the influence of pulmonary artery banding. J Thorac Cardiovasc Surg 91:732,1986.

27. Graham TP, Atwood GF, Boerth RC, Boucek RJ, Smith CW: Right and left heart size and function in infants with symptomatic coarctation. Circulation 56:641,1977.

28. Herrmann VM, Laks H, Fagan L, Terschluse D, Willman VL: Repair of aortic coarctation in the first year of life. Ann Thorac Surg 25:57,1978.

29. Ho ECK, Moss AJ: The syndrome of ''mesenteric arteritis'' following surgical repair of aortic coarctation. Pediatrics 49:40,1972.

30. Hughes RK, Reemtsma K: Correction of coarctation of the aorta: manometric determination of safety during test occlusion. J Thorac Cardiovasc Surg 62:31,1971.

31. Hujazi ZM, Fahey JT, Kleinman CS, Hellenbrand WE: Balloon angioplasty for recurrent coarctation of the aorta: immediate and long-term results. Circulation 84:1150,1991.

32. Jacob T, Cobanoglu A, Starr A: Late results of ascending aorta-descending aorta bypass grafts for recurrent coarctation of the aorta. J Thorac Cardiovasc Surg 95:78,1988.

33. James FW, Kaplan S: Systolic hypertension during submaximal exercise after correction of coarctation of aorta. Circulation 49,50(Suppl II):II-27,1974.

34. Johnson MC, Canter CE, Strauss AW, Spray TL: Repair of coarctation of the aorta in infancy: comparison of surgical and balloon angioplasty. Am Heart J 125: 464,1993.

35. Keith JD, Rowe RD, Vlad P: Heart Disease in Infancy and Childhood, 2nd ed. New York, Macmillan, 1967, p 216.

36. Kron IL, Flanagan TL, Rheuban KS, Carpenter MA, Gutgesell HP, Blackbourne LH, Nolan SP: Incidence and risk of reintervention after coarctation repair. Ann Thorac Surg 49:920,1990.

37. Lababidi ZA, Daskalopoulos DA, Stoeckle H: Transluminal balloon coarctation angioplasty: experience with 27 patients. Am J Cardiol 54:1288,1984.

38. Lacour-Gayet F, Conte S, Serraf A, Bruniaux J, Sousa-Uva M, Planche C: Surgical management of neonatal coarctation: a study of 221 patients. Presented at the American Association for Thoracic Surgery, 1993.

39. Lansman S, Shapiro AJ, Schiller MS, Ritter S, Cooper R, Galla JD, Lowery RC, Golinko R, Ergin A, Griepp RB: Extended aortic arch anastomosis for repair of coarctation in infancy. Circulation 74(Suppl I):I-37,1986.

40. Leandro J, Smallhorn JF, Benson L, Musewe N, Balfe JW, Dyck JD, West L, Freedom R: Ambulatory blood pressure monitoring and left ventricular mass and function after successful surgical repair of coarctation of the aorta. J Am Coll Cardiol 20:197,1992.

41. Lock JE, Bass JL, Amplatz K, Fuhrman BP, Castaneda-Zuniga W: Balloon dilatation angioplasty of aortic coarctations in infants and children. Circulation 68: 109,1983.

42. Lock JE, Niemi T, Burke BA, Einzig S, Castaneda-Zuniga WR: Transcutaneous angioplasty of experimental aortic coarctation. Circulation 68:1280,1982.

43. Macmanus Q, Starr A, Lambert LE, Grunkemeier GL: Correction of aortic coarctation in neonates: mortality and late results. Ann Thorac Surg 24:544,1977.

44. Maron BJ, Humphries JO, Rowe RD, Mellits ED: Prognosis of surgically corrected coarctation of the aorta. Circulation 47:119,1973.

45. Mays ET, Sergeant CK: Postcoarctectomy syndrome. Arch Surg 91:58,1965.

46. Meier MA, Lucchese FA, Jazbik W, Nesralla IA, Mendonca JT: A new technique for repair of aortic coarctation: subclavian flap aortoplasty with preservation of arterial blood flow to the left arm. J Thorac Cardiovasc Surg 92:1005,1986.

47. Metzdorff MT, Cobanoglu A, Grunkemeier GL, Sunderland CO, Starr A: Influence of age at operation on late results with subclavian flap aortoplasty. J Thorac Cardiovasc Surg 89:235,1985.

48. Morrow WR, Huhta JC, Murphy DJ, McNamara DG: Quantitative morphology of the aortic arch in neonatal coarctation. J Am Coll Cardiol 8:616,1986.

49. Moulaert AJ, Bruins CC, Oppenheimer-Decker A: Anomalies of the aortic arch and ventricular septal defects. Circulation 53:1011,1976.

50. Myers JL, Campbell DB, Waldhausen JA: The use of absorbable monofilament polydioxanone suture in pediatric cardiovascular operations. J Thorac Cardiovasc Surg 92:771,1986.

51. Myers JL, Waldhausen JA, Pae WE, Abt AB, Prophet GA, Pierce WS: Vascular anastomoses in growing vessels: the use of absorbable sutures. Ann Thorac Surg 34:529,1982.

52. Palatianos GM, Thurer RJ, Kaiser GA: Comparison of operations for coarctation of the aorta in infants. J Cardiovasc Surg 28:128,1987.

53. Park JK, Dell RB, Ellis K, Gersony WM: Surgical management of the infant with coarctation of the aorta and ventricular septal defect. J Am Coll Cardiol 20: 176,1992.

54. Rao PS: Balloon angioplasty for coarctation of the aorta in infancy. J Pediatr 110: 713,1987.

55. Rao PS, Chopra PS: Role of balloon angioplasty in the treatment of aortic coarctation. Ann Thorac Surg 52:621,1991.

56. Redington AN, Booth P, Shore DF, Rigby ML: Primary balloon dilatation of coarctation of the aorta in neonates. Br Heart J 64:277,1990.

57. Reifenstein GH, Levine SA, Gross RE: Coarctation of the aorta: a review of 104 autopsied cases of the ''adult type,'' 2 years of age or older. Am Heart J 33: 146,1947.

58. Rocchini AP, Rosenthal A, Barger AC, Castaneda AR, Nadas AS: Pathogenesis of paradoxical hypertension after coarctation resection. Circulation 54:382,1976.

59. Sanchez GR, Balsara RK, Dunn JM, Mehta AV, O'Riordan AC: Recurrent obstruction after subclavian flap repair of coarctation of the aorta in infants: can it be predicted or prevented? J Thorac Cardiovasc Surg 91:738,1986.

60. Sciolaro C, Copeland J, Cork R, Barkenbush M, Donnerstein R, Goldberg S: Long-term follow-up comparing subclavian flap angioplasty to resection with modified end-to-end anastomosis. J Thorac Cardiovasc Surg 101:1,1991.

61. Sealy WC: Coarctation of the aorta and hypertension. Ann Thorac Surg 3:15,1967.

62. Sealy WC: Paradoxical hypertension after repair of coarctation of the aorta: a review of its causes. Ann Thorac Surg 50:323,1990.

63. Shaddy RE, Boucek MM, Sturtevant JE, Ruttenberg HD, Jaffe RB, Tani LY, Judd VE, Veasy LG, McGough EC, Orsmond GS: Comparison of angioplasty and surgery for unoperated coarctation of the aorta. Circulation 87:793,1993.

64. Shenberger JS, Prophet SA, Waldhausen JA, Davidson WR, Sinoway LI: Left subclavian flap aortoplasty for coarctation of the aorta: effects on forearm vascular function and growth. J Am Coll Cardiol 14:953,1989.

65. Sinha SN, Kardatzke ML, Cole RB, Muster AJ, Wessel JU, Paul MH: Coarctation of the aorta in infancy. Circulation 40:385,1969.

66. Smerling A, Gersony WM: Esmolol for severe hypertension following repair of aortic coarctation. Crit Care Med 18:1288,1990.

67. Sos T, Sniderman KW, Rettek-Sos B, Strupp A, Alonso DR: Percutaneous transluminal dilatation of coarctation of thoracic aorta post mortem. Lancet 2:970,1979.

68. Stansel HC, Tabry IF, Poirier RA, Berman MA, Hellenbrand WE: One hundred consecutive coarctation resections followed from one to thirteen years. J Pediat Surg 12:279,1977.

69. Trinquet F, Vouhe PR, Vernant F, Touati G, Roux P-M, Pome G, Leca F, Neveux J-Y: Coarctation of the aorta in infants: which operation? Ann Thorac Surg 45:186,1988.

70. van Son JAM, Daniels O, Vincent JG, van Lier HJJ, Lacquet LK: Appraisal of resection and end-to-end anastomosis for repair of coarctation of the aorta in infancy: preference for resection. Ann Thorac Surg 48:496,1989.

71. Vincent RN, Click LA, Williams HM, Plauth WH, Williams WH: Esmolol as an adjunct in the treatment of systemic hypertension after operative repair of coarctation of the aorta. Am J Cardiol 65:941,1990.

72. Vouhe PR, Trinquet F, Lecompte Y, Vernant F, Roux P-M, Touati G, Pome G, Leca F, Neveux J-Y: Aortic coarctation with hypoplastic aortic arch: results of extended end-to-end aortic arch anastomosis. J Thorac Cardiovasc Surg 96:557,1988.

73. Waldhausen JA, Nahrwold DL: Repair of coarctation of the aorta with a subclavian flap. J Thorac Cardiovasc Surg 51:532,1966.

74. Waldman JD: Make balloon dilatation an approved procedure for recurrent coarctation in children (editorial). Circulation 84:1440,1991.

75. Waldman JD, Karp RB: How should we treat coarctation of the aorta? (editorial). Circulation 87:1043,1993.

76. Watterson KG, Dhasmana JP, O'Higgins JW, Wisheart JD: Distal aortic pressure during coarctation operation. Ann Thorac Surg 49:987,1990.

77. Weldon CS, Hartmann AF, Steinhoff NG, Morrissey JD: A simple, safe and rapid technique for the management of recurrent coarctation of the aorta. Ann Thorac Surg 15:510,1973.

78. Will RJ, Walker OM, Traugott RC, Treasure RL: Sodium nitroprusside and propranolol therapy for management of postcoarctectomy hypertension. J Thorac Cardiovasc Surg 75:722,1978.

79. Ziemer G, Jonas RA, Perry SB, Freed MD, Castaneda AR: Surgery for coarctation of the aorta in the neonate. Circulation 74(Suppl I):I-25,1986.

17

Systemic-Pulmonary Shunts

The dramatic performance of an anastomosis between the left subclavian artery and the left pulmonary artery by Alfred Blalock on November 29, 1944, inaugurated the age of surgical treatment of cyanotic congenital heart disease.[4] This operation, performed in a 15-month-old girl, was strongly encouraged by Helen Taussig and was stimulated by research being carried out in Blalock's research laboratory.[24] In the ensuing decades, a number of additional operations have been developed to improve deficient pulmonary blood flow by constructing a communication between the systemic and pulmonary circulations.

This chapter describes the historical evolution of the shunting procedures, the advantages and disadvantages of the different operations, and the indications, techniques, and results of the three operations we consider most pertinent today: the Classic Blalock-Taussig shunt, the Modified Blalock-Taussig shunt, and the Central shunt using the prosthetic material polytetrafluoroethylene.

History

In spite of Blalock's initial success in a small child, it soon became apparent that thrombosis of the shunt was a problem in small children. The surgical instruments, sutures, and techniques used in that period were poorly suited for anastomosis of small vessels. The troublesome occurrence of thrombosis with the Blalock-Taussig shunt stimulated development of other operations, some of which had more dependable patency, but also introduced complications not usually found with the Blalock-Taussig shunt.

Potts, Smith, and Gibson[21] developed the anastomosis between the descending thoracic aorta and left pulmonary artery and reported it in 1946. Although this shunt decreased the incidence of thrombosis, it is seldom used any longer because it has a high incidence of excessive pulmonary blood flow and development of pulmonary vascular disease. The Potts shunt is also difficult to close at the time of corrective surgery.[15]

Waterston[28] in 1962 reported his construction of a shunt between the ascending aorta and the right pulmonary artery. This report appeared in a non-English-language journal of limited circulation. Widespread use of the Waterston shunt was stimulated by the report of Cooley and Hallman[7] in 1966. The Waterston shunt has serious disadvantages: high pulmonary blood flow may cause secondary congestive heart failure and pulmonary vascular disease[3,20]; kinking can occur at the anastomosis with almost all the flow going to the right lung with inadequate growth of the left pulmonary artery; closure of the anastomosis at total repair may require detachment and patching of the pulmonary artery.[8,9,11,29] Waterston himself preferred the Blalock-Taussig shunt, having stated in 1972: "Because of the low incidence of cardiac decompensation, we generally prefer the Blalock-Taussig shunt whenever the anatomy or size of the subclavian artery permits."[27] We have performed the Waterston shunt occasionally in the past, but have since abandoned it.

The development of microporous expanded polytetrafluoroethylene grafts has made available an additional method of creating communication between the systemic and pulmonary circuits,[12,14,17] including the Modified Blalock-Taussig shunt and the Central shunt, both of which will be shown in this chapter.

The ideal systemic-pulmonary shunt (1) is suitable for all anatomic variations, (2) can be performed quickly and easily, (3) is free of early and late morbidity and mortality, (4) does not result in excessive pulmonary blood flow causing congestive heart failure and pulmonary vascular disease, (5) has good longevity in that it maintains adequate pulmonary blood flow with growth of the child, (6) is easy to close at the time of total repair, and (7) leaves no residual abnormality after closure. No shunt has all these desirable attributes. Therefore, the choice of shunt in a given patient depends upon the anatomic possibilities and the short- and long-term objectives of management of the malformation.

Classic Blalock-Taussig Shunt

Indications for Surgery

The Classic Blalock-Taussig shunt has always had the following advantages: (1) an extremely low incidence of secondary congestive heart failure and pulmonary vascular disease, (2) ease of closure at reparative surgery, (3) lack of residual abnormality after closure, and (4) possibility of growth of the anastomosis. The predominant disadvantages of the Blalock-Taussig shunt— early and late failure, especially when performed in the neonate or infant— have largely been overcome with the advent of microsurgical techniques. The potential disadvantage of longer operating time has been overcome by improvement in perioperative oxygenation by pharmacologic dilatation of the ductus with prostaglandin.[5,13,19] Additional potential complications of the Blalock-Taussig shunt include Horner's syndrome and arm growth abnormalities. Severe arm ischemia from division of the subclavian artery is extremely rare.[2]

Improvements in surgical technique and the shunt's basic value contributed to a renascence of the Blalock-Taussig shunt during the 1970s. Reports of a high degree of success in neonates and infants have shown that a properly constructed Blalock-Taussig shunt can function well regardless of age or size.[2,6,16,25] The Classic Blalock-Taussig shunt remains an option for most cyanotic malformations requiring palliation, although in recent years we have generally preferred the Modified Blalock-Taussig shunt, since it is more predictable in avoiding overcirculation, or a Central shunt.

Surgical Technique

The success of the Blalock-Taussig shunt in the neonate or infant appears to depend on (1) use of the subclavian artery before its branches, (2) extensive dissection of the innominate and right common carotid arteries to improve downward mobility of the subclavian, (3) spatulating the subclavian artery to enlarge the anastomosis, and (4) meticulous suture techniques with fine suture material (6–0 polydioxanone or 6–0 or 7–0 polypropylene). The shunt should be performed on the side opposite the aortic arch to avoid kinking at

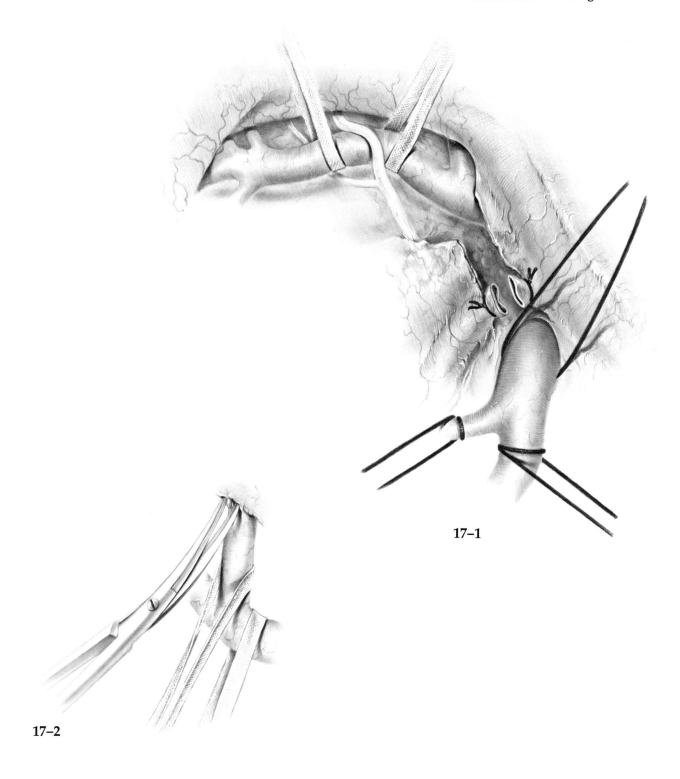

17–1

17–2

the takeoff of the subclavian artery. Although Blalock performed the shunt through an anterolateral thoracotomy, we prefer a full lateral thoracotomy through the fourth interspace. The main pulmonary artery and its branches are dissected and encircled (Fig. 17–1). Division of the azygos vein may improve mobility of the main pulmonary artery.

The mediastinal pleura is incised between the vagus and phrenic nerves, and the subclavian artery dissected out to its branches, taking care to avoid injury to the phrenic nerve, recurrent laryngeal nerve, and ansa subclavia. Dissection down the innominate artery and up the right common carotid artery (Fig. 17–2) is an essential step. This increases the mobility of the subcla-

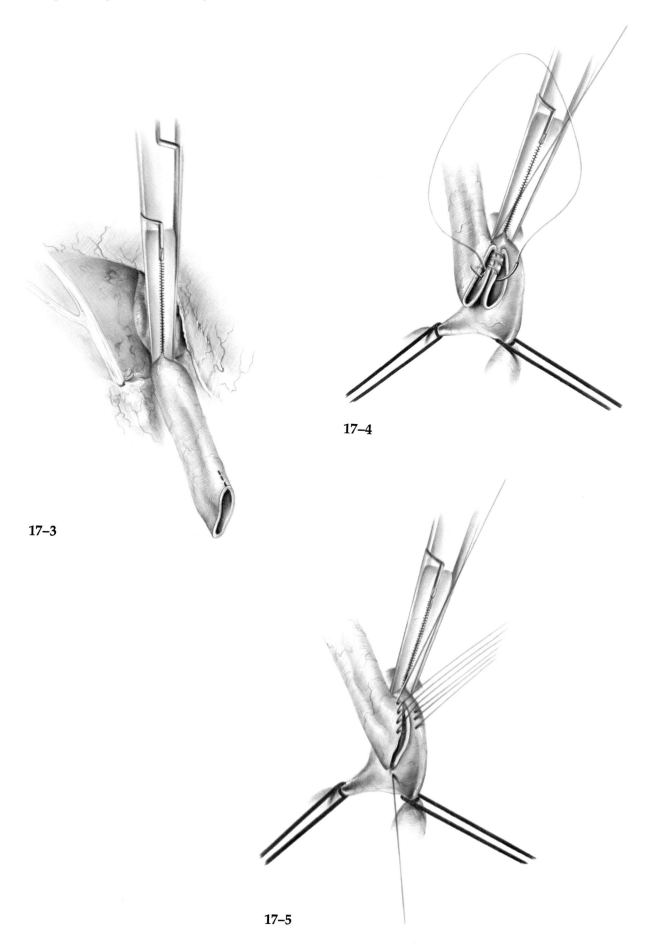

17–3

17–4

17–5

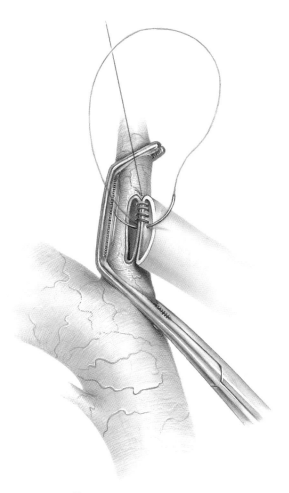

17-6

vian artery toward the hilum. The subclavian is clamped near its origin, tied distally, and divided. The subclavian artery is then brought carefully through the recurrent laryngeal nerve sling, and the end of the artery is spatulated (Fig. 17-3).

The main pulmonary artery is clamped proximally, distal loops are tightened, and a transverse or longitudinal incision is made. The posterior suture line is running (Fig. 17-4). The anterior suture line is interrupted (Fig. 17-5) if prolene is used, running if absorbable polydioxanone is used. The resulting anastomosis is larger than the diameter of the subclavian artery.

Results

The Classic Blalock-Taussig shunt has always been an excellent shunt for children. With the advent of initial corrective procedures during infancy for most cyanotic malformations, there are fewer indications for a shunt during childhood. The patient group requiring shunting at present are those with disorders not suitable for initial corrective surgery, such as tricuspid atresia or tetralogy of Fallot with pulmonary atresia or small pulmonary arteries. These patients usually require shunting during infancy or the neonatal period.

The Classic Blalock-Taussig shunt can give good results in these small patients. Arciniegas and co-workers[2] reported 63 patients operated on at less than 1 year of age, with only 4.2% of the hospital survivors requiring another operation before they were 3 years old. Tyson and colleagues[25] reported 12 patients less than 1 year of age with no late shunt failures.

Modified Blalock-Taussig Shunt

Expanded polytetrafluoroethylene (PTFE) grafts began to be used in the 1970s as alternative methods of creating communications between the systemic and pulmonary circulations.[12,14,17] The Modified Blalock-Taussig shunt is a connection between the subclavian artery and pulmonary artery using a PTFE graft, usually from 4 to 6 mm in size. The Modified Blalock-Taussig shunt is easier to perform, requires less dissection and has a lower risk of phrenic nerve injury, and, if no subclavian stenosis is produced, maintains normal arm blood flow. The Modified Blalock-Taussig shunt can be performed with patency as good as or better than the Classic Blalock-Taussig shunt, in all age groups, and has a very low incidence of pulmonary artery distortion.[18,22,26] For these reasons we perform the Modified Blalock-Taussig shunt more frequently than the Classic Blalock-Taussig shunt.

Surgical Technique

The shunt is usually performed on the same side as the aortic arch. A posterolateral thoracotomy incision is made and the fourth intercostal space is entered. The pulmonary artery and its branches are dissected and encircled as shown in Figure 17–1. The proximal subclavian artery is dissected. Heparin is administered.

A partial occluding clamp is placed so it clamps the proximal and distal subclavian artery, and a longitudinal incision is made. A PTFE graft is cut diagonally and sutured to the subclavian artery, usually with 6-0 polypropylene (Figs. 17–6, 17–7). The proximal pulmonary artery is clamped and the

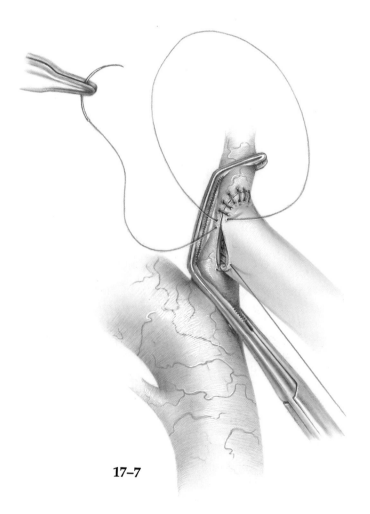

17–7

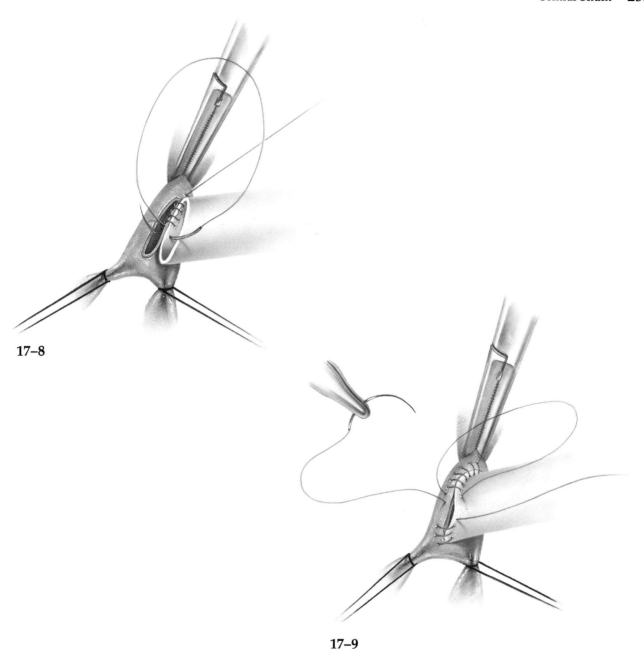

17–8

17–9

ligatures on the branches tightened. The pulmonary artery is incised longitudinally on its superior aspect, and the PTFE graft is cut to length and sutured to the pulmonary artery with polypropylene (Figs. 17-8, 17-9).

Results

With the use of modern microsurgical techniques and contemporary perioperative management of these critically ill patients, operative mortality as low as 6% can be obtained.[10,23] Patency rates can be excellent, as high as 89% at 3 years.[22]

Central Shunt

Construction of a shunt between the ascending aorta and the main pulmonary artery is useful when the branch pulmonary arteries are very small, a previously constructed Modified Blalock-Taussig shunt has failed, or a con-

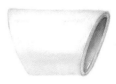

17–10

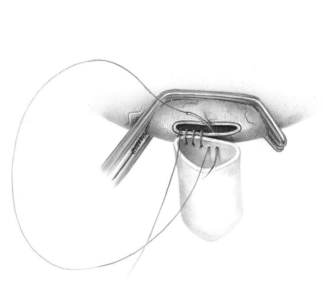

17–11

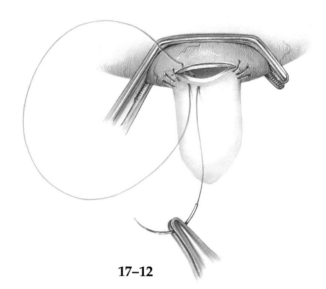

17–12

comitant procedure, such as a transventricular closed pulmonary valvotomy, requires a median sternotomy. A central shunt with a PTFE graft can be performed with low operative mortality and a patency rate equal or superior to the Blalock-Taussig shunt.[1]

Surgical Technique

A median sternotomy is performed and the pericardium is opened and suspended. Heparin is administered. A short piece of PTFE graft, 4 mm for the neonate, is cut with a bevel on each end (Fig. 17–10), so it will fit between the ascending aorta and main pulmonary artery without kinking. A portion of the pulmonary artery is excluded with a partial occluding clamp, and a longitudinal incision is made. The posterior suture line is performed inside-out the pulmonary artery and outside-in the graft (Fig. 17–11), usually with 6–0 polypropylene. The anterior suture line is performed outside-in the pulmonary artery and inside-out the graft (Fig. 17–12).

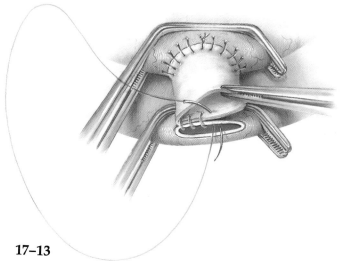

17–13

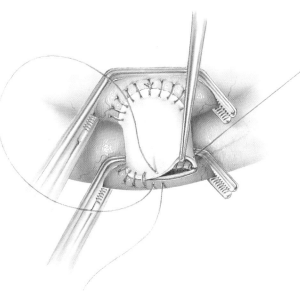

17–14

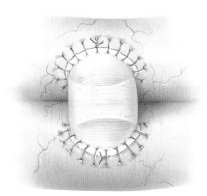

17–15

A second partial occluding clamp is used to exclude a portion of ascending aorta, and a longitudinal incision is made. The posterior suture line is performed inside-out the graft and outside-in the aorta (Fig. 17–13). The anterior suture line is performed outside-in the graft and inside-out the aorta (Fig. 17–14). The air is flushed out of the graft, the suture tied, and the clamps released (Fig. 17–15).

References

1. Amato JJ, Marbey ML, Bush C, Galdieri RJ, Cotroneo JV, Bushong J: Systemic-pulmonary polytetrafluoroethylene shunts in palliative operations for congenital heart disease: revival of the central shunt. J Thorac Cardiovasc Surg 95:62,1988.

2. Arciniegas E, Blackstone EH, Pacifico AD, Kirklin JW: Classic shunting operations as part of a two-stage repair of tetralogy of Fallot. Ann Thorac Surg 27:514,1979.

3. Bernhard WF, Jones JE, Friedberg DZ, Litwin SB: Ascending aorta-right pulmonary artery shunt in infants and older patients with certain types of cyanotic congenital heart disease. Circulation 43:580,1971.

4. Blalock A, Taussig HB: The surgical treatments of malformations of the heart in which there is pulmonary stenosis or pulmonary atresia. JAMA 128:189,1945.

5. Browdie DA, Norberg W, Agnew R, Altenburg B, Ignacio R, Hamilton C: The use of prostaglandin E_1 and Blalock-Taussig shunts in neonates with cyanotic congenital heart disease. Ann Thorac Surg 27:508,1979.

6. Chopra PS, Levy JM, Dacumos GC Jr, Berkoff HA, Loring LL, Kahn DR: The Blalock-Taussig operation: the procedure of choice in the hypoxic infant with tetralogy of Fallot. Ann Thorac Surg 22:235,1976.

7. Cooley DA, Hallman GL: Intrapericardial aortic-right pulmonary arterial anastomosis. Surg Gynec Obstet 122:1084,1966.

8. Cooley DA, Smith JM: Repair of pulmonary arterial stenosis after Waterston-Cooley anastomosis. J Thorac Cardiovasc Surg 77:474,1979.

9. Ebert PA, Gay WA Jr, Oldham HN: Management of aorta-right pulmonary artery anastomosis during total correction of tetralogy of Fallot. Surgery 71:231,1972.

10. Fermanis GG, Ekangaki AK, Salmon AP, Keeton BR, Shore DF, Lamb RK, Monro JL: Twelve year experience with the modified Blalock-Taussig shunt in neonates. Eur J Cardio-thorac Surg 6:586,1992.

11. Gay WA Jr, Ebert PA: Aorta-to-right pulmonary artery anastomosis causing obstruction of the right pulmonary artery: management during correction of tetralogy of Fallot. Ann Thorac Surg 16:402,1973.

12. Gazzaniga AB, Lamberti JJ, Siewers RD, Sperling DR, Dietrick WR, Arcilla RA, Replogle RL: Arterial prosthesis of microporous expanded polytetrafluoroethylene for construction of aorta-pulmonary shunt. J Thorac Cardiovasc Surg 72:357,1976.

13. Heymann MA, Rudolph AM: Ductus arteriosus dilatation by prostaglandin E_1 in infants with pulmonary atresia. Pediatrics 59:325,1977.

14. Jennings RB, Innes BJ, Brickman RD: Use of microporous expanded polytetrafluoroethylene grafts for aorta-pulmonary shunts in infants with complex cyanotic heart disease. J Thorac Cardiovasc Surg 76:489,1978.

15. Kirklin JW, Devloo RA: Hypothermic perfusion and circulatory arrest for surgical correction of tetralogy of Fallot with previously constructed Potts anastomosis. Dis Chest 39:87,1961.

16. Marbarger JP, Sandza JG Jr, Hartmann AF, Weldon CS: Blalock-Taussig anastomosis: the preferred shunt in infants and newborns. Circulation 58(Suppl I):I-73,1978.

17. Miyamoto K, Zavanella C, Lewin AN, Subramanian S: Aorta-pulmonary artery shunts with expanded polytetrafluoroethylene (PTFE) tube. Ann Thorac Surg 27:414,1979.

18. Moulton AL, Brenner JI, Ringel R, Nordenberg A, Berman MA, Ali S, Burns J: Classic versus modified Blalock-Taussig shunts in neonates and infants. Circulation 72(Suppl II):II-35,1985.

19. Neutze JM, Starling MB, Elliott RB, Barratt-Boyes BG: Palliation of cyanotic congenital heart disease in infancy with E-type prostaglandins. Circulation 55:238,1977.

20. Norberg WJ, Tadavarthy M, Knight L, Nicoloff DM, Moller JH: Late hemodynamic and angiographic findings after ascending aorta-pulmonary artery anastomosis. J Thorac Cardiovasc Surg 76:345,1978.

21. Potts WJ, Smith S, Gibson S: Anastomosis of the aorta to a pulmonary artery. JAMA 132:627,1946.

22. Sakai K, Goh K, Gohda T, Sakuma M, Matsunami O, Yasuda K, Tanabe T, Murakami T: Modified versus classical Blalock-Taussig shunts for congenital cyanotic heart diseases: a comparison of long-term results. Jpn J Surg 17:470,1987.

23. Smith VC, Caggiano AV, Knauf DG, Alexander JA: The Blalock-Taussig shunt in the newborn infant. J Thorac Cardiovasc Surg 102:602,1991.
24. Thomas V: Pioneering Research in Surgical Shock and Cardiovascular Surgery: Vivian Thomas and His Work with Alfred Blalock. Philadelphia, University of Pennsylvania Press, 1985.
25. Tyson KRT, Larrieu AJ, Kirchmer JT: The Blalock-Taussig shunt in the first two years of life: a safe and effective procedure. Ann Thorac Surg 26:38,1978.
26. Ullom RL, Sade RM, Crawford FA Jr, Ross BA, Spinale F: The Blalock-Taussig shunt in infants: standard versus modified. Ann Thorac Surg 44:539,1987.
27. Waterston DJ, Stark J, Ashcraft KW: Ascending aorta-to-right pulmonary artery shunts: experience with 100 patients. Surgery 72:897,1972.
28. Waterston DJ: Treatment of Fallot's tetralogy in children under one year of age. Rozhl Chir 41:181,1962.
29. Yamamoto N, Reul GJ Jr, Kidd JN, Cooley DA, Hallman GL: A new approach to repair of pulmonary branch stenosis following ascending aorta-right pulmonary artery anastomosis. Ann Thorac Surg 21:237,1976.

18

Pulmonary Valve Stenosis

This chapter deals with obstruction at the level of the pulmonary valve with an intact ventricular septum. The obstruction may be caused by valvular stenosis or atresia and is often accompanied by a variable degree of infundibular muscular stenosis. Pulmonary stenosis or atresia presenting in the neonatal period can be a difficult problem. Moderate to severe pulmonary stenosis presenting in the child or adult can usually be managed by a percutaneous balloon valvuloplasty. If surgery for pulmonary valvar stenosis is required in the child or adult, it can be performed at very low risk.

Percutaneous Balloon Valvuloplasty

Percutaneous balloon valvuloplasty was first reported by Semb and colleagues[35] in 1979 and Kan and colleagues[18] in 1982. Since then balloon valvuloplasty has become the treatment of choice for pulmonary valvar stenosis. It can be performed at very low risk and effectively reduces the transvalvar gradient.[21,30,32,37] These good results persist for at least 4 to 5 years.[23,28] O'Connor and co-workers[28] compared a group of patients who had balloon valvuloplasty with a similar group of patients who had surgery, although the mean time of follow-up was 5.3 years for the valvuloplasty group and 11.7 years for the surgical group. They found that balloon valvuloplasty provided nearly equivalent long-term gradient relief with less valvular insufficiency and less late ventricular ectopic activity.

Pulmonary Valvotomy

Indications for Surgery and Choice of Operation

Neonate
Pulmonary stenosis or atresia with intact ventricular septum presenting in the first days of life is lethal without surgical treatment. Pulmonary blood flow is dependent upon the ductus; and as the ductus closes, these patients present with severe cyanosis and acidosis. The difficulty in management of this condition is reflected in the number and variety of surgical approaches.[2,7,9,10,13,14,15,22]

A wide variety of operations have been described for the initial procedure, including a number of different types of open valvotomy[17,19] and closed valvotomy,[15,25] with transanular patching[10,24] and without transanular patching,[22,25] with systemic-pulmonary shunting[17,19,22] and without systemic-pulmonary shunting.[10,24] Rarer initial operations have been described for patients with severely hypoplastic right ventricles, including thromboexclusion of the right ventricle[38] and avulsion of the tricuspid valve.[36] Definitive procedures are either biventricular repair with a right ventricular outflow tract patch and take-down of systemic-pulmonary shunts,[1,9] usually with partial or complete closure of the atrial septal defect or patent foramen ovale, and univentricular repair with total cavopulmonary connection (Fontan procedure).[1,9] Biventricular repair with a bidirectional cavopulmonary shunt has also been described.[2]

The broad heterogeneity of morphology in this condition affects the selection of initial and subsequent surgical management.[14] The size and morphology of the right ventricle spans the spectrum of near normal size with an open infundibulum to a severely hypoplastic chamber with only an inlet portion and no trabecular or infundibular portion. Approximately half of the patients will have right ventricular to coronary connections,[7,14] and a small portion will have coronary circulation that is dependent on the right ventricle.[6,12,14] There is a wide variation in size of the tricuspid valve, which correlates with right ventricular size.[14]

A number of methods have evolved to assess tricuspid valve size and right ventricular size and morphology and thereby guide selection of initial and subsequent surgical intervention. Bull and co-workers[5] have described a classification system based on a tripartite division of the right ventricle into inlet, trabecular, and infundibular portions. The right ventricle is categorized depending on how many of the three parts are present. A system of subjective assessment has been described dividing the degree of right ventricular hypoplasia into mild, moderate, and severe.[26] Measurement of the tricuspid valve diameter has been performed during catheterization, using the known dimension of the catheter as a reference point. The tricuspid valve size is then compared to the normal.[9,25] A recent multiinstitutional study by the Congenital Heart Surgeons Society[14] measured the tricuspid size by two-dimensional echocardiography and then compared it to mean normal diameters and their standard deviations from the anatomic studies of Rowlatt, Rimoldi, and Lev.[33] The right ventricular cavity size was estimated from echocardiography or angiocardiography.

Our initial operation for management of pulmonary stenosis or pulmonary atresia with presence of an infundibulum that is patent up to the valve is closed valvotomy with a central shunt (Sutter/Sacramento) or closed pulmonary valvotomy with postoperative continuation of prostaglandin E_1 with performance of a subsequent shunt depending on the ability to wean the prostaglandin E_1 (Children's Cardiac Center of Oregon/Portland). If there is no patent infundibulum, only a central shunt is performed.

It is not necessary, nor is it always possible, to drop right ventricular pressure to below systemic levels or to raise arterial oxygen levels to normal. After valvotomy alone, the oxygen tension gradually rises as right ventricular compliance increases, right ventricular volume increases, and right ventricular filling pressure drops—all resulting in a reduction in the right-to-left shunt at the atrial level.

Valvotomy in the neonatal period seldom results in permanent relief of stenosis. Repeat valvotomy, frequently with patch enlargement of the pulmonary anulus (a low-risk procedure at that time), is usually necessary within the first 3 years of life.[13] Decision as to whether a biventricular repair or a univentricular repair is chosen is determined either by subjective assessment of right ventricular morphology and size[26] or by measurement of tricuspid valve dimension.[25]

Child and Adult
Pulmonary stenosis can cause easy fatigability, dyspnea on exertion, or cyanosis on exertion or at rest. It also may be asymptomatic.[8] We consider a gradient of 80 mm Hg or more or right ventricular pressure over 100 mm Hg to be an indication for surgery. Gradients between 50 and 80 must be considered on an individual basis. Gradients less than 50 mm Hg can be tolerated well for years and are not usually an indication for surgery.[16]

Surgical Strategy

Myocardial Preservation
Cold blood cardioplegia is used.

Management of the Foramen Ovale
A small foramen ovale is seldom closed. However, a significant atrial defect should be excluded, either preoperatively by echocardiography or at the time of operation by palpation or inspection. The foramen ovale is never closed in neonates, since closure would prevent decompression of the right side of the heart.

Transanular Patch
The method of determining the necessity of a transanular patch during tetralogy of Fallot repair (Chapter 22), as described by Pacifico, Kirklin, and Blackstone,[29] is also applicable to isolated pulmonary stenosis. This method bases the decision for enlargement of the pulmonary valve ring on a weight-related or surface area-related "minimum pulmonary valve ring diameter." This method is based on the studies of normal pulmonary anulus size by Rowlatt, Rimoldi, and Lev.[33]

Calibrated dilators are passed through the pulmonary valve from above. If valvotomy does not result in a normal or near-normal pulmonary diameter, the incision is extended across the anulus and a patch is placed. The chart of Pacifico and colleagues is also useful for determining the size of the patch. We do not usually place transanular patches in neonates, expecting that they will need a second operation.

Infundibular Resection
Marked infundibular hypertrophy occurs in approximately 50% of cases of pulmonary stenosis. However, infundibular resection or patching is rarely needed. The infundibular stenosis is usually dynamic and resolves after relief of the valvular stenosis.

The ventriculogram should be carefully assessed to determine the state of the infundibulum throughout the cardiac cycle. The dynamic basis of the infundibular stenosis is demonstrated by relaxation and wide opening of the infundibular region during diastole.

At operation the infundibulum is exposed through the valve after valvotomy. Inspection usually reveals no evidence of infundibular fibrosis or fixed narrowing. The probes that are passed through the valve are also passed through the infundibulum into the right ventricle. They should pass with little, if any, resistance. If fibrosis or fixed resistance is found, infundibular muscle is resected through the pulmonary valve or, more likely, by ventriculotomy with patch graft. We have found resection to be necessary in less than 10% of cases.

Surgical Technique

Closed Valvotomy
Closed valvotomy was the original surgical approach for pulmonary stenosis.[3,4,34] The instruments that we use for closed valvotomy are shown in Figure

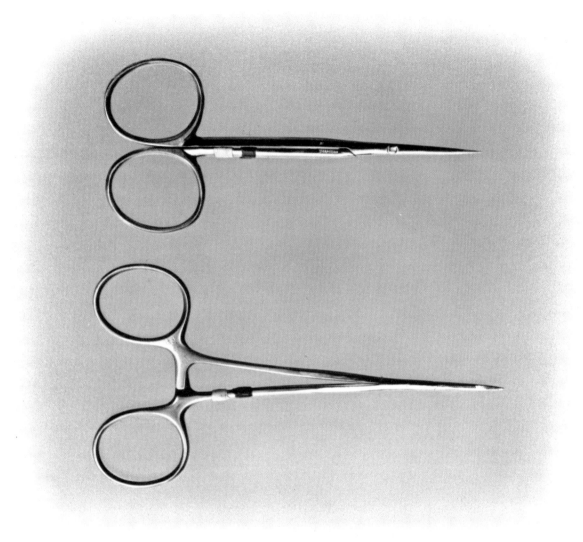

18-1

18-1. These include a sharp instrument to perforate the valve and clamps that are spread to tear open the valve.

A purse-string suture of polypropylene is placed in the infundibulum. The sharp instrument is used to perforate the valve if the valve is atretic. The spreading instrument is then placed in the valve. Proper position can be confirmed by palpation through the pulmonary artery. The instrument is then opened. A ''pop'' or tearing of the valve can usually be felt. Closed valvotomy should create an easily palpable thrill over the pulmonary artery.

Open Valvotomy
After the administration of cold blood cardioplegia, retraction sutures are placed in the infundibulum just below the valve, and the main pulmonary artery is opened longitudinally. Leaflet retractors are placed exposing the valve, which is usually tricuspid with fusion of all three commissures. The

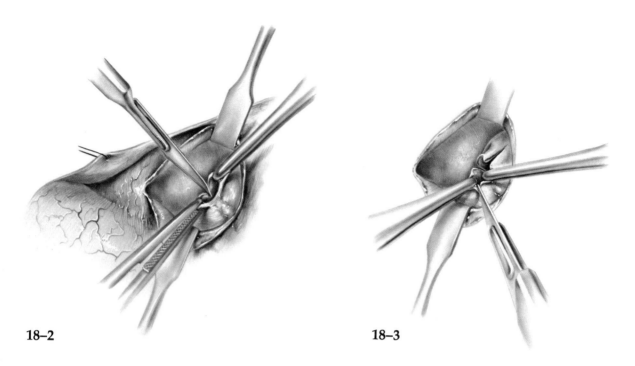

18–2   18–3

commissures are incised sharply back to the anulus (Figs. 18–2, 18–3). The infundibulum is then inspected, and the valve diameter and infundibulum are calibrated as previously discussed.

Results

Neonate

The range of operative mortality reported in the literature reflects the different patient mix from series to series, since no single institution can assemble a group of patients matching the spectrum of morphology in the disease. Operative mortality will be lowest in patients with a near normal-sized right ventricle and highest in patients with a severely hypoplastic right ventricle and right ventricular dependent coronary circulation. In patients who are suitable for closed valvotomy and central shunt, operative mortality as low as 7% has been reported.[15] Most series have mortality between 15% and 25%.[10,22] Growth of the right ventricle can be dramatic, with as much as doubling in size.[11,27,31] As noted earlier, a second operation during the first 3 years of life is frequently necessary.[13]

Child and Adult

The operative risk of open valvotomy in acyanotic patients is less than 1%. Symptom relief and late survival are excellent.[8] Patients who have pulmonary valvotomy before the age of 21 years have long-term survival the same as the general population.[20]

References

1. Alboliras ET, Juisrud PR, Danielson GK, Puga FJ, Schaff HV, McGoon DC, Hagler DJ, Edwards WD, Driscoll DJ: Definitive operation for pulmonary atresia with intact ventricular septum: results in twenty patients. J Thorac Cardiovasc Surg 93: 454,1987.
2. Billingsley AM, Laks H, Boyce SW, George B, Santulli T, Williams RG: Definitive repair in patients with pulmonary atresia and intact ventricular septum. J Thorac Cardiovasc Surg 97:746,1989.

3. Brock RC: Pulmonary valvulotomy for the relief of congenital pulmonary stenosis: report of three cases. Br Med J 1:1121,1948.
4. Brock RC, Campbell M: Valvulotomy for pulmonary valvular stenosis. Br Heart J 12:377,1950.
5. Bull C, de Laval M, Mercanti C, Macartney FJ, Anderson RH: Pulmonary atresia and intact ventricular septum: a revised classification. Circulation 66:266,1982.
6. Burrows PE, Freedom RM, Benson LN, Moes CAF, Wilson G, Koike K, Williams WG: Coronary angiography of pulmonary atresia, hypoplastic right ventricle, and ventriculocoronary communications. AJR 154:789,1990.
7. Coles JG, Freedom RM, Lightfoot NE, Dasmahapatra HK, Williams WG, Trusler GA, Burrows PE: Long-term results in neonates with pulmonary atresia and intact ventricular septum. Ann Thorac Surg 47:213,1989.
8. Danielson GK, Exarhos ND, Weidman WH, McGoon DC: Pulmonic stenosis with intact ventricular septum. J Thorac Cardiovasc Surg 61:228,1971.
9. de Laval M, Bull C, Hopkins R, Rees P, Deanfield J, Taylor JFN, Gersony W, Stark J, Macartney FJ: Decision making in the definitive repair of the heart with a small right ventricle. Circulation 72(Suppl II):II-52,1985.
10. Foker JE, Braunlin EA, St Cyr JA, Hunter D, Molina JE, Moller JH, Ring WS: Management of pulmonary atresia with intact ventricular septum. J Thorac Cardiovasc Surg 92:706,1986.
11. Freed MD, Rosenthal A, Bernhard WF, Litwin SB, Nadas AS: Critical pulmonary stenosis with diminutive right ventricle in neonates. Circulation 48:875,1973.
12. Gittenberger-de Groot AC, Sauer U, Bindl L, Babic R, Essed CE, Buhlmeyer K: Competition of coronary arteries and ventriculo-coronary arterial communications in pulmonary atresia with intact ventricular septum. Int J Cardiol 18:243,1988.
13. Gomez-Engler HE, Grunkemeier GL, Starr A: Critical pulmonary valve stenosis with intact ventricular septum. Thorac Cardiovasc Surg 27:160,1979.
14. Hanley FL, Sade RM, Blackstone EH, Kirklin JW, Freedom RM, Nanda NC: Outcomes in neonatal pulmonary atresia with intact ventricular septum: a multiinstitutional study. J Thorac Cardiovasc Surg 105:406,1993.
15. Hawkins JA, Thorne JK, Boucek MM, Orsmond GS, Ruttenbery HD, Veasy LG, McGough EC: Early and late results in pulmonary atresia and intact ventricular septum. J Thorac Cardiovasc Surg 100:492,1990.
16. Johnson LW, Grossman W, Dalen JE, Dexter L: Pulmonic stenosis in the adult: long-term follow-up results. N Engl J Med 287:1159,1972.
17. Joshi SV, Brawn WJ, Mee RBB: Pulmonary atresia with intact ventricular septum. J Thorac Cardiovasc Surg 91:192,1986.
18. Kan JS, White RI Jr, Mitchell SE, Gardner TJ: Percutaneous balloon valvuloplasty: a new method for treatment of congenital pulmonary valve stenosis. N Engl J Med 307:540,1982.
19. Kanter KR, Pennington DG, Nouri S, Chen S-U, Jureidini S, Balfour I: Concomitant valvotomy and subclavian-main pulmonary artery shunt in neonates with pulmonary atresia and intact ventricular septum. Ann Thorac Surg 43:490,1987.
20. Kopecky SL, Gersh BJ, McGoon MD, Mair DD, Porter CJ, Ilstrup DM, McGoon DC, Kirklin JW, Danielson GK: Long-term outcome of patients undergoing surgical repair of isolated pulmonary valve stenosis: follow-up at 20–30 years. Circulation 78:1150,1988.
21. Lababidi Z, Wu JR: Percutaneous balloon pulmonary valvuloplasty. Am J Cardiol 52:560,1983.
22. Lewis AB, Wells W, Lindesmith GG: Right ventricular growth potential in neonates with pulmonary atresia and intact ventricular septum. J Thorac Cardiovasc Surg 91:835,1986.
23. Masura J, Burch M, Deanfield JE, Sullivan ID: Five-year follow-up after balloon pulmonary valvuloplasty. J Am Coll Cardiol 21:132,1993.
24. McCaffrey FM, Leatherbury L, Moore HV: Pulmonary atresia and intact ventricular septum: definitive repair in the neonatal period. J Thorac Cardiovasc Surg 102:617,1991.
25. Metzdorff MT, Pinson CW, Grunkemeier GL, Cobanoglu A, Starr A: Late right ventricular reconstruction following valvotomy in pulmonary atresia with intact ventricular septum. Ann Thorac Surg 42:45,1986.
26. Milliken JC, Laks H, Hellenbrand W, George B, Chin A, Williams RG: Early and

late results in the treatment of patients with pulmonary atresia and intact ventricular septum. Circulation 72(Suppl II):II-61,1985.

27. Moller JH, Girod D, Amplatz K, Varco RL: Pulmonary valvotomy in pulmonary atresia with hypoplastic right ventricle. Surgery 68:730,1970.

28. O'Connor BK, Beekman RH, Lindauer A, Rocchini A: Intermediate outcome after pulmonary balloon valvuloplasty: comparison with a matched surgical control group. J Am Coll Cardiol 20:169,1992.

29. Pacifico AD, Kirklin JW, Blackstone EH: Surgical management of pulmonary stenosis in tetralogy of Fallot. J Thorac Cardiovasc Surg 74:382,1977.

30. Radtke W, Keane JF, Fellows KE, Lang P, Lock JE: Percutaneous balloon valvulotomy of congenital pulmonary stenosis using oversized balloons. J Am Coll Cardiol 8:909,1986.

31. Rao PS, Liebman J, Borkat G: Right ventricular growth in a case of pulmonic stenosis with intact ventricular septum and hypoplastic right ventricle. Circulation 53:389,1976.

32. Rocchini AP, Kveselis DA, Crowley DC, Dick M, Rosenthal A: Percutaneous balloon valvuloplasty for treatment of congenital pulmonary valvular stenosis in children. J Am Coll Cardiol 3:1005,1984.

33. Rowlatt UF, Rimoldi HJA, Lev M: The quantitative anatomy of the normal child's heart. Pediatr Clin North Am 10:499,1963.

34. Sellors TH: Surgery of pulmonary stenosis: a case in which the pulmonary valve was successfully divided. Lancet 1:988,1948.

35. Semb BHK, Tjonneland S, Stake G, Aabyholm G: "Balloon valvulotomy" of congenital pulmonary valve stenosis with tricuspid valve insufficiency. Cardiovasc Radiol 2:239,1979.

36. Squitieri C, di Carlo D, Giannico S, Marino B, Giamberti A, Marcelletti C: Tricuspid valve avulsion or excision for right ventricular decompression in pulmonary atresia with intact ventricular septum. J Thorac Cardiovasc Surg 97:779,1989.

37. Stanger P, Cassidy SC, Girod DA, Kan JS, Shapiro SR: Balloon pulmonary valvuloplasty: results of the Valvuloplasty and Angioplasty of Congenital Anomalies Registry. Am J Cardiol 65:775,1990.

38. Williams WG, Burrows P, Freedom RM, Trusler GA, Coles JG, Moes CAF, Smallhorn J: Thromboexclusion of the right ventricle in children with pulmonary atresia and intact ventricular septum. J Thorac Cardiovasc Surg 101:222,1991.

19

Atrial Septal Defects

Atrial septal defect (ASD) was the first cardiac malformation to be successfully treated surgically using the mechanical pump oxygenator. Following Gibbon's pioneering report,[14] surgical risk for closure of most defects became minimal and has been near 0% for the past three decades. Indications for surgery and surgical techniques for the three main types of defects—sinus venosus, ostium secundum, and ostium primum—are straightforward and widely accepted.

Indications for Surgery

Ostium secundum defects account for approximately 70% of ASDs, ostium primum defects for approximately 20%, and sinus venosus defects for approximately 10%.[46] Ostium primum defects usually cause symptoms in childhood,[41] but all types usually become symptomatic by the fourth decade of life,[7,35] usually associated with massive right ventricular dilatation, right ventricular failure, and chronic atrial fibrillation. Premature death during the fourth and fifth decades is common.[5-7,12,42]

The extremely low risk of surgical closure and excellent results justify closure if a left-to-right shunt of 1.5 : 1 or more is present. Closure should be performed during the first decade, preferably before school age, even in the absence of symptoms. Rarely, an isolated secundum ASD will require closure in infancy.[30]

Preoperative cardiac catheterization and angiography are not necessary in many patients with ASD.[18] Two-dimensional echocardiography can give an accurate diagnosis. Shub and colleagues[40] and Lipshulz and colleagues[24] had no false-positive two-dimensional echocardiographic studies. Contrast echocardiography, radionuclide shunt studies, and doppler echocardiography can be used as additional confirmatory tests.[32,40]

ASD is the most common congenital cardiac lesion presenting in adulthood. The vast majority of adults with ASDs should have closure and good results should be achieved.[15] However, pulmonary hypertension (pulmonary artery systolic pressure over 60 mm Hg) may have developed and may affect the decision regarding surgery. In the presence of pulmonary hypertension, a shunt of at least 1.5 : 1 should be present for closure.[2] Closure should probably not be performed if the pulmonary vascular resistance is over 8 units. A continuous right-to-left shunt is an absolute contraindication to closure.

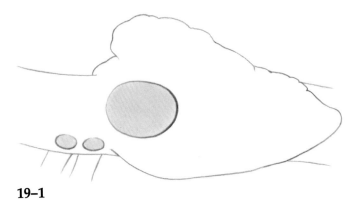

19–1

Sinus Venosus Defect

Surgical Anatomy

The sinus venosus defect[38] is in the upper atrial septum, above the fossa ovalis and separate from it[11] (Fig. 19–1). Anomalous pulmonary veins from the right upper lobe are almost always present and usually empty into the superior vena cava.

Surgical Technique

Our technique is similar to that described by Kirklin, Ellis, and Wood.[21] Proper surgical technique will result in complete closure while avoiding the complications of sinus node injury, pulmonary vein obstruction, and obstruction of the SVC.[43]

The SVC is carefully dissected to well above the pericardium prior to cannulation, identifying the site of entry of the anomalous pulmonary veins and the azygos vein. The azygos vein is encircled and tied. The SVC is encircled with a tape above the azygos vein. Placement of the tape above the azygos vein avoids injury to the sinus node and provides adequate exposure of the upper margin of the defect and the orifices of the pulmonary veins. Cannulation is performed using a small cannula in the SVC. A right-angled cannula placed directly in the vena cava above the entrance of the anomalous veins can also be used. The method of myocardial preservation is cold blood cardioplegia.

The right atriotomy is made and extended laterally up the SVC; lateral incision is important to avoid injury to the sinus node (Fig. 19–2). The SVC cannula is retracted anteriorly.

A patch of Dacron or pericardium is then cut to provide a baffle for closure of the defect and direction of pulmonary venous blood into the left atrium via the ASD. The ASD may need enlarging in some cases. A running suture of 4-0 or 5-0 polypropylene is started medially and carried along the upper portion of the defect and laterally (Fig. 19–3). Large bites medially can injure the sinus node or sinus node artery.

The inferior suture line is then brought laterally to complete the repair (Fig. 19–4). If there is any question about SVC obstruction by the baffle, the SVC should be patched with pericardium.[39]

An alternative technique is described by Williams and colleagues.[47] The high SVC or innominate vein is cannulated with a right-angled cannula and the SVC is transected above the site of entry of the anomalous veins. The cardiac end of the SVC is oversewn and a pericardial patch is sewn in the right atrium well away from the sinus node and cavoatrial junction, directing blood to the left atrium through the atrial defect. Continuity between the

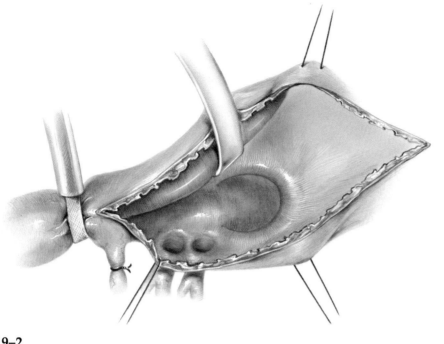

19–2

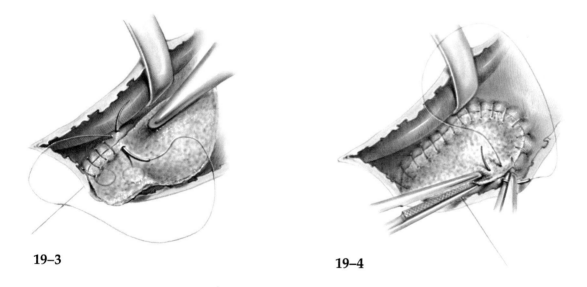

19–3

19–4

cephalad end of the SVC and the right atrium is established by direct anastomosis to the right atrial appendage or by creation of a pedicle conduit of right atrial appendage, right atrial free wall, and pericardium.

Results

Results vary, probably due to differences in surgical technique. Clark and colleagues[9] reported sinus node dysfunction in 70%, with 60% residual defects and 20% SVC obstruction in a group undergoing recatheterization. However, Trusler and co-workers[43] reported only minor electrocardiographic abnormalities, with normal sinus node recovery times, small residual defects in 22%, and SVC obstruction in 6%. Kyger and colleagues[22] reported similarly good results. Excellent results are more likely to be achieved if repair is performed before age 15 years.

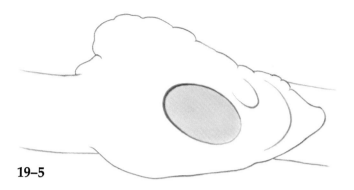

19–5

Ostium Secundum Defects

Surgical Anatomy

Secundum defects are located in the middle of the septum (Fig. 19–5). They may simply be large foramen ovale defects. They can extend toward the inferior vena cava (IVC) as well as posteriorly.[4] A large secundum defect may lack any ridge at the inferior caval junction.

Surgical Technique

The defect is exposed through a lateral atriotomy (Fig. 19–6) after institution of total bypass. The method of myocardial preservation is cold blood cardioplegia.

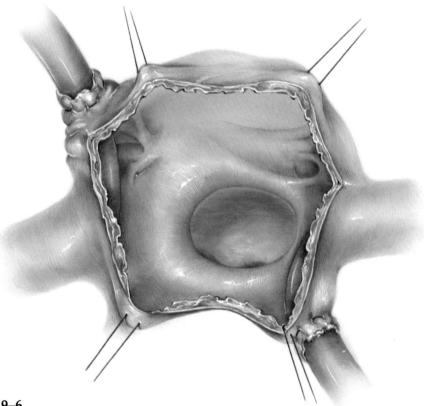

19–6

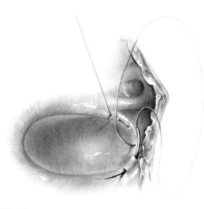
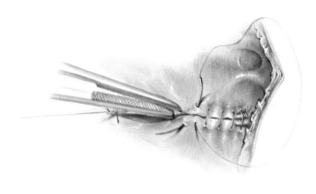

19–7

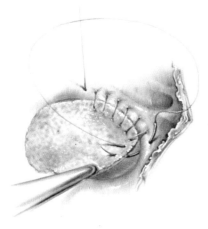
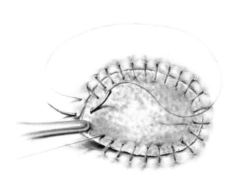

19–9   **19–10**

Some secundum defects can be closed primarily. The suture line is begun near the IVC orifice, frequently with a partial purse-string suture (Fig. 19–7). Such a suture closes the inferior margin of the defect securely and avoids the potential complication of creating a channel directing some IVC blood into the left atrium. The suture line is brought superiorly (Fig. 19–8), completing the closure. If the defect is large, it is closed with a Dacron patch or pericardium (Figs. 19–9, 19–10). A Valsalva maneuver is performed, evacuating air from the left atrium, and the suture is tied.

Results

Closure of secundum defects in children and young adults is associated with uniformly excellent results. Operative mortality is usually 0%, and 90% to 100% of patients are asymptomatic postoperatively.[10,48] Murphy and co-workers,[28] reporting on those patients from the early years of ASD repair at the Mayo Clinic, found that the 27-year survival rates of those patients repaired before the age of 25 years were the same as that of the general population. Results are also good in adults, with usual relief of symptoms of dyspnea on exertion and fatigue.[13,15] Horvarth and colleagues[17] found 5- and 10-year survival rates of 98% and 94% in adults undergoing ASD repair. In the elderly patient with congestive heart failure, there is improvement, but not return to normal. Arrhythmias in adults are frequently unaffected by surgery.

Transcatheter Closure

Transcatheter closure of ASDs, using a double-disc device, was reported by King and Mills[20] in 1976 and by Rashkind[36] in 1983. Lock and co-workers[37] have developed a device with lengthened arms and a hinge allowing them to fold back against themselves, creating a double umbrella with a "clamshell" configuration. Transcatheter closure has been effective, but it is complicated by device embolization and residual leaks.[37] More clinical experimentation will be required to determine the role of transcatheter ASD closure. As of mid-1993, clinical experimentation using the Lock Clamshell Occluder was on hold pending modification of the device.[44]

Unroofed Coronary Sinus Defect

The unroofed coronary sinus or coronary sinus septal defect is a rare anomaly.[23,34] Left-to-right shunting occurs from the left atrium to the right atrium via the coronary sinus. The defect is usually associated with a left superior vena cava (LSVC). If temporary occlusion of the LSVC and measurement of pressure shows that ligation of the LSVC can be tolerated, repair consists of closing or patching the orifice of the coronary sinus, with care to avoid the conduction system. If ligation of the LSVC cannot be tolerated, the roof of the coronary sinus is patched from within the left atrium.[23,34]

Ostium Primum Defect

Surgical Anatomy

Ostium primum defect is located in the inferior atrial septum and results from abnormal growth of the endocardial cushions (Fig. 19–11). Ostium primum defect has also been called partial atrioventricular canal[19] and partial atrioventricular septal defect.[3,31] The left ventricular chamber, mitral valve, and papillary muscles are all abnormal in ostium primum ASD. The outlet is longer than the inlet, resulting in the "goose-neck" deformity seen angiographically.[29,31] The posteromedial papillary muscle is more anterior.[27] The anterior leaflet of the mitral valve has a cleft, and the mural leaflet makes up a smaller proportion of the anular circumference.[29] There is considerable controversy about definition and nomenclature, with Carpentier[8] and Anderson[1] calling the cleft a commissure.

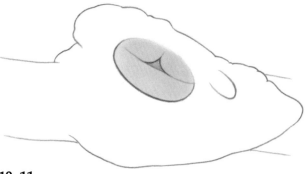

19–11

Surgical Technique

Myocardial preservation is cold blood cardioplegia.

Repair of the Mitral Valve

There has been controversy for the past three decades concerning management of the cleft.[8,45] Carpentier[8] in 1978 advanced the concept of the mitral valve as a trifoliate structure that should not be altered if there is no regurgitation. We adopted this approach for a period during the 1980s but were discouraged by patients requiring reoperation for subsequent development of mitral regurgitation, who were found to have regurgitation through the unclosed cleft. For this reason we and others[33] resumed the closure of the cleft in all patients. King and colleagues[19] have shown that routine closure of the cleft in all patients results in a low incidence of reoperation (93% free from reoperation at 10 years) and does not cause mitral stenosis.

A suture is placed in the leading edge (free margin) of the anterior leaflet for alignment of closure of the cleft (Fig. 19–12). A fine running suture closes the cleft. Interrupted suture technique is also used. Pledgets are not used since they may stiffen the leaflet. Competence of the valve is checked by injecting cold saline through the valve with a large bulb syringe. Anuloplasty at one or both commissures is performed if necessary.

Closure of the Septal Defect: Coronary Sinus to the Right

The technique of Dacron patch closure leaving the coronary sinus to the right is used at the Children's Cardiac Center of Oregon/Portland. Precise suture placement near the base of the mitral valve and around the coronary sinus is necessary to avoid heart block. The inferior sutures are placed in the thick-

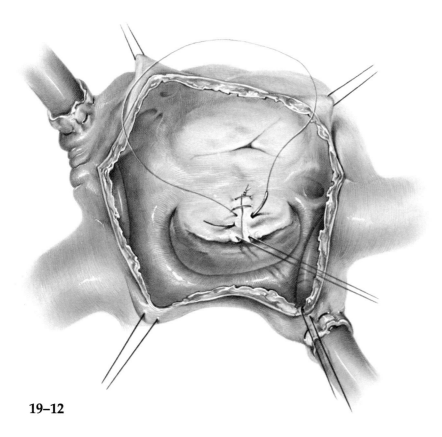

19–12

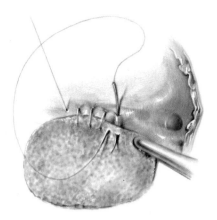

19–13

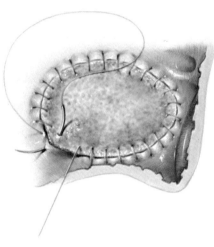

19–14

ened tissue at the base of the anterior leaflet of the mitral valve[16] (Fig. 19–13). The suture line is carried toward the coronary sinus. At the transition point from the mitral leaflet to the atrial ridge near the coronary sinus, the sutures are placed right on the ridge or on the underside of the ridge. They should not be placed on the right atrial side of the ridge or near the coronary sinus, where injury to the atrioventricular node and bundle of His can occur.

The suture line is then carried laterally and superiorly to complete the closure (Fig. 19–14).

Closure of the Septal Defect: Coronary Sinus to the Left

The technique of pericardial patch closure leaving the coronary sinus to the left is used at Sutter/Sacramento. Since the conduction system is behind the repair, there is little or no chance of creating atrioventricular block. A suture of polypropylene is placed through the base of the septal leaflet of the tricuspid valve and through the pericardial patch (Fig. 19–15). This suture line is then carried toward the coronary sinus (Fig. 19–16). At the edge of the valve

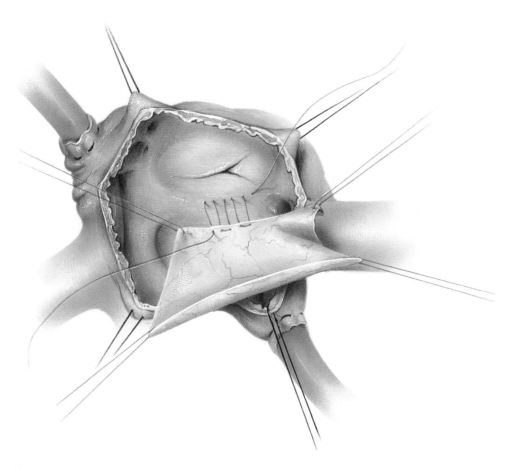

19–15

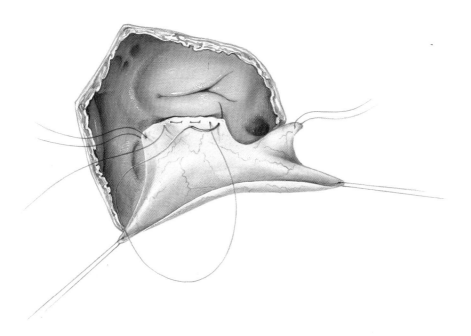

19–16

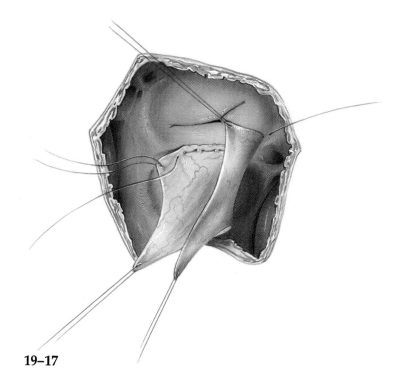

19–17

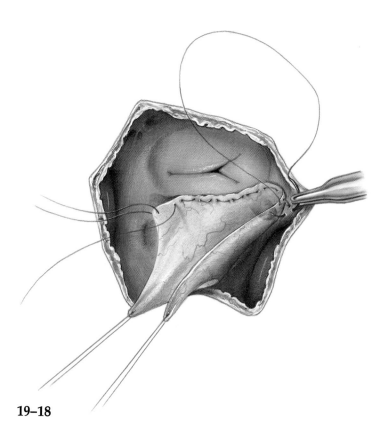

19–18

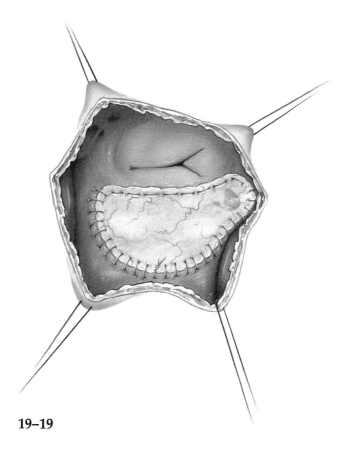

19–19

the suture is carried onto the atrium with the suture line progressing around the coronary sinus (Figs. 19-17, 19-18). The other end of the suture is then brought around to complete the repair (Fig. 19-19). If the base of the tricuspid valve is extremely delicate, horizontal mattress sutures with pledgets can be brought from below the valve and then through the pericardial patch.

Results

Operative mortality for closure of ostium primum defects can approach 0%.[25] Approximately 80% of patients are asymptomatic. Late survival is excellent, with 5-year survival of 95%.[26]

References

1. Anderson RH, Zuberbuhler JR, Penkoske PA, Neches WH: Of cleft, commissures, and things. J Thorac Cardiovasc Surg 90:605,1985.
2. Beck W, Swan HJC, Burchell HB, Kirklin JW: Pulmonary vascular resistance after repair of atrial septal defects in patients with pulmonary hypertension. Circulation 22:938,1960.
3. Becker AE, Anderson RH: Atrioventricular septal defects: What's in a name? J Thorac Cardiovasc Surg 83:461,1982.
4. Bedford DE, Sellors TH, Sommerville W, Belcher JR, Besterman EMM: Atrial septal defect and its surgical treatment. Lancet 1:1255,1957.
5. Braudo JL, Nadas AS, Rudolph AM, Neuhauser EBD: Atrial septal defects in children: a clinical study with special emphasis on indications for operative repair. Pediatrics 14:618,1954.
6. Burrett JB, White PD: Large interauricular septal defect with particular reference to diagnosis and longevity. Am J Med Sci 209:355,1945.
7. Campbell M, Neill C, Suzman S: Prognosis of atrial septal defect. Br Med J 1: 1375,1957.

8. Carpentier A: Surgical anatomy and management of the mitral component of atrioventricular canal defects. *In* Anderson RH, Shinebourne EA (eds): Pediatric Cardiology 1977. Edinburgh, Churchill Livingstone, 1978, p 477.

9. Clark EB, Roland JMA, Varghese PJ, Neill CA, Haller JA: Should the sinus venosus type ASD be closed? A review of the atrial conduction defects and surgical results in twenty-eight children (abstr). Am J Cardiol 35:127,1975.

10. Cooley DA: Results of surgical treatment of atrial septal defects. Am J Cardiol 6:605,1960.

11. Davia JE, Cheitlin MD, Bedynek JL: Sinus venosus atrial septal defect: analysis of fifty cases. Am Heart J 85:177,1973.

12. Dexter L: Atrial septal defect. Br Heart J 18:209,1956.

13. Forgang K, Simonsen S, Andersen A, Efskind L: Atrial septal defect of secundum type in the middle-aged. Am Heart J 94:44,1977.

14. Gibbon JH Jr: Application of a mechanical heart and lung apparatus to cardiac surgery. Minn Med 37:171,1954.

15. Hairston P, Parker EF, Arrants JE, Bradham RR, Lee WH: The adult atrial septal defect. Ann Surg 179:799,1974.

16. Hallman GL, Cooley DA: Surgical Treatment of Congenital Heart Disease, 2nd ed. Philadelphia, Lea & Febiger, 1975, p 85.

17. Horvarth KA, Burke RP, Collins JJ Jr, Cohn LH: Surgical treatment of adult atrial septal defect: early and long-term results. J Am Coll Cardiol 20:1156,1992.

18. Huhta JC, Glasgow P, Murphy DJ Jr, Gutgesell HP, Ott D, McNamara DG, Smith EO: Surgery without catheterization for congenital heart defects: management of 100 patients. J Am Coll Cardiol 9:823,1987.

19. King RM, Puga FJ, Danielson GK, Schaff HV, Julsrud PR, Feldt RH: Prognostic factors and surgical treatment of partial atrioventricular canal. Circulation 74(Suppl I):I-42,1986.

20. King TD, Mills NL: Secundum atrial septal defects: nonoperative closure during cardiac catheterization. JAMA 235:2506,1976.

21. Kirklin JW, Ellis FH, Wood EH: Treatment of anomalous pulmonary venous connections in association with interatrial communications. Surgery 39:389,1956.

22. Kyger ER III, Frazier OH, Cooley DA, Gillette PC, Reul GJ Jr, Sandiford FM, Wukasch DC: Sinus venosus atrial septal defect: early and late results following closure in 109 patients. Ann Thorac Surg 75:248,1978.

23. Lee ME, Sade RM: Coronary sinus septal defect: surgical considerations. J Thorac Cardiovasc Surg 78:563,1979.

24. Lipshultz SE, Sanders SP, Mayer JE, Colan SD, Lock JE: Are routine preoperative cardiac catheterization and angiography necessary before repair of ostium primum atrial septal defect? J Am Coll Cardiol 11:373,1988.

25. Losay J, Rosenthal A, Castaneda AR, Bernhard WH, Nadas AS: Repair of atrial septal defect primum. J Thorac Cardiovasc Surg 75:248,1978.

26. McMullan MH, McGoon DC, Wallace RB, Danielson GK, Weidman WH: Surgical treatment of partial atrioventricular canal. Arch Surg 107:705,1973.

27. Meijboom EJ, Ebels T, Anderson RH, Schasfoort-van Leeuwen MJM, Deanfield JE, Eijgelaar A, Homan JN, van der Heide JNH: Left atrioventricular valve after surgical repair in atrioventricular septal defect with separate valve orifices ("Ostium primum atrial septal defect"): an echo-doppler study. Am J Cardiol 57:433,1986.

28. Murphy JG, Gersh BJ, McGoon MD, Mair DD, Porter CJ, Ilstrup DM, McGoon DC, Puga FJ, Kirklin JW, Danielson GK: Long-term outcome after surgical repair of isolated atrial septal defect: follow-up at 27 to 32 years. N Engl J Med 323:1645,1990.

29. Penkoske PA, Neches WH, Anderson RH, Zuberbuhler JR: Further observations on the morphology of atrioventricular septal defects. J Thorac Cardiovasc Surg 90:611,1985.

30. Phillips SJ, Okies JE, Henken D, Sunderland CO, Starr A: Complex of secundum atrial septal defect and congestive heart failure in infants. J Thorac Cardiovasc Surg 70:696,1975.

31. Piccoli GP, Gerlis LM, Wilkinson JL, Lozsadi K, Macartney FJ, Anderson RH: Morphology and classification of atrioventricular defects. Br Heart J 42:621,1979.

32. Pollick C, Sullivan H, Cujec B, Wilansky S: Doppler color-flow imaging assessment of shunt size in atrial septal defect. Circulation 78:522,1988.

33. Pozzi M, Remig J, Fimmers R, Urban AE: Atrioventricular septal defects: analysis of short- and medium-term results. J Thorac Cardiovasc Surg 101:138,1991.
34. Quaegebeur J, Kirklin JW, Pacifico AD, Bargeron LM: Surgical experience with unroofed coronary sinus. Ann Thorac Surg 27:418,1979.
35. Rahimtoola SH, Kirklin JW, Burchell HB: Atrial septal defect. Circulation 37(Suppl V):V-2,1968.
36. Rashkind WJ: Transcatheter treatment of congenital heart disease. Circulation 67:711,1983.
37. Rome JJ, Keane JF, Perry SB, Spevak PJ, Lock JE: Double-umbrella closure of atrial defects: initial clinical application. Circulation 82:751,1990.
38. Ross DN: The sinus venosus type of atrial septal defect. Guys Hosp Rep 105:376,1956.
39. Schuster SR, Gross RE, Colodny AH: Surgical management of anomalous right pulmonary venous drainage to the superior vena cava, associated with superior marginal defect of the atrial septum. Surgery 51:805,1962.
40. Shub C, Tajik AJ, Seward JB, Hagler DJ, Danielson GK: Surgical repair of uncomplicated atrial septal defect without "routine" preoperative cardiac catheterization. J Am Coll Cardiol 6:49,1985.
41. Somerville J: Ostium primum defect: factors causing deterioration in the natural history. Br Heart J 27:413,1965.
42. Swan HJC, Zapata-Diaz J, Burchell HB, Wood EH: Pulmonary hypertension in congenital heart disease. Am J Med 16:12,1954.
43. Trusler GA, Kazenelson G, Freedom RM, Williams WG, Rowe RD: Late results following repair of partial anomalous pulmonary venous connection with sinus venosus atrial septal defect. J Thorac Cardiovasc Surg 79:776,1980.
44. USCI/Bard: Personal communication. 1993.
45. Van Mierop LHS, Alley RD: The management of the cleft mitral valve in endocardial cushion defects. Ann Thorac Surg 2:416,1966.
46. Watson H (ed): Paediatric Cardiology. St Louis, CV Mosby Co, 1968.
47. Williams WH, Zorn-Chelton S, Raviele AA, Michalik RE, Guyton RA, Dooley KJ, Hatcher CR: Extracardiac atrial pedicle conduit repair of partial anomalous pulmonary venous connection to the superior vena cava in children. Ann Thorac Surg 38:345,1984.
48. Young D: Later results of closure of secundum atrial septal defect in children. Am J Cardiol 31:14,1973.

20

Complete Atrioventricular Canal

The pioneering work in the 1960s by Rastelli and his colleagues[31,32] at the Mayo Clinic defined the anatomy of atrioventricular (AV) canal defects and developed a rational approach to surgical correction. Continued refinement of their basic principles has resulted in a surgical approach that is reproducible and predictable in its outcome.[16]

Indications for Surgery

The history of complete AV canal medically treated is associated with high mortality in the first months of life. Congestive heart failure secondary to large left-to-right shunting and/or AV valve incompetence results in death in 46% by 6 months of age, 65% by 12 months, and 85% by 24 months.[4] The development of pulmonary vascular disease is rapid and common.[18] Newfeld and colleagues,[28] in a combined autopsy and lung biopsy study, found that two-thirds of patients had severe (Heath-Edwards[19] grade 3 or greater) pulmonary vascular disease by age 12 months. Clapp and colleagues[12] found that Down's syndrome patients with complete AV canal have a greater degree of elevation of pulmonary vascular resistance in the first year of life and more rapid progression to fixed pulmonary vascular obstructive disease than children with normal chromosomes.

The poor prognosis with medical treatment and the rapid development of pulmonary vascular disease have been the basis for recommending early total correction.[5,13,24] Correction before 1 year of age can be performed with an operative mortality of 15% or less[9,11,35]—a mortality that is much lower than that of nonsurgical treatment. It is our policy to repair all complete AV canals by age 6 months or at the time of diagnosis.[1] Any patient in persistent congestive heart failure or failing to grow is repaired regardless of age or weight.

Pulmonary artery banding has been recommended as a preliminary surgical approach to AV canal in patients with a large ventricular shunt and minimal mitral insufficiency.[15] We do not agree with this approach, since banding is usually associated with a high mortality.[5,22] Banding may be indicated in very unusual situations, such as AV canal with multiple ventricular septal defects (VSDs).

Surgical Strategy

Operation is performed with standard bypass and hypothermia of 24°–26°C. Cold blood cardioplegia is the method of myocardial preservation.

Surgical Anatomy

Atrioventricular Defect

The septal defect in complete AV canal consists of an ostium primum type of atrial septal defect, a single common AV orifice, a deficiency in the upper ventricular septum, and a bare area on the crest of the ventricular septum. Between 30% and 50% of the expected surface area of the ventricular septum in usually missing.[14]

Atrioventricular Valves

The common AV orifice is bridged by anterior and posterior common leaflets that are not connected to each other. Rastelli and co-workers[31] based their classic classification on the configuration, relationships, and attachments of the anterior common leaflet, proposing three types: A, B, and C. Type A has an anterior common leaflet that is divided into two distinct portions, both of which are attached by chordae to the rim of the ventricular septum. In type B the anterior common leaflet is divided, but attached to chordae arising from an anomalous papillary muscle originating in the right ventricle from the ventricular septum. Type B is uncommon. In type C the anterior common leaflet is undivided and free floating, with essentially no chordal attachments to the septum. The posterior common leaflet varies widely in configuration, without any definite relationship to the anatomy of the anterior leaflet.[14,31]

The Rastelli classification is helpful, but is overly simple. There is enormous variability of the anterior and posterior leaflets that Rastelli's classification does not take into account.[5–7,30,34]

As discussed in the previous chapter, there has been a considerable amount written during the 1980s regarding alternate concepts and nomenclature of the abnormal structures of complete AV canal.[2,3,10,29,30]

Conduction System

Knowledge of the conduction system anatomy is critical to prevent complete heart block as a complication of repair. Our knowledge of conduction system anatomy is based on the classic studies of Lev.[23]

The AV node is posteriorly displaced and is frequently directly adjacent to the coronary sinus ostium.[17] The bundle of His passes along the rim of the ventricular septum, dividing into the left and right bundle branches.

Ventricular Size and Dominance

Complete AV canal is usually associated with biventricular hypertrophy and increased volume of both ventricles.[20,33] However, hypoplasia of a ventricle may exist, with one ventricle being dominant, as described by Bharati and Lev.[7] The valve leaflets tend to be preferentially distributed into the larger ventricle. It is doubtful that such anatomy is suitable for correction. Echocardiography is valuable in assessing ventricular size in complete AV canal.[26]

Surgical Technique

The atrium is opened and suspended. The anatomy of the atrium, ventricles, and atrioventricular valves is carefully and thoroughly inspected. Cold saline injected into the ventricles will float the valve leaflets and help to show their anatomy and relationships. This method is used to determine the location of incision of the common leaflets. A common location of incision of the anterior and posterior leaflets is shown in Figure 20–1.

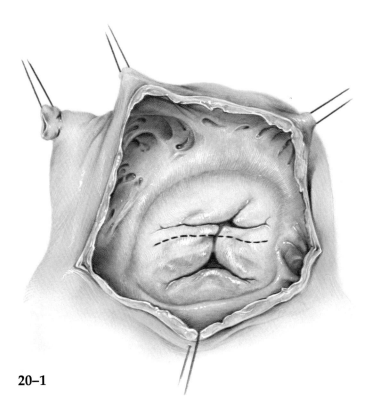

20–1

The anterior (Fig. 20–2) and posterior leaflets are divided as necessary. The most important principle of dividing the leaflets is to provide for an adequate amount of valve tissue on the left ventricular side. In special instances where a cleft is present in the anterior leaflet and division at the site of the cleft would leave deficient tissue, the cleft may be closed and the incision made further to the right.[5]

A single patch of Dacron double-velour is cut and carefully sized. Too large a patch will distort the AV valves by making the mitral anulus too large. A running suture of polypropylene is begun at the inferior portion of the ven-

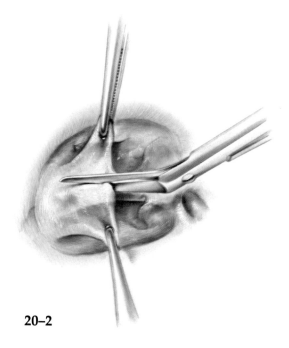

20–2

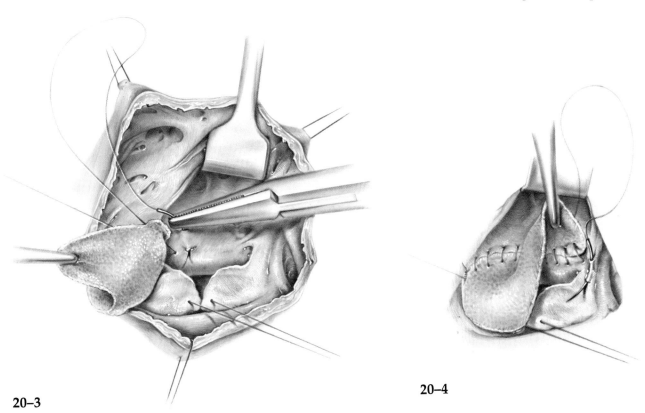

20–3

20–4

tricular defect and brought up, staying off the ridge on the right ventricular side in order to avoid injury to the conduction tissue (Fig. 20-3). As the suture line comes near the coronary sinus, superficial bites should be taken (Fig. 20-4) to avoid injury to the AV node.

The mitral valve is assessed to determine whether a bicuspid valve is to be constructed. This is determined by the size of the mural cusp. The cleft is usually closed, but the valve is left tricuspid if rendering it bicuspid might make it stenotic.

For a bicuspid repair, the mitral components of the anterior and posterior common leaflets are joined, approximating the edges of the leaflets (Fig. 20-5). The height at which the valve is to be attached to the patch is then assessed. Short chordae connecting the ventricular septum may require cutting to release the leaflet for proper positioning (Fig. 20-6).

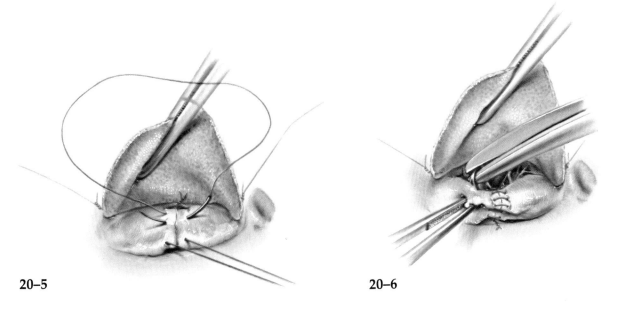

20–5

20–6

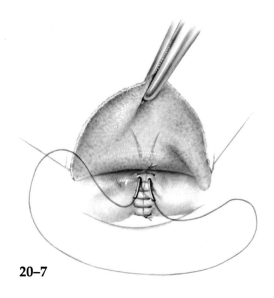

20–7

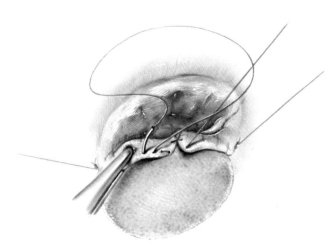

20–8

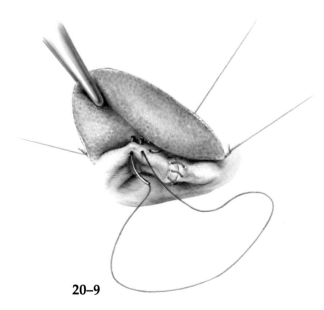

20–9

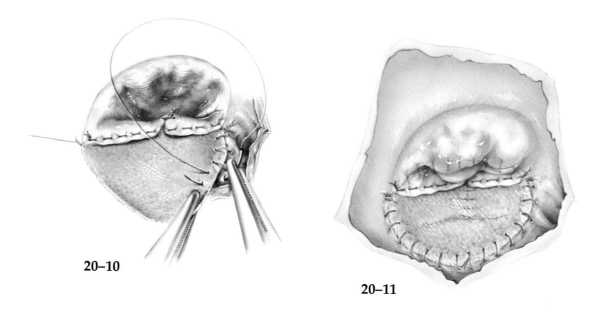

20–10

20–11

The proper height for attachment of the valve can be judged by a combination of factors, including the point at which the major chordae appear to be in proper alignment and the level of lateral attachment of the common leaflets. The midportion of the divided leaflets is usually attached to the patch at about the same level as their lateral attachments.

The leaflets are attached with a horizontal running mattress suture of fine polyester, placed well back from the cut edge of the leaflets, beginning with the mitral leaflet (Fig. 20–7) and working laterally (Figs. 20–8, 20–9).

The valve is then checked for competence, and sutures are added as necessary to shorten the free edge of the leaflet, thereby increasing apposition of the leaflets. An anuloplasty at one or both commissures is performed if necessary.

The atrial portion of the repair is then completed (Figs. 20–10, 20–11). Alternative methods of repair, without dividing the anterior common leaflet and using separate patches, have been described, with satisfactory results.[8]

Results

Operative mortality in infancy can be less than 10%.[9,35] Two series of patients repaired during childhood have been reported with 0% operative mortality.[21,27]

Functional and hemodynamic results are good. Hemodynamically significant mitral regurgitation occurs in fewer than 20% of patients.[35] Elevated pulmonary vascular resistance usually returns to normal.[21]

Late survival is excellent.[25] Berger and colleagues[5] report a 5-year survival rate of 91% among hospital survivors.

Reoperation may be necessary for mitral regurgitation, residual VSD, or subaortic stenosis.

References

1. Abbruzzese PA, Kirby WC, Sunderland CO, Starr A: Primary repair of complete A-V canal during the first 6 months of life. Unpublished data.

2. Anderson RH, Zuberbuhler JR, Penkoske PA, Neches WH: Of clefts, commissures, and things. J Thorac Cardiovasc Surg 90:605,1985.

3. Becker AE, Anderson RH: Atrioventricular septal defects: What's in a name? J Thorac Cardiovasc Surg 83:461,1982.

4. Berger TJ, Blackstone EH, Kirklin JW, Bargeron LM, Hazelrig JB, Turner ME: Survival and probability of cure without and with operation in complete atrioventricular canal. Ann Thorac Surg 27:104,1979.

5. Berger TJ, Kirklin JW, Blackstone EH, Pacifico AD, Kouchoukos NT: Primary repair of complete atrioventricular canal in patients less than 2 years old. Am J Cardiol 41:906,1978.

6. Bharati S, Lev M, McAllister HA, Kirklin JW: Surgical anatomy of the atrioventricular valve in the intermediate type of common atrioventricular orifice. J Thorac Cardiovasc Surg 79:884,1980.

7. Bharati S, Lev M: The spectrum of common atrioventricular orifice (canal). Am Heart J 86:553,1973.

8. Bove EL, Sondheimer HM, Kavey RW, Byrum CJ, Blackman MS: Results with the two-patch technique for repair of complete atrioventricular septal defect. Ann Thorac Surg 38:157,1984.

9. Capouya ER, Laks H, Drinkwater DC, Pearl JM, Milgalter E: Management of the left atrioventricular valve in the repair of complete atrioventricular septal defects. J Thorac Cardiovasc Surg 104:196,1992.

10. Carpentier A: Surgical anatomy and management of the mitral component of atrioventricular canal defects. In Anderson RH, Shinebourne EA (eds): Pediatric Cardiology 1977. Edinburgh, Churchill Livingstone, 1978, p 477.

11. Castaneda AR, Mayer JE, Jonas RA: Repair of complete atrioventricular canal in infancy. World J Surg 9:590,1985.

12. Clapp S, Perry BL, Farooki ZQ, Jackson WL, Karpawich PP, Hakimi M, Arcinegas E, Green EW, Pinsky WW: Down's syndrome, complete atrioventricular canal, and pulmonary vascular obstructive disease. J Thorac Cardiovasc Surg 100: 115,1990.

13. Culpepper W, Kolff J, Chung-Yuan L, Vitullo D, Lamberti J, Arcilla RA, Replogle R: Complete common atrioventricular canal in infancy—surgical repair and postoperative hemodynamics. Circulation 58:550,1978.

14. Ebert P, Goor DA: Complete atrioventricular canal malformation: further clarification of the anatomy of the common leaflet and its relationship to the VSD in surgical correction. Ann Thorac Surg 25:134,1978.

15. Epstein ML, Moller JH, Amplatz K, Nicoloff DM: Pulmonary artery banding in infants with complete atrioventricular canal. J Thorac Cardiovasc Surg 78:28,1979.

16. Feldt RH (ed): Atrioventricular Canal Defects. Philadelphia, London, Toronto, WB Saunders Co, 1976.

17. Feldt RH, DuShane JW, Titus JL: The atrioventricular conduction system in persistent common atrioventricular canal defect: correlations with the electrocardiogram. Circulation 42:437,1970.

18. Fyfe DA, Buckles DS, Gillette PC, Crawford FC: Preoperative prediction of postoperative pulmonary arteriolar resistance after surgical repair of complete atrioventricular canal. J Thorac Cardiovasc Surg 102:784,1991.

19. Heath D, Edwards JE: Pathology of hypertensive vascular disease: a description of six grades of structural changes in the pulmonary arteries with special reference to congenital cardiac defects. Circulation 43:533,1958.

20. Jarmakani JM, George B, Wheeler J: Ventricular volume characteristics in infants and children with endocardial cushion defects. Circulation 43:533,1958.

21. Kahn DR, Levy J, France NE, Chung KJ, Dacumos GD: Recent results after repair of atrioventricular canal. J Thorac Cardiovasc Surg 73:413,1977.

22. Kirklin JW, Blackstone EH: Management of the infant with complete atrioventricular canal. J Thorac Cardiovasc Surg 78:32,1979.

23. Lev M: The architecture of the conduction system in congenital heart disease. I. Common atrioventricular orifice. Arch Pathol 65:174,1958.

24. Mair DD, McGoon DC: Surgical correction of atrioventricular canal during the first year of life. Am J Cardiol 40:66,1977.

25. McMullan MH, Wallace RB, Weidman WH, McGoon DC: Surgical treatment of complete atrioventricular canal. Surgery 72:905,1972.

26. Mehta S, Hirshfield S, Riggs T, Liebman J: Echocardiographic estimation of ventricular hypoplasia in complete atrioventricular canal. Circulation 59:888,1979.

27. Mills NL, Ochsner JL, King TD: Correction of Type C complete atrioventricular canal: surgical considerations. J Thorac Cardiovasc Surg 71:20,1976.

28. Newfeld EA, Sher M, Paul MH, Nidaidoh H: Pulmonary vascular disease in complete atrioventricular canal defect. Am J Cardiol 39:721,1977.

29. Penkoske PA, Neches WH, Anderson RH, Zuberbuhler JR: Further observations on the morphology of atrioventricular septal defects. J Thorac Cardiovasc Surg 90: 611,1985.

30. Piccoli GP, Wilkinson JL, Macartney FJ, Gerlis LM, Anderson RH: Morphology and classification of complete atrioventricular defects. Br Heart J 42:633,1979.

31. Rastelli GC, Kirklin JW, Titus JL: Anatomic observations on complete form of persistent common atrioventricular canal with special reference to atrioventricular valves. Mayo Clin Proc 41:296,1966.

32. Rastelli GC, Ongley PA, Kirklin JW, McGoon DC: Surgical repair of the complete form of persistent common atrioventricular canal. J Thorac Cardiovasc Surg 55: 299,1968.

33. Thanopoulos BD, Fisher EA, DuBrow IW, Hastreiter AR: Right and left ventricular volume characteristics in common atrioventricular canal. Circulation 57:991,1978.

34. Ugarte M, de Salamanca FE, Quero M: Endocardial cushion defects: an anatomical study of 54 specimens. Br Heart J 38:674,1976.

35. Weintraub RG, Brawn WJ, Venables AW, Mee RBB: Two-patch repair of complete atrioventricular septal defect in the first year of life. J Thorac Cardiovasc Surg 99: 320,1990.

21

Ventricular Septal Defects

Isolated ventricular septal defect (VSD) is the most common congenital cardiac defect, with an incidence of approximately 2 per 1000 live births.[22] Isolated VSD accounts for 25% of all congenital heart disease.[26] The wide range of physiology and natural history of VSDs necessitates careful consideration of operative indications and timing. Understanding of the anatomic variations and applicable surgical techniques is necessary to achieve the excellent results that are possible today.

Indications for Surgery

The indications for surgery of VSDs are influenced by the wide variation in natural history. Some defects close or decrease in size early in life. Approximately one-third of all defects will spontaneously close, and another third will become smaller during the first 2 years of life.[21,22,26,36] Other defects follow a benign course for many years. However, some follow a course of congestive heart failure (CHF), failure to thrive, recurrent pulmonary infections, or development of pulmonary vascular disease. Timely intervention with surgical treatment is necessary in the latter group to prevent development of irreversible pulmonary vascular disease or death secondary to CHF.

Infants with clinically small defects should be followed. Infants with CHF should have medical treatment instituted and the response assessed. Those who have persistence of CHF or intractable respiratory distress should have early catheterization and surgery.[27] Those with good response to medical treatment should be followed, at least until age 6 months, to determine whether there is any evidence of spontaneous closure or decrease in the size of the defect. It must be remembered that clinical evidence of decreasing left-to-right shunt may also be caused by development of infundibular stenosis or rising pulmonary vascular resistance (PVR). Echocardiography is useful for following these patients.[44]

If evidence of a large shunt persists or rise in pulmonary artery pressure is suggested, catheterization should be performed. Patients with shunts less than 2 : 1 and pulmonary artery pressure less than one-third systemic pressure should be managed conservatively. Patients with shunts over 2 : 1 must be carefully considered for surgery, taking into account their overall clinical status and pulmonary vascular resistance.

Blackstone, Kirklin, and colleagues[6] have performed a careful study of the optimal age related to late results in elective repair of large VSDs. They found that the age at operation, the preoperative pulmonary vascular resistance, and preoperative pulmonary artery pressure were directly related to the mean pulmonary artery pressure 5 or more years later. For such elective or semi-elective patients, they recommend waiting until about 2 years of age if the PVR is low (less than 4 units/m^2). If the PVR is moderately elevated (8 units/m^2), operation should be done at about 6 months of age, hopefully to avoid established pulmonary vascular disease. If PVR is markedly elevated (12 units/m^2), but pulmonary blood flow is 1.3 or more times systemic blood flow, operation should be done promptly, even before 6 months of age. We agree with these recommendations for elective surgery. As stated earlier, urgent operation is recommended regardless of age or size for infants who are severely symptomatic, have serious growth retardation, or have intractable CHF.

Older children or adults with VSD should undergo closure if a pulmonary-to-systemic flow ratio of 2 : 1 or more is present.[39] Patients with a smaller shunt should also be considered for surgery under some circumstances, such as recurrent bacterial endocarditis, fear of progressive aortic insufficiency with supracristal defects, or disparity between symptoms and calculated shunt.

Choice of Operation

The high mortality of open repair of VSD in infancy during the 1950s and early 1960s prompted the adoption of two-stage management, consisting of initial palliation by pulmonary artery banding[37] followed by later open closure of the VSD and debanding of the pulmonary artery.[17,45] This approach became inappropriate once excellent results could be achieved by primary total correction, regardless of age or size. The cumulative mortality of the two-stage approach was 20%–30% in most series.[11,34] This mortality greatly exceeded the 5% or lower mortality that could be achieved by primary total correction.[1,3,53] Pulmonary artery banding for isolated VSD is obsolete.[16] However, in unusual situations, such as multiple VSDs or complex anomalies, we continue to employ pulmonary artery banding on a selective basis.

Surgical Strategy

Method of Cardiopulmonary Bypass

The technique of profound hypothermia and low flow is used for most infants weighing less than 6 kg. In all other patients, standard cardiopulmonary bypass with moderate systemic hypothermia is used (Chapter 5).

Myocardial Preservation

Cold blood cardioplegia is the method in all cases (Chapter 6).

Management of Aortic Insufficiency

The association of aortic insufficiency (AI) with VSD is rare, with a reported incidence of 2%–4%.[40,42] The AI is most often caused by prolapse of the right coronary cusp.[13,47,64] Hypotheses regarding causation of the AI include trauma to the valve by the surge of blood through the VSD[55] and a deficiency in anatomic structures supporting the aortic valve anulus and the sinus of Valsalva.

Many approaches to management of aortic insufficiency have been recommended, from doing nothing to the valve to replacement of the valve. Although minimal AI may be corrected by simply closing the VSD, moderate to severe AI requires valvuloplasty or valve replacement.

Many techniques of valvuloplasty have been described, most involving suspension and/or shortening of the free margin of the prolapsing leaflet.[19,23,38,50,51,60,62] Because of the small number of patients in any one series, it is impossible to determine whether any specific technique of valvuloplasty is clearly superior.[50] Failure of valvuloplasty appears to be more likely if the AI is severe and of long duration. Valve repair should be attempted in all patients, although a few will require valve replacement.[42]

Surgical Anatomy

Defect Location (Fig. 21–1)

The classic studies of Becu[4] and Kirklin[28] formed the basis for a widely used classification of VSDs. This classification utilizes the major anatomic landmarks of the interior of the right ventricle as reference points, the most important being the crista supraventricularis. Other classifications[33] use the trabecula septomarginalis, as defined by Tandler,[54] as the main reference point.

Becu and Kirklin divide the right ventricle into an inflow tract and an outflow tract. The outflow tract is that part which lies between the pulmonary valve above and the tricuspid valve below. The four major anatomic landmarks of the outflow tract of the right ventricle are the tricuspid ring, the papillary muscle of the conus, the crista supraventricularis, and the anulus fibrosus of the pulmonary valve. Most of the outflow tract of the right ventricle and the pulmonary valve lies more cephalad and anterior than the left ventricular outflow tract and aortic valve, so the crista supraventricularis overlies a portion of the root of the aorta. These anatomic characteristics explain the frequent intimate relationship of VSDs in the right ventricular outflow tract with portions of the aortic valve.

The most common location of VSDs is just inferior to the crista supraventricularis in the region of the membranous septum—the "membranous defect"[17,28,33]—or perimembranous.[48,49] These defects usually involve more than just absence of membranous septum and have variable amounts of muscular

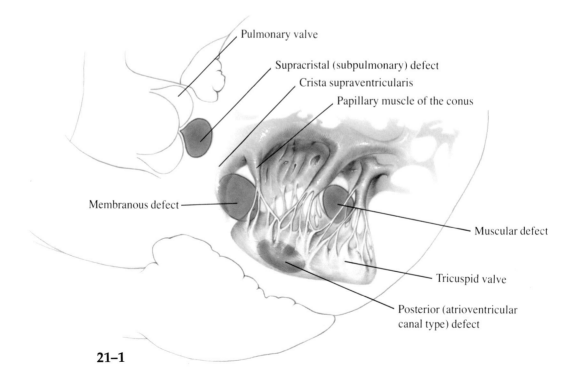

Pulmonary valve

Supracristal (subpulmonary) defect

Crista supraventricularis

Papillary muscle of the conus

Membranous defect

Muscular defect

Tricuspid valve

Posterior (atrioventricular canal type) defect

21–1

septal deficiency. Membranous defects account for approximately 75%–85% of VSDs. They have also been termed subaortic or conoventricular.[41] From the left ventricular side they are under the right coronary cusp and noncoronary cusp.

The other location of defects in the right ventricular outflow tract is above the crista supraventricularis, just below the pulmonary valve—"supracristal type." The anulus fibrosus of the pulmonary valve usually forms the upper border of these defects. From the left ventricular side the supracristal defect is under the left coronary cusp.

Defects in the inflow are either posterior under the septal leaflet or in the midportion or apical portion of the muscular septum. Defects high and posterior have been termed "atrioventricular canal type," but we prefer "posterior," since this terminology is less confusing. From the left ventricular side, posterior defects are between the posteromedial papillary muscle and the mitral valve.

The last major type of defect is "muscular," lying either in the midportion of the septum or near the apex.[66] Muscular defects may be multiple.

Conduction System

Knowledge of the anatomy of the conduction system and its relationship to the various types of defects is important to avoid surgical injury to conduction tissue.[30,31]

In the normal heart the major portion of the atrioventricular (AV) node is located in the lower right atrium, to the left of the coronary sinus.[43,56-59] The terminal portion of the AV node is in the atrial septum at its attachment to the central fibrous body. The central fibrous body is at the confluence of the AV valves, atrial septum, membranous ventricular septum, and aortic valve ring.

The bundle of His begins as a continuation of the AV node at the right fibrous trigone and pierces the membranous ventricular septum or skirts the septum posteriorly to enter the summit of the muscular ventricular septum, where it gives off multiple left branches. The bundle of His continues as the right bundle branch on the right side of the muscular septum.

The location of the VSD usually determines the relationship of the bundle of His and bundle branches.[30,31,35,56-58] In the most common type of VSD, the membranous, the conduction tissue is usually on the posterior-inferior aspect of the defect and may be on the rim or the left or right side of the rim. In the posterior defects the conduction tissue may pass in the superior aspect of the defect.[35] The conduction tissue is usually distant from supracristal defects and muscular defects.

Milo[35] and Lincoln[33] have recommended that the apex of the triangle of Koch[29] be used as the guide to the location of the conduction tissue. The "base" of the triangle is the coronary sinus. The apex of the triangle is where the tendon of Todaro (a rim of tissue from the top of the coronary sinus to the septal leaflet) meets the attachment of the septal leaflet. As examined from the right atrium, the membranous defects will generally be to the left of this apex; the posterior defects will be to the right.[20] Sutures can therefore be placed in a manner to avoid the conduction tissue.

Surgical Technique

A number of approaches to repair of VSDs have been described.[12] In addition to the usual right atrial or right ventricular approaches, closure through the aortic valve[15,18] or pulmonary valve[24] has also been described. Our standard approach to supracristal defects is through the pulmonary artery and to membranous, posterior, and muscular defects is via the right atrium.

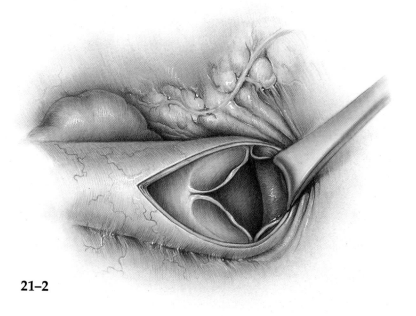

21–2

Supracristal Type

Closure through the pulmonary artery provides excellent exposure of the defect and the pulmonary and aortic valves and avoids a right ventriculotomy and its attendant potential for decreasing ventricular function and causing late ventricular arrhythmia.[2,24] A longitudinal arteriotomy is made in the pulmonary artery and a vein retractor is placed across the pulmonary valve to expose the defect (Fig. 21-2). A patch in the shape of a teardrop is cut from knitted Dacron. Horizontal mattress sutures, usually 4-0 polyester, with pledgets are placed along the inferior rim of the defect and through the base of the patch with the point of the teardrop patch oriented so it will fit under the posterior commissure of the pulmonary valve (Fig. 21-3). Horizontal mattress sutures are then placed through the patch and then through the base of the posterior leaflets of the pulmonary valve with careful visualization of the

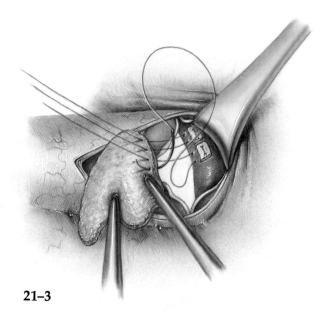

21–3

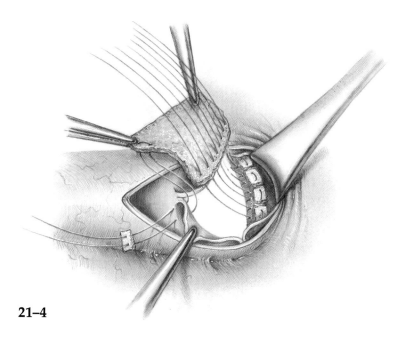

21–4

aortic valve. The sutures are then passed through pledgets. The patch is then seated and tied (Fig. 21–5).

Perimembranous Type

Running Suture Technique

Transatrial closure was suggested during the early years of VSD surgery,[10] particularly in the case of defects with high pulmonary vascular resistance,[5,9,25,32] since this approach avoided the deleterious hemodynamic effects of a right ventriculotomy.[52] With the effect of experience and especially with the improved exposure provided by the flaccid heart of cold cardioplegic arrest, the atrial approach is our approach of choice. The atrial approach can be used for all membranous defects.

The running suture technique is used at the Children's Cardiac Center of Oregon/Portland. The atrium is opened from below the appendage to near the inferior caval junction. A suture can be placed in the anterior leaflet of the

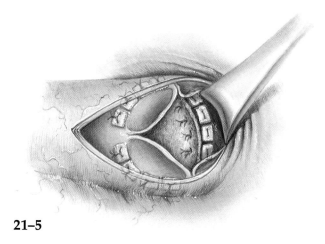

21–5

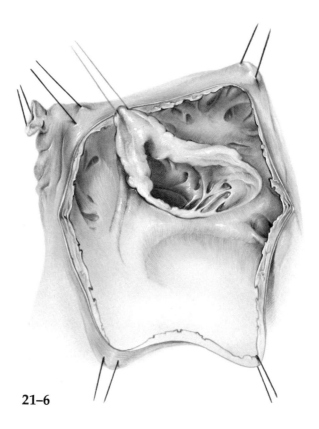

21-6

tricuspid valve to help expose the defect (Fig. 21-6). One or two chordae to the septal leaflet may be cut to obtain good exposure. In the presence of aneurysm of the membranous septum, exposure is enhanced by cutting chordae, which are reattached to the margin of the Dacron patch in their anatomic location. Although small defects may be closed by simple suture, most defects are closed using a Dacron patch. The suture line of polypropylene is begun on the right side of the inferior rim and carried in a counterclockwise direction to penetrate the septal leaflet. The other arm is carried clockwise (Fig. 21-7) and brought around (Fig. 21-8). The upper portion of the patch is then sutured to the base of the septal leaflet (*not* through the anulus) with pledgets or a single strip of Teflon buttressing the repair on the atrial

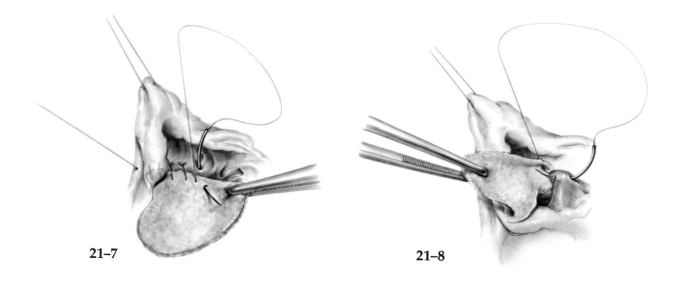

21-7   21-8

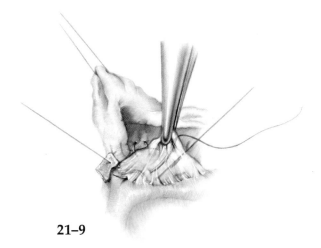

21–9

side of the leaflet (Fig. 21–9). Horizontal mattress sutures are used and are tied after they have all been placed.

Interrupted Suture Technique

The interrupted suture technique is used at Sutter/Sacramento. The anterior leaflet of the tricuspid valve is retracted with a vein retractor. Horizontal mattress sutures with pledgets, usually of 4-0 polyester, are placed below and on the right side of the inferior rim of the defect and through the Dacron patch (Fig. 21–10). Sutures are then placed anteriorly and superiorly with careful visualization and avoidance of the aortic valve (Fig. 21–11). Horizontal

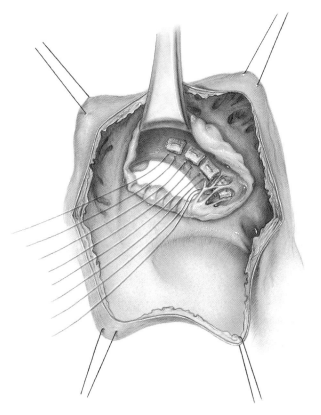

21–10

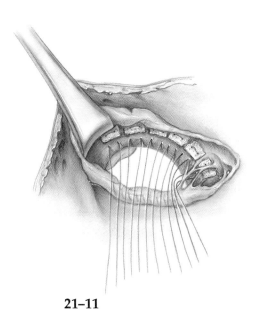

21–11

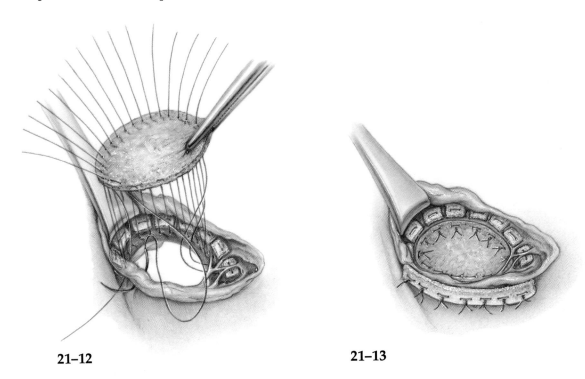

21–12

21–13

mattress sutures are then placed through the patch, through the base of the septal leaflet of the tricuspid valve, and through pledgets or a strip of Teflon (Fig. 21–12). The patch is then seated and tied (Fig. 21–13).

Posterior Defects

Posterior defects may be overlaid by papillary muscles and chordae (Fig. 21–14). Many are suitable for primary repair with buttressed horizontal mattress sutures. The sutures are placed through the right side of the defect and the base of the septal leaflet (Fig. 21–15) and tied (Fig. 21–16). Larger defects are

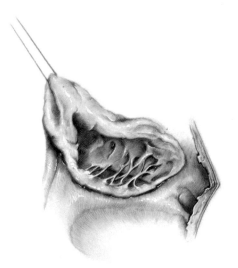

21–14

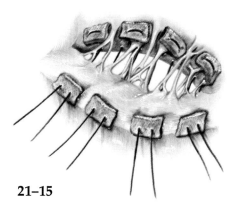

21–15

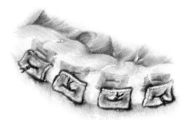

21–16

closed with a patch, remembering that the bundle of His is usually on the anterior-superior border of these defects.

Muscular Defects

Most defects in the midportion of the septum can be exposed through the tricuspid valve (Fig. 21–17) and closed primarily or with a patch (Fig. 21–18). If the defect is toward the apex, a limited left ventriculotomy is made between the distal left anterior descending and diagonal coronary arteries, and the defect is closed from the left ventricular side.[46] Such a ventriculotomy can cause late ventricular dysfunction. Transcatheter closure of apical muscular defects has been described and may well become more widespread in the future.[7] An alternative operative technique, which avoids a left ventriculotomy, is to expose the defect through the tricuspid valve, place horizontal mattress sutures with pledgets through the posterior and inferior rim of the defect, and bring them through the free wall of the right ventricle, tying them over pledgets, using intraoperative echocardiography to assure adequate closure of the defect.

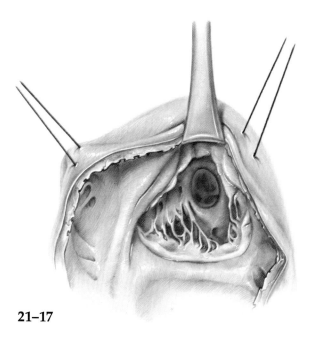

21–17

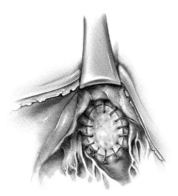

21–18

Results

Operative mortality for closure of VSD during infancy can be as low as 2%–4%.[1,3,14] Late survival is excellent and growth usually returns to normal.[8,41,65] Pulmonary artery pressure and pulmonary vascular resistance are usually normal 1 year postoperatively.[41] Closure of VSD in childhood can be associated with operative mortality as low as 0% and excellent late survival.[6]

Pulmonary Artery Banding

In the case of normally related great arteries, a left lateral thoracotomy is made through the fourth interspace. The pericardium is incised longitudinally anterior to the phrenic nerve and suspended. The plane between the pulmonary artery and aorta is opened, and a right angle is passed around the pulmonary artery. A silicone-coated strip of Teflon or a band of nylon is then brought around the pulmonary artery.

There are several methods of determining the degree of banding, including pressure measurements and predetermination of band circumference. Pressure measurement has not been completely reliable as a means of evaluating adequacy of a pulmonary artery band. This may be due to the variations in pulmonary vascular resistance and systemic vascular resistance during and after pulmonary artery banding.[63] An alternate method of determining the proper degree of banding is the use of a premarked measured band, with the size of the band being calculated from the patient's body weight.[61] We have used the technique of a premarked measured band and find it to be a good initial guideline. Any method must take into account the immediate clinical effect of the band, with appropriate adjustments being made as necessary.

References

1. Agosti J, Chiarello L, Wagner H, Subramanian S: Intracardiac repair of isolated ventricular septal defects below two years of age. J Cardiovasc Surg 17:147,1976.
2. Backer CL, Idriss FS, Zales VR, Ilbawi MN, DeLeon SY, Muster AJ, Mavroudis C: Surgical management of the conal (supracristal) ventricular septal defect. J Thorac Cardiovasc Surg 102:288,1991.
3. Barratt-Boyes BG, Neutze JM, Clarkson PM, Shardey GC, Brandt PWT: Repair of ventricular septal defect in the first two years of life using profound hypothemia-circulatory arrest techniques. Ann Surg 184:376,1976.
4. Becu LM, Fontana RS, DuShane JW, Kirklin JW, Burchell HB, Edwards JE: Anatomic and pathologic studies in ventricular septal defect. Circulation 14:349,1956.
5. Bjork VO: The transatrial approach to ventricular septal defect. J Thorac Cardiovasc Surg 47:178,1964.
6. Blackstone EH, Kirklin JW, Bradley EL, DuShane JW, Appelbaum A: Optimal age and results in repair of large ventricular septal defects. J Thorac Cardiovasc Surg 72:661,1976.
7. Bridges ND, Perry SB, Keane JF, Goldstein SAN, Mandell V, Mayer JE, Jonas RA, Castaneda AR, Lock JE: Preoperative transcatheter closure of congenital muscular ventricular septal defects. N Engl J Med 324:1312,1991.
8. Cartmill TB, DuShane JW, McGoon DC, Kirklin JW: Results of repair of ventricular septal defect. J Thorac Cardiovasc Surg 52:486,1966.
9. Castaneda AR, Zamora R, Nicoloff DM, Moller JH, Hunt CE, Lucas RV: High-pressure, high-resistance ventricular septal defect. Ann Thorac Surg 12:29,1971.
10. Cooley DA, Belmonte BA, DeBakey ME, Latson JR: Temporary extracorporeal circulation in the surgical treatment of cardiac and aortic disease. Ann Surg 145:898,1957.
11. Dooley KJ, Parisi-Buckley L, Fyler DC, Nadas AS: Results of pulmonary arterial banding in infancy: survey of 5 years' experience in the New England Regional Infant Cardiac Program. Am J Cardiol 36:484,1975.
12. Doty DB: Closure of perimembranous ventricular septal defect. J Thorac Cardiovasc Surg 85:781,1983.

13. Ellis FH, Ongley PA, Kirklin JW: Ventricular septal defect with aortic valvular incompetence. Surgical considerations. Circulation 27:789,1963.
14. Fisher RD, Faulkner SL, Sell CG, Graham TP Jr, Bender HW Jr: Operative closure of isolated defects of the ventricular septum: planned delay. Ann Thorac Surg 26:351,1978.
15. Galioto FM Jr, Cooley DA, El-Said G, Mullins CE, Sandiford FM: Closure of ventricular septal defect through the aortic valve. Chest 64:683,1973.
16. Griepp RE, French JW, Shumway NE, Baum D: Is pulmonary artery banding for ventricular septal defects obsolete? Circulation 48,50(Suppl II):II-14,1974.
17. Hallman GL, Cooley DA, Bloodwell RD: Two-stage surgical treatment of ventricular septal defect: results of pulmonary banding in infants and subsequent open-heart repair. J Thorac Cardiovasc Surg 52:476,1966.
18. Harlan BJ, Cooley DA: Transaortic repair of double-outlet right ventricle with situs inversus, l-loop, l-malposition (I,L,L), subaortic ventricular septal defect, and associated anomalies. J Thorac Cardiovasc Surg 72:547,1976.
19. Hitchcock JF, Suijker WJL, Ksiezycka E, Harinck E, van Mill JG, Ruzyllo W, Borman R, Meijboom EJ: Management of ventricular septal defect with associated aortic incompetence. Ann Thorac Surg 52:70,1991.
20. Ho SY, Anderson RH: Conduction tissue in congenital heart surgery. World J Surg 9:550,1985.
21. Hoffman JIE: Natural history of congenital heart disease. Circulation 37:97,1968.
22. Hoffman JIE, Rudolph AM: Natural history of ventricular septal defect in infancy. Am J Cardiol 16:634,1965.
23. Kawashima Y, Danno M, Shimizu Y, Matsuda H, Miyamoto T, Fujita T, Kozuka T, Manabe H: Ventricular septal defect associated with aortic insufficiency. Anatomic classification and method of operation. Circulation 47:1057,1973.
24. Kawashima Y, Fujita T, Mori T, Ihara K, Manabe H: Trans-pulmonary arterial closure of ventricular septal defect. J Thorac Cardiovasc Surg 74:191,1977.
25. Kay JH, Anderson RM, Tolentino P, Dykstra P, Shapiro MJ, Meihaus JE, Magidson O: The surgical repair of high pressure ventricular septal defect through the right atrium. Surgery 48:65,1960.
26. Keith JD, Rose V, Collins G, Kidd BSL: Ventricular septal defect: incidence, morbidity, and mortality in various age groups. Br Heart J 33:81,1971(Suppl).
27. Kirklin JW, DuShane JW: Repair of ventricular septal defect in infancy. Pediatrics 27:961,1961.
28. Kirklin JW, Harshbarger HG, Donald DE, Edwards JE: Surgical correction of ventricular septal defect: anatomic and technical considerations. J Thorac Surg 33:45,1957.
29. Koch W: Weitere Mitteilungen über den Sinusknoten des Herzens. Verh Dtsch Ges Pathol 13:85,1909.
30. Lev M: The architecture of the conduction system in congenital heart disease. III. Ventricular septal defect. Arch Pathol 70:529,1970.
31. Lev M, Fell EH, Arcilla R, Weinberg MH: Surgical injury to the conduction system in ventricular septal defect. Am J Cardiol 14:464,1964.
32. Lillehei CW, Levy MJ, Adams P, Anderson RC: High-pressure ventricular septal defects. JAMA 188:949,1964.
33. Lincoln C, Jamieson S, Joseph M, Shinebourne E, Anderson RH: Transatrial repair of ventricular septal defects with reference to their anatomic classification. J Thorac Cardiovasc Surg 74:183,1977.
34. McNicholas KW, Bowman FO Jr, Hayes CJ, Edie RN, Malm JR: Surgical management of ventricular septal defects in infants. J Thorac Cardiovasc Surg 75:346,1978.
35. Milo S, Yen HS, Wilkinson JL, Anderson RH: Surgical anatomy and atrioventricular conduction tissues of hearts with isolated ventricular septal defects. J Thorac Cardiovasc Surg 79:244,1980.
36. Mitchell SC, Korones SB, Berendes HW: Congenital heart disease in 56,109 births. Incidence and natural history. Circulation 43:323,1971.
37. Muller WH Jr, Damman JF Jr: The treatment of certain congenital malformations of the heart by creation of pulmonic stenosis to reduce pulmonary hypertension and pulmonary flow. Surg Gynecol Obstet 95:312,1952.
38. Murphy DA, Poirier N: A technique of aortic valvuloplasty for aortic insufficiency associated with ventricular septal defect. J Thorac Cardiovasc Surg 64:800,1972.
39. Nadas AS, Blount SG Jr: Management of ventricular septal defects in adults. Chest 74:3,1978.

40. Nadas AS, Thilenius OG, LaFarge CG, Hauck AJ: Ventricular septal defect with aortic regurgitation. Medical and pathologic aspects. Circulation 29:862,1964.

41. Rein JG, Freed MD, Norwood WI, Castaneda AR: Early and late results of closure of ventricular septal defect in infancy. Ann Thorac Surg 24:19,1977.

42. Sanfelippo PM, DuShane JW, McGoon DC, Danielson GK: Ventricular septal defect and aortic insufficiency. Ann Thorac Surg 17:213,1974.

43. Sealy WC, Hackel DB, Seaber AV: A study of methods for interruption of the His bundle. J Thorac Cardiovasc Surg 73:424,1977.

44. Serwer GA, Armstrong BE, Anderson PAW, Sherman D, Benson DW Jr, Edwards SB: Use of contrast echocardiography for evaluation of right ventricular hemodynamics in the presence of ventricular septal defects. Circulation 58:327,1978.

45. Seybold-Epting W, Reul GJ Jr, Hallman GL, Cooley DA: Repair of ventricular septal defect after pulmonary artery banding. J Thorac Cardiovasc Surg 71:392,1976.

46. Singh AK, deLeval MR, Stark J: Left ventriculotomy for closure of muscular ventricular septal defects: treatment of choice. Ann Surg 186:577,1977.

47. Somerville J, Brandao A, Ross DN: Aortic regurgitation with ventricular septal defect. Surgical management and clinical features. Circulation 41:317,1970.

48. Soto B, Becker AE, Moulaert AJ, Lie JT, Anderson RH: Classification of ventricular septal defects. Br Heart J 43:332,1980.

49. Soto B, Ceballos R, Kirklin JW: Ventricular septal defects: a surgical viewpoint. J Am Coll Cardiol 14:1291,1989.

50. Spencer FC, Doyle EF, Danilowicz DA, Bahnson HT, Weldon CS: Long-term evaluation of aortic valvuloplasty for aortic insufficiency and ventricular septal defect. J Thorac Cardiovasc Surg 65:15,1973.

51. Starr A, Menashe V, Dotter C: Successful correction of aortic insufficiency associated with ventricular septal defect. Surg Gynecol Obstet 111:71,1960.

52. Stirling GR, Stanley PH, Lillehei CW: The effects of cardiac bypass and ventriculotomy upon right ventricular function. Surg Forum 8:433,1957.

53. Suzuki Y, Ishizawa E, Tanaka S, Itoh T, Satoh K, Koizumi S, Tadokoro M, Horiuchi T, Satoh T, Kanoh I: Surgical treatment of large ventricular septal defect with pulmonary hypertension in the first 24 months of life. Ann Thorac Surg 22:228,1976.

54. Tandler J: Anatomie des Herzens, Jena, Gustav Fischer, 1913, p 64.

55. Tatsuno K, Konno S, Ando M, Sakakibara S: Pathogenetic mechanisms of prolapsing aortic valve and aortic regurgitation associated with ventricular septal defect. Anatomical, angiographic and surgical considerations. Circulation 48:1028,1973.

56. Titus JL: Normal anatomy of the human cardiac conduction system. Mayo Clin Proc 48:24,1973.

57. Titus JL, Daugherty GW, Edwards JE: Anatomy of the atrioventricular conduction system in ventricular septal defect. Circulation 28:72,1963.

58. Truex RC, Bishof JK: Conduction system in human hearts with interventricular septal defects. J Thorac Surg 35:421,1958.

59. Truex RC, Smythe MQ: Reconstruction of the human atrioventricular node. Anat Rec 158:11,1964.

60. Trusler GA, Moes CAF, Kidd BSL: Repair of ventricular septal defect with aortic insufficiency. J Thorac Cardiovasc Surg 66:394,1973.

61. Trusler GA, Mustard WT: A method of banding the pulmonary artery for large isolated ventricular septal defect with and without transposition of the great arteries. Ann Thorac Surg 13:351,1972.

62. Trusler GA, Williams WG, Smallhorn JF, Freedom RM: Late results after repair of aortic insufficiency associated with ventricular septal defect. J Thorac Cardiovasc Surg 103:276,1992.

63. Utley JR: Hemodynamic observations during and after pulmonary artery banding. Ann Thorac Surg 13:351,1972.

64. Van Praagh R, McNamara JJ: Anatomic types of ventricular septal defect with aortic insufficiency: diagnostic and surgical considerations. Am Heart J 75:604,1968.

65. Weintraub RG, Menahem S: Early surgical closure of a large ventricular septal defect: influence on long-term growth. J Am Coll Cardiol 18:552,1991.

66. Wenink ACG, Oppenheimer-Dekker A, Moulaert AJ: Muscular ventricular septal defects: a reappraisal of anatomy. Am J Cardiol 43:259,1979.

22

Tetralogy of Fallot

It is now almost four decades since total correction of tetralogy of Fallot was first reported by Lillehei[43] and demonstrated to be a feasible, low-risk operation by Kirklin.[35] During that time significant advances have occurred. Primary total correction can now be performed with low mortality in most infants regardless of size or weight. Surgery has an extremely important role in tetralogy of Fallot. The life expectancy without surgery is extremely poor: one-third of patients will die before 1 year, half before 3 years, and only one-quarter will live to 10 years.[3]

Indications for Surgery

Initial Palliation Versus Primary Total Correction

Alfred Blalock,[7] in his discussion of Lillehei's paper in 1955, correctly predicted that "the mortality accompanying the anastomotic procedure in the treatment of tetralogy of Fallot will remain lower for quite some time than that accompanying the direct attack under vision." Such was the case for many years in many institutions.

In the early 1970s a number of reports[1,2,12,16,52,56,67] documented the fact that primary total correction of tetralogy of Fallot during infancy could be performed in properly selected patients with a mortality below 10% and with excellent late results. Since that time early primary total correction has become the approach of choice in properly selected patients.

Proper timing of surgical intervention and proper choice of surgical procedure in tetralogy of Fallot are based on an understanding of the spectrum of anatomy and physiology that can occur.[8] The anatomic variability in tetralogy of Fallot occurs in the pulmonary outflow tract and pulmonary arteries: the anatomy that does not cause symptoms until childhood usually consists of infundibular stenosis with mild or no stenosis at the pulmonary anulus, main pulmonary arteries, or branch pulmonary arteries; the anatomy that causes symptoms and severe hypoxemia during infancy usually consists of stenosis at the pulmonary anulus[12] and frequently is associated with some hypoplasia of the main pulmonary artery as well. Hypoplasia of the branch pulmonary arteries may also be present. Infundibular stenosis often is mild in this latter subset of tetralogy of Fallot.[62]

Although small size,[33,34] young age,[17] and severity of hypoxemia may correlate with increased risk of primary total correction, the most significant variable appears to be the degree of hypoplasia of the main and branch pulmonary arteries and therefore the capacitance of the pulmonary artery system. A

301

poorly developed pulmonary artery system will not accommodate the total cardiac output resulting from closure of the ventricular septal defect (VSD). This causes right ventricular failure and death from low cardiac output. Therefore, it has been our objective for years to identify those patients with underdeveloped pulmonary artery systems and to perform initial palliation in this group in infancy.[62] Patients who have an adequate main pulmonary artery and adequate branch pulmonary arteries undergo total correction at the onset of cyanosis or hypoxic spells.

A number of methods have been described to define those patients with a hypoplastic pulmonary arterial system. We and others have used the ratio of the main pulmonary artery to the ascending aorta and perform a palliative operation if the ratio is less than 0.3. Blackstone, Kirklin, and colleagues[5] have described a formula using the ratio of the right and left pulmonary arteries to the descending thoracic aorta. Tucker, Ebert, and co-workers[65] use the ratio of the right pulmonary artery to the ascending aorta, choosing initial palliation if the ratio is less than 0.3. Nakata and colleagues[51] have described an index, the pulmonary artery index (PA index), which is a quantitative standardization of cross-sectional area of bilateral pulmonary arteries. The normal PA index is $330 \pm 30 \ mm^2/m^2$ of body surface area. DiDonato and co-workers,[17] in a study of patients undergoing neonatal repair of tetralogy of Fallot at Boston Children's Hospital, found that all deaths occurred in patients with a PA index less than $150 \ mm^2/m^2$.

In the presence of adequate pulmonary arteries, our only general contraindication to total correction of tetralogy of Fallot in the infant is an anomalous anterior descending coronary artery arising from the right coronary artery. However, others[66] do not consider this a contraindication.

The symptomatic patient with tetralogy of Fallot therefore undergoes total correction regardless of size or age if the main pulmonary artery/ascending aorta ratio is over 0.3 and if the origin of the anterior descending is normal. This encompasses the majority of patients. The remaining patients undergo a palliative procedure.

Reoperation

Reoperation is indicated if a hemodynamically significant VSD is present (Q_p/Q_s over 2 : 1),[57] a large right ventricular outflow gradient persists (over 60 mm Hg), or there is an aneurysm of the right ventricular outflow patch. An aneurysm of the outflow patch is usually associated with an outflow gradient. Some patients with marked pulmonary regurgitation and progressive right ventricular dilatation and drop in right ventricular function require insertion of a homograft valve in the right ventricular outflow tract.[21,49] Reoperation for residual lesions after tetralogy repair can be performed with the same low mortality and morbidity associated with the original operation,[13] if serious deterioration of right ventricular function has not occurred. Periodic follow-up of all patients postoperatively and early performance of studies if hemodynamic abnormality is suspected will prevent neglected situations.

Surgical Strategy

Choice of Palliative Procedure

We have detailed the reasoning underlying our choice of systemic-pulmonary shunts in Chapter 17. Our preference is to perform a Modified Blalock-Taussig shunt on the same side as the aortic arch. A properly performed shunt results in growth of the pulmonary arteries.[22]

Closure of Systemic-Pulmonary Shunts

The patency of shunts should be confirmed at catheterization. A continuous murmur may be due to bronchial collaterals and does not invariably indicate the presence of a patent shunt. The right-sided Blalock-Taussig shunt is usually easy to close at the time of total correction. The approach is intrapericardial.[36] The subclavian artery is located just above its junction with the right main pulmonary artery; this is usually medial to the superior vena cava. The superior vena cava is dissected, encircled, and retracted laterally. The aorta is retracted medially. An incision is made in the posterior pericardium over the palpated subclavian artery, and the artery is dissected and encircled; it is tied after cardiopulmonary bypass is begun. The polytetrafluoroethylene (PTFE) graft of a Modified Blalock-Taussig shunt is divided after cardiopulmonary bypass is begun.

Dissection and encirclement or division of the left-sided Blalock-Taussig shunt are more formidable. The approach is outside the pericardium over the left pulmonary artery, with dissection guided by the palpable thrill.[36]

Closure of a properly constructed Waterston shunt can usually be accomplished through the ascending aorta. If the right pulmonary artery is kinked or narrowed, it should be detached from the aorta and patched with pericardium if necessary.[25]

Myocardial Preservation

Cold blood cardioplegic arrest is our method of myocardial preservation.

Decision Regarding Transanular Patch

Relief of resistance to right ventricular emptying is an essential component of successful repair. It is desirable, if possible, to achieve this without producing pulmonary insufficiency. However, the relief of outflow obstruction is more important than avoidance of pulmonary insufficiency. A number of methods have been used for predicting the necessity of a transanular patch.

Empirical estimates at the time of repair and measuring the ratio of right ventricular to left ventricular pressure while temporarily discontinuing cardiopulmonary bypass following repair have both been used. However, a more scientific and predictable method of determining the necessity of a transanular patch during the initial repair was desirable. Such a method was described by Pacifico, Kirklin, and Blackstone,[53] basing the decision for primary enlargement of the pulmonary valve ring on a weight-related or surface area-related "minimum pulmonary valve ring diameter." This method is based on the studies of normal pulmonary anulus circumference by Rowlatt, Rimoldi, and Lev[59] and is a predictable method.[6]

At operation we pass calibrated dilators through the pulmonary valve from below and generally seek a normal anulus diameter, using the weight-related chart of Pacifico and colleagues,[53] patching across the anulus whenever indicated. We keep the chart posted in our operating room and find it useful for assessing all forms of pulmonary stenosis as well as determining the size of the patch. If there is any question, we are liberal in our use of a patch, since a transanular patch has little if any effect on early or late results.[31,45]

Associated Anomalies

Patent Ductus Arteriosus
This is ligated at the time of open repair, as described in Chapter 15.

Anomalous Coronary Artery
The anterior descending artery arises from the right coronary artery in approximately 5% of patients with tetralogy of Fallot,[15] crossing the right ven-

tricular outflow tract in a position where it can be transected by a vertical ventriculotomy. Such transection frequently results in myocardial infarction and death. As noted earlier, we consider an anomalous anterior descending artery a contraindication to repair in infancy.

Injury to an anomalous anterior descending artery can be avoided by repair through the right atrium[18] or by performing a transverse ventriculotomy caudal to the artery.[55] If the outflow tract cannot be adequately enlarged through such a ventriculotomy, a conduit can be placed over the anomalous artery to the pulmonary artery.[30,47]

Atrial Septal Defect or Patent Foramen Ovale
Atrial septal communications should be searched for and closed if present.

Single Pulmonary Artery
This condition can be congenital or can be caused by a systemic-pulmonary shunt. Successful repair is possible. Some recommend a valved conduit as a standard component of repair.[50]

Absent Pulmonary Valve
This condition is usually associated with dilation of the pulmonary arteries and tracheobronchial obstruction. Pulmonary difficulties are often more serious than the intracardiac pathophysiology.[39,48] Repair involving insertion of a tube graft between the main pulmonary artery and distal pulmonary arteries has been recommended,[44] although often this is not necessary.[61] Our practice has been to treat tetralogy with absent pulmonary valve the same as the more common forms of tetralogy.

Complete Atrioventricular Canal
This lesion can be corrected, when it occurs in association with tetralogy of Fallot, by a combined approach through the atrium and ventricle.[71]

Surgical Anatomy

Fallot[19,20] described the tetralogy in 1888: ventricular septal defect, infundibular pulmonic stenosis, dextroposition of the aorta, right ventricular hypertrophy. There is a variation in the anatomy of tetralogy of Fallot, which can cause controversy over the proper classification of some anatomic subsets. For most cases, however, there is little question over proper classification.

The anatomic defects as described by Fallot invariably result in equal ventricular pressures. Right-to-left shunting at the ventricular level usually occurs and may be constant or intermittent.

Ventricular Septal Defect

The VSD is large, usually the diameter of the ascending aorta or larger. It is subaortic in location, in the anterior portion of the muscular septum, anterior to the pars membranacea (Fig. 22–1). It is below the posterior part of the right coronary cusp and the anterior part of the noncoronary cusp.[42]

The VSD, as viewed by the surgeon through an infundibular incision, is bordered anteriorly, inferiorly, and superiorly by septal musculature. The posterior border is often formed by tissue at the base of the septal leaflet of the tricuspid valve, and may also contain some of the pars membranacea as well as a portion of the aortic anulus. The superior border is the crista supraventricularis, also referred to as the conus septum.

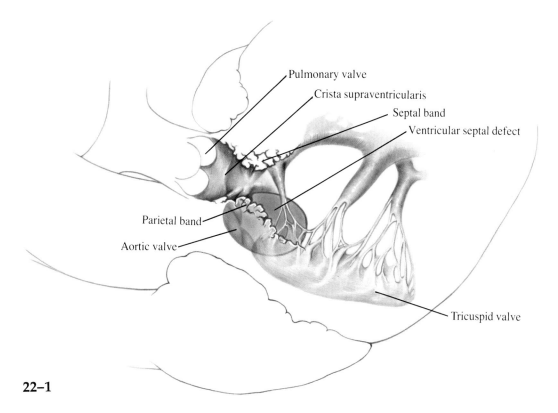

Pulmonary valve

Crista supraventricularis

Septal band

Ventricular septal defect

Parietal band

Aortic valve

Tricuspid valve

22–1

Conduction System

Lev's[40,41] careful studies of the architecture of the conduction system in congenital heart disease, particularly tetralogy of Fallot, have greatly contributed to our knowledge. He has shown that, in tetralogy of Fallot, the atrioventricular bundle penetrates the central fibrous body as the conus musculature inserts on the central fibrous body. If there is an upward extension of the central fibrous body (pars membranacea), then the bundle lies on the left side of the septum as it reaches the level of the ventricular septal defect. Here it is flattened and widened out, lying on the left side of the septum below the defect.

Right Ventricular Outflow Obstruction

A variable amount of pulmonic stenosis is always present at the infundibular level. The next most frequent location of pulmonic stenosis is at the valvar or anular level. The pulmonic valve is often bicuspid. A small main pulmonary artery is common.[60] Stenotic or hypoplastic branch pulmonary arteries are rare.[60]

Surgical Technique

Repair via Ventriculotomy

This technique is used at the Children's Cardiac Center of Oregon/Portland. A vertical incision is made in the infundibulum (Fig. 22–2). A vertical incision is preferred because it exposes the infundibular stenosis and the VSD well and, in contrast to a transverse incision, can easily be extended across the pulmonary anulus if necessary.

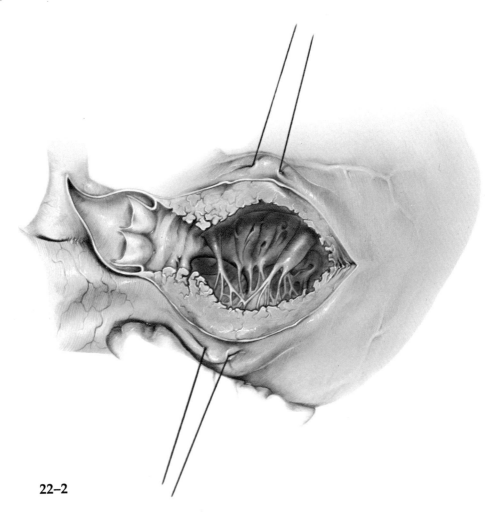

22–2

The constricting septal bands (Fig. 22–3) and parietal bands (Fig. 22–4) are incised and excised (Fig. 22–5). The bands are frequently tightly packed, but a right-angle clamp can be insinuated behind them, aiding incision and excision. The parietal band is not excised if it is small or the aortic valve is in close proximity, so as to avoid damage to the aortic valve and so as to leave adequate tissue for placing sutures.

None of the crista supraventricularis (conus septum) is excised; such excision can injure the underlying aortic valve and also jeopardizes secure anchoring of sutures around the superior border of the VSD patch.

The pulmonary valve and anulus are inspected from below, and Bakes or Hegar dilators are passed to calibrate the valve and anulus diameter,[53] as discussed earlier in this chapter. If the pulmonary anulus and pulmonary artery are of good size but there is valvular stenosis, a pulmonic commissurotomy is performed through a separate pulmonary arteriotomy. In the presence of a small anulus and main pulmonary artery, the ventriculotomy is extended across the anulus onto the pulmonary artery as far as necessary, frequently into the left pulmonary artery.

Incision and excision of the septal and parietal bands help expose the VSD. Exposure is further aided by placing a small intracardiac sucker through the defect, with retraction to the left (Fig. 22–6).

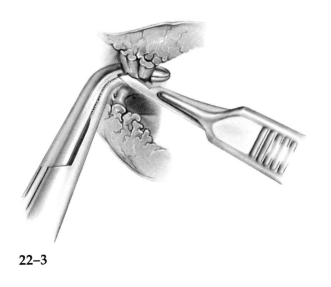

22–3

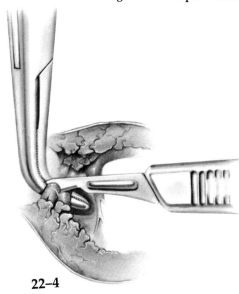

22–4

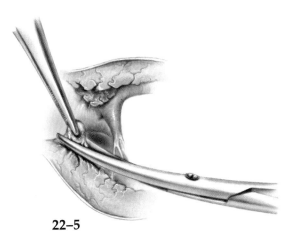

22–5

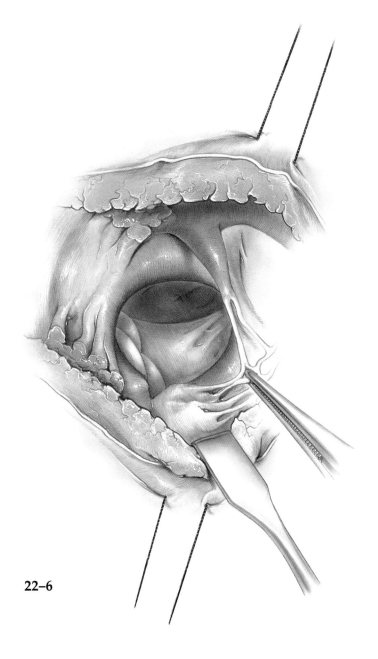

22–6

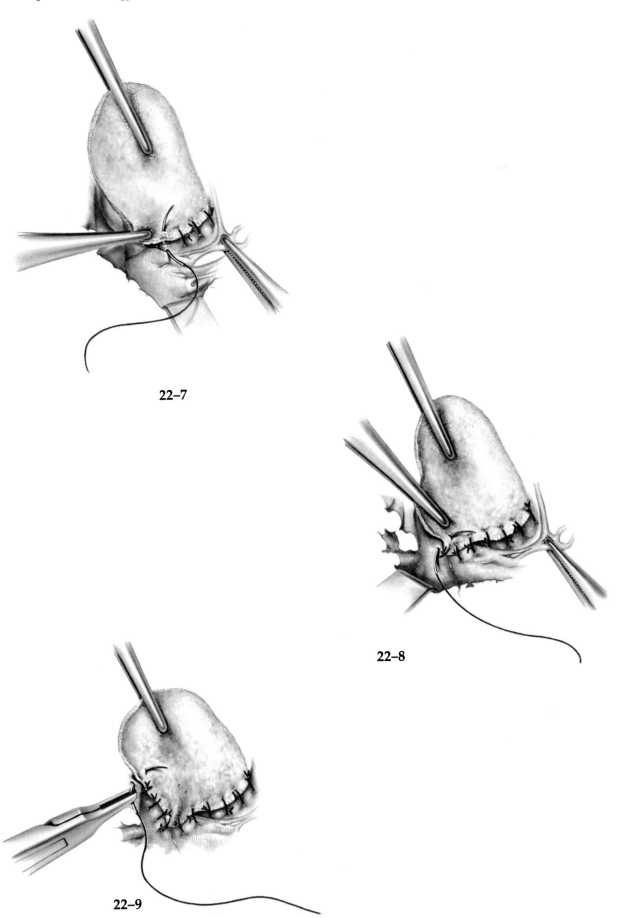

22–7

22–8

22–9

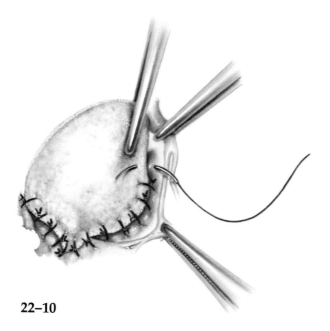

22–10

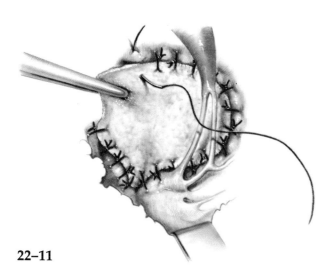

22–11

Closure of the VSD is with a patch of knitted Dacron double-velour, using interrupted 4-0 silk sutures on small half-circle needles.

The first suture is placed in the midportion of the caudal rim of the defect (Fig. 22–7). Forceps never grasp the defect margin. The patch, slightly larger in diameter than the aortic root, is tied into place.

Sutures are placed in a clockwise direction, into the tricuspid anulus (Fig. 22–8) and the aortic anulus if extreme overriding is present. Sutures are placed in the parietal limb of the crista supraventricularis (Fig. 22–9).

Closure then begins again at the first suture and moves counterclockwise up to the crista, with deep sutures in the muscular margin (Fig. 22–10). Sutures are then placed attaching the patch to the crista (Fig. 22–11).

If the pulmonary valve diameter is adequate, the infundibular outflow area is assessed. If the ventricular edges cannot be approximated easily over a Hegar dilator the size of the patient's pulmonary valve orifice, a patch of pericardium or woven Dacron, cut from a tubular graft, is placed over the infundibulum. If transanular patching is necessary, it is frequently begun on

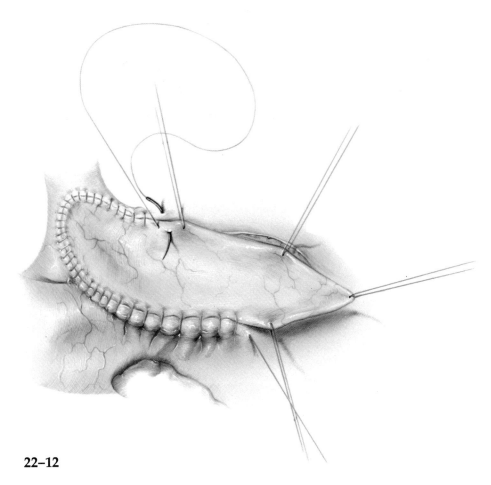

22–12

or at the base of the left pulmonary artery and carried across the anulus onto the ventricle (Fig. 22–12).

After cardiopulmonary bypass is terminated, prior to decannulation, pressures are measured in the right ventricle. A desirable right ventricle-systemic artery pressure ratio is 0.65 or less.[33]

Repair via Right Atrium and Limited Ventriculotomy

The transatrial approach to repair of tetralogy was described by Hudspeth and colleagues[29] in 1963. It was not until the late 1970s and 1980s that the use of this approach, often combined with a transpulmonary approach or a limited ventriculotomy, became more widespread.[4,18,32,46,54] This approach has the hypothetical advantage of better postoperative ventricular function because of a smaller ventricular incision or no ventricular incision. Relief of right ventricular outflow tract obstruction can be as effective through the transatrial and transpulmonary approach as through the transventricular approach.[14] The repair of the VSD is often easier from the atrium, especially when there is marked overriding of the aorta. This is the approach most often used at Sutter/Sacramento.

The VSD and right ventricular outflow tract are explored through the right atrium. If it is clear that a transanular patch will be needed, a short infundibular incision is made and carried across the pulmonary anulus onto the pulmonary artery. Infundibular muscle is resected either from above or from below. The VSD is closed with interrupted horizontal mattress sutures as shown in the previous chapter (Figs. 21–14 to 21–17). The transanular patch is then placed.

Late Results

Clinical Status

Late survival at 5 to 10 years following correction of tetralogy of Fallot is 95%.[11,27,37,55] The vast majority of patients are asymptomatic. Sunderland and co-workers,[64] in a study of 27 survivors of correction in infancy, found all to be asymptomatic. Similarly excellent results have been reported by others.[37,55,68] Garson and colleagues[23] have shown that over 80% of adults who underwent correction during childhood can lead a normal life without impairment of intellect, exercise tolerance, or fertility.

Hemodynamic Status

Most patients have minor hemodynamic abnormalities after correction. They still are able, however, to have normal or nearly normal cardiovascular responses to maximal exercise as measured by cardiac output, maximal oxygen consumption, and left ventricular ejection fraction.[58] The most common hemodynamic abnormalities are mild right ventricular hypertension (30–45 mm Hg), a small gradient between the right ventricle and pulmonary artery (10–20 mm Hg), and pulmonary regurgitation.[9,10,64] Bristow and colleagues[9] have demonstrated a stable hemodynamic status in patients for up to 10 years.

Electrophysiologic Changes

Minor electrophysiologic changes are the rule after repair of tetralogy of Fallot. More severe changes are much less frequent but are an area of controversy, regarding both their significance and their proper management.

Right bundle branch block (RBBB) occurs in 85%–95% of patients after repair of tetralogy of Fallot.[26,63] As an isolated electrophysiologic change it is entirely benign.

Right bundle branch block with left anterior hemiblock (RBBB + LAH) occurs much less frequently, in 8%–18% of patients.[28,63,70] There are conflicting reports regarding the prognosis of RBBB + LAH. Wolff and co-workers[69] reported sudden death in 12.5% of patients with RBBB + LAH and in 2% of patients without the pattern. However, Gillette[26] and Steeg[63] reported two separate series of patients with RBBB + LAH without any late deaths. The different prognoses may be due to different sites of conduction injury.[38]

Gillette and colleagues[26] reported premature ventricular contractions (PVCs) to be associated with sudden death. In addition, all of the patients who died had significant congestive heart failure. They recommend treating postoperative patients who have PVCs. Garson and colleagues,[24] in a study of the treatment of ventricular arrhythmias after repair of tetralogy of Fallot, found that sudden death did not occur in any patient with successful antiarrhythmic treatment.

References

1. Adams P, Radley-Smith R, Yacoub M: Primary total correction of Fallot's tetralogy below the age of 2 years. Br Heart J 36:1036,1974.
2. Barratt-Boyes BG, Neutze JM: Primary repair of tetralogy of Fallot in infancy using profound hypothermia with circulatory arrest and limited cardiopulmonary bypass: a comparison with conventional two stage management. Ann Surg 178: 406,1973.
3. Bertanou EG, Blackstone EH, Hazelrig JB, Turner ME Jr, Kirklin JW: Life expectancy without surgery in tetralogy of Fallot. Am J Cardiol 41:458,1978.
4. Binet J-P: Correction of tetralogy of Fallot with combined transatrial and pulmonary approach: experience with 184 consecutive cases. J Card Surg 3:97,1988.
5. Blackstone EH, Kirklin JW, Bertranou EG, Labrosse CJ, Soto B, Bargeron LM:

Preoperative prediction from cineangiograms of post-repair right ventricular pressure in tetralogy of Fallot. J Thorac Cardiovasc Surg 78:542,1979.

6. Blackstone EH, Kirklin JW, Pacifico AD: Decision-making in repair of tetralogy of Fallot based on intraoperative measurements of pulmonary arterial outflow tract. J Thorac Cardiovasc Surg 77:526,1979.

7. Blalock A: Discussion of Lillehei et al: Direct vision intracardiac surgical correction of the tetralogy of Fallot, pentalogy of Fallot and pulmonary atresia defects. Ann Surg 142:418,1955.

8. Bonchek LI, Starr A, Sunderland CO, Menashe VD: Natural history of tetralogy of Fallot in infancy: clinical classification and therapeutic implications. Circulation 48:392,1973.

9. Bristow JD, Kloster FE, Lees MH, Menashe VD, Griswold HE, Starr A: Serial cardiac catheterizations and exercise hemodynamics after correction of tetralogy of Fallot: average follow-up 13 months and 7 years after operation. Circulation 41: 1057,1970.

10. Burnell RH, Woodson RD, Lees MH, Bristow JD, Starr A: Results of correction of tetralogy of Fallot in children under four years of age. J Thorac Cardiovasc Surg 57:153,1969.

11. Calder AL, Barratt-Boyes BG, Brandt PWT, Neutze JM: Postoperative evaluation of patients with tetralogy of Fallot repaired in infancy: including criteria for use of outflow patching and radiologic assessment of pulmonary regurgitation. J Thorac Cardiovasc Surg 77:704,1979.

12. Castaneda AR, Freed MD, Williams RG, Norwood WI: Repair of tetralogy of Fallot in infancy. J Thorac Cardiovasc Surg 74:372,1977.

13. Castaneda AR, Sade RM, Lamberti J, Nicoloff DM: Reoperation for residual defects after repair of tetralogy of Fallot. Surgery 76:1010,1974.

14. Coles JG, Kirklin JW, Pacifico AD, Kirklin JK, Blackstone EH: The relief of pulmonary stenosis by a transatrial versus a transventricular approach to the repair of tetralogy of Fallot. Ann Thorac Surg 45:7,1988.

15. Dabizzi RP, Caprioli G, Aiazzi L, Castelli C, Baldrighi G, Parenzan L, Baldrighi V: Distribution and anomalies of coronary arteries in tetralogy of Fallot. Circulation 61:95,1980.

16. Daily PO, Stinson EB, Griepp RB, Shumway NE: Tetralogy of Fallot: choice of surgical procedure. J Thorac Cardiovasc Surg 75:338,1978.

17. DiDonato RM, Jonas RA, Lang P, Rome JJ, Mayer JE Jr, Castaneda AR: Neonatal repair of tetralogy of Fallot with and without pulmonary atresia. J Thorac Cardiovasc Surg 101:126,1991.

18. Edmunds LH Jr, Saxena NC, Friedman S, Rashkind JW, Dodd PF: Transatrial repair of tetralogy of Fallot. Surgery 80:681,1976.

19. Fallot A: Contribution de l'anatomie pathologique de la maladie bleue (cyanose cardiaque). Marseille Med 25:77,138,207,341,403,1888.

20. Fallot A: Contribution to the pathologic anatomy of morbus caeruleus (translated summary). *In* Willins, Keys (eds): Cardiac Classics. St Louis, CV Mosby Co, 1941, pp 689,690.

21. Finck SJ, Puga FJ, Danielson GK: Pulmonary valve insertion during reoperation for tetralogy of Fallot. Ann Thorac Surg 45:610,1988.

22. Gale AW, Arcinegas E, Green EW, Blackstone EH, Kirklin JW: Growth of the pulmonary anulus and pulmonary arteries after the Blalock-Taussig shunt. J Thorac Cardiovasc Surg 77:459,1979.

23. Garson A Jr, Nihill MR, McNamara DG, Cooley DA: Status of the adult and adolescent after repair of tetralogy of Fallot. Circulation 59:1232,1979.

24. Garson A Jr, Randall DC, Gillette PC, Smith RT, Moak JP, McVey P, McNamara DG: Prevention of sudden death after repair of tetralogy of Fallot: treatment of ventricular arrhythmias. J Am Coll Cardiol 6:221,1985.

25. Gay WA Jr, Ebert PA: Aorta-to-right pulmonary artery anastomosis causing obstruction of the right pulmonary artery: management during correction of tetralogy of Fallot. Ann Thorac Surg 16:402,1973.

26. Gillette PC, Yeoman MA, Mullins CE, McNamara DG: Sudden death after repair of tetralogy of Fallot: electrocardiographic and electrophysiologic abnormalities. Circulation 56:566,1977.

27. Horneffer PJ, Zahka KG, Rowe SA, Manolio TA, Gott VL, Reitz BA, Gardner TJ:

Long-term results of total repair of tetralogy of Fallot in childhood. Ann Thorac Surg 50:179,1990.

28. Howe A, Rastelli GC, Ritter DG, DuShane JW, McGoon DC: Management of the right ventricular outflow tract in severe tetralogy of Fallot. J Thorac Cardiovasc Surg 60:131,1970.

29. Hudspeth AS, Cordell AR, Johnston FR: Transatrial approach to total correction of tetralogy of Fallot. Circulation 27:796,1963.

30. Humes RA, Driscoll DJ, Danielson GK, Puga FJ: Tetralogy of Fallot with anomalous origin of left anterior descending coronary artery: surgical options. J Thorac Cardiovasc Surg 94:784,1987.

31. Jones EL, Conti CR, Neill CA, Gott VL, Brawley RK, Haller JA: Long-term evaluation of tetralogy patients with pulmonary valvular insufficiency resulting from outflow-patch correction across the pulmonic annulus. Circulation 48(Suppl III)III-11,1973.

32. Kawashima Y, Matsuda H, Hirose H, Nakano S, Shirakura R, Kobayashi J: Ninety consecutive corrective operations for tetralogy of Fallot with or without minimal right ventriculotomy. J Thorac Cardiovasc Surg 90:856,1985.

33. Kirklin JW, Blackstone EH, Jonas RA, Shimazaki Y, Kirklin JK, Mayer JE Jr, Pacifico AD, Castaneda AR: Morphologic and surgical determinants of outcome events after repair of tetralogy of Fallot and pulmonary stenosis. J Thorac Cardiovasc Surg 103:706,1992.

34. Kirklin JW, Blackstone EH, Pacifico AD, Brown RN, Bargeron LM: Routine primary repair vs two-stage repair of tetralogy of Fallot. Circulation 60:373,1979.

35. Kirklin JW, Ellis FH, McGoon DC, DuShane JW, Swan JC: Surgical treatment for the tetralogy of Fallot by open intracardiac repair. J Thorac Cardiovasc Surg 37:22,1959.

36. Kirklin JW, Payne WS: Surgical treatment for tetralogy of Fallot after previous anastomosis of systemic to pulmonary artery. Surg Gynecol Obstet 110:707,1960.

37. Kirklin JW, Wallace RB, McGoon DC, DuShane JW: Early and late results after intracardiac repair of tetralogy of Fallot. Ann Surg 162:578,1965.

38. Krongard E: Prognosis for patients with congenital heart disease and postoperative intraventricular conduction defects. Circulation 57:867,1978.

39. Lakier JB, Stanger P, Heymann MA, Hoffman JIE, Rudolph AM: Tetralogy of Fallot with absent pulmonary valve: natural history and hemodynamic considerations. Circulation 50:167,1974.

40. Lev M: The architecture of the conduction system in congenital heart disease. II. Tetralogy of Fallot. Arch Pathol Lab Med 67:572,1959.

41. Lev M: Conduction system in congenital heart disease. Am J Cardiol 21:619,1968.

42. Lev M, Eckner RAO: The pathologic anatomy of tetralogy of Fallot and its variations. Dis Chest 45:251,1964.

43. Lillihei CW, Cohen M, Warden HE, Reed RC, Aust JB, Dewall RA, Varco RL: Direct vision intracardiac surgical correction of the tetralogy of Fallot, pentalogy of Fallot and pulmonary artresia defects. Ann Surg 142:418,1955.

44. Litwin SB, Rosenthal A, Fellows K: Surgical management of young infants with tetralogy of Fallot, absence of pulmonary valve, and respiratory distress. J Thorac Cardiovasc Surg 65:552,1973.

45. McGoon DC: Discussion of Pacifico et al: Surgical management of pulmonary stenosis in tetralogy of Fallot. J Thorac Cardiovasc Surg 74:382,1977.

46. McGrath LB, Gonzalez-Lavin L: Determination of the need for a ventriculotomy in the repair of tetralogy of Fallot. J Thorac Cardiovasc Surg 96:947,1988.

47. Meyer J, Chiarello L, Hallman GL, Cooley DA: Coronary artery anomalies in patients with tetralogy of Fallot. J Thorac Cardiovasc Surg 69:373,1975.

48. Miller RA, Lev M, Paul MH: Congenital absence of the pulmonary valve: the clinical syndrome of tetralogy of Fallot with pulmonary regurgitation. Circulation 26:266,1962.

49. Misbach GA, Turley K, Ebert PA: Pulmonary valve replacement for regurgitation after repair of tetralogy of Fallot. Ann Thorac Surg 36:684,1983.

50. Mistrot JJ, Bernhard WF, Rosenthal A, Castaneda AR: Tetralogy of Fallot with a single pulmonary artery: operative repair. Ann Thorac Surg 23:249,1977.

51. Nakata S, Imai Y, Takanashi Y, Kurosawa H, Tezuka K, Nakazawa M, Ando M, Takao A: A new method for the quantitative standardization of cross-sectional

areas of the pulmonary arteries in congenital heart diseases with decreased pulmonary blood flow. J Thorac Cardiovasc Surg 88:610,1984.

52. Pacifico AD, Bargeron LM, Kirklin JW: Primary total correction of tetralogy of Fallot in children less than four years of age. Circulation 48:1085,1973.

53. Pacifico AD, Kirklin JW, Blackstone EH: Surgical management of pulmonary stenosis in tetralogy of Fallot. J Thorac Cardiovasc Surg 74:382,1977.

54. Pacifico AD, Sand ME, Bargeron LM Jr, Colvin EC: Transatrial-transpulmonary repair of tetralogy of Fallot. J Thorac Cardiovasc Surg 93:919,1987.

55. Poirer RA, McGoon DC, Danielson GK, Wallace RB, Ritter DG, Moodie DS, Wiltse CG: Late results after repair of tetralogy of Fallot. J Thorac Cardiovasc Surg 73:900,1977.

56. Rees GM, Starr A: Total correction of Fallot's tetralogy in patients aged less than 1 year. Br Heart J 35:898,1973.

57. Rocchini AP, Rosenthal A, Freed M, Castaneda AR, Nadas AS: Chronic congestive heart failure after repair of tetralogy of Fallot. Circulation 56:305,1977.

58. Rosing DR, Borer JS, Kent KM, Maron BJ, Seides SF, Morrow AG, Epstein SE: Long-term hemodynamic and electrocardiographic assessment following operative repair of tetralogy of Fallot. Circulation 58(Suppl III)III-209,1978.

59. Rowlatt UR, Rimoldi HJA, Lev M: The quantitative anatomy of the normal child's heart. Pediatr Clin North Am 10:499,1963.

60. Shimazaki Y, Blackstone EH, Kirklin JW, Jonas RA, Mandell V, Colvin EV: The dimensions of the right ventricular outflow tract and pulmonary arteries in tetralogy of Fallot and pulmonary stenosis. J Thorac Cardiovasc Surg 103:692,1992.

61. Stafford EG, Mair DD, McGoon DC, Danielson GK: Tetralogy of Fallot with absent pulmonary valve. Circulation 48(Suppl III):III-24,1973.

62. Starr A, Bonchek LI, Sunderland CO: Total correction of tetralogy of Fallot in infancy. J Thorac Cardiovasc Surg 65:45,1973.

63. Steeg CN, Krongrad E, Davachi F, Bowman FO Jr, Malm JR, Gersony WM: Postoperative left anterior hemiblock and right bundle branch block following repair of tetralogy of Fallot. Circulation 51:1026,1975.

64. Sunderland CO, Matarazzo RG, Lees MH, Menashe VD, Bonchek LI, Rosenberg JA, Starr A: Total correction of tetralogy of Fallot: postoperative hemodynamic evaluation. Circulation 48:398,1973.

65. Tucker WY, Turley K, Ullyot DJ, Ebert PA: Management of symptomatic tetralogy of Fallot in the first year of life. J Thorac Cardiovasc Surg 78:494,1979.

66. Turley K, Tucker WY, Ebert PA: The changing role of palliative procedures in the treatment of infants with congenital heart disease. J Thorac Cardiovasc Surg 79:194,1980.

67. Venugopal P, Subramanian S: Intracardiac repair of tetralogy of Fallot in patients under five years of age. Ann Thorac Surg 18:228,1974.

68. Walsh EP, Rockenmacher S, Keane JF, Hougen TJ, Lock JE, Castaneda AR: Late results in patients with tetralogy of Fallot repaired during infancy. Circulation 77:1062,1988.

69. Wolff GS, Rowland TW, Ellison RC: Surgically induced right bundle-branch block with left anterior hemiblock: an ominous sign in postoperative tetralogy of Fallot. Circulation 46:587,1972.

70. Yabek SM, Jarmakani JM, Roberts NK: Diagnosis of trifascicular damage following tetralogy of Fallot and ventricular septal defect repair. Circulation 55:23,1977.

71. Zavanella C, Matsuda H, Subramanian S: Successful correction of a complete form of atrioventricular canal associated with tetralogy of Fallot. J Thorac Cardiovasc Surg 74:195,1977.

23

Transposition of the Great Arteries

The first approach to physiologic correction of transposition of the great arteries, based on transposing venous inflow, was conceived by Albert,[2] using animal experiments, and reported in 1954. Senning[73] reported in 1959 a successful intraatrial operation in humans utilizing the walls and septum of the atria. Shumacker[79] described in 1961 an operation using a bipedicled atrial flap. Mustard's[55] report in 1964 of an intraatrial transposition operation in a human using pericardium led to its almost universal use during the late 1960s and early 1970s. The 1970s saw a widespread return to the Senning operation in hopes of decreasing or eliminating some of the complications seen with the Mustard operation.[8,20,59,63]

Anatomic correction of transposition of the great arteries, based on transposing the great arteries and coronary arteries, was tried unsuccessfully as early as the 1950s.[5,34,41,56,73] Successful anatomic repair, the arterial switch procedure, reported by Jatene[38] in 1976 and Yacoub[98] in 1977, stimulated once again a strong interest in the possibilities of repair involving outflow correction, with its advantage of returning the left ventricle to the status of the systemic ventricle and avoiding extensive surgery within the atria with the resultant rhythm problems.

The experience of the 1980s has established the arterial switch procedure as the procedure of choice for surgical treatment of transposition of the great arteries.[92] This chapter presents the arterial switch procedure, the Senning procedure, and the Mustard procedure. The Senning procedure and the Mustard procedure are presented primarily for historical interest.

Indications for Surgery

The outcome of transposition of the great arteries without intervention to increase systemic and pulmonary venous admixture is death for 80%–90% of infants by age 1 year.[60,75] This high mortality made search for an operative approach intense. A palliative procedure, atrial septectomy, was introduced by Blalock and Hanlon[10] in 1950. This was an effective means of increasing systemic oxygen saturation in a large proportion of patients, but was associated with a mortality of at least 20%–30%.[19,82]

In the middle 1960s Rashkind[65] introduced the technique of balloon atrial septostomy, performed by tearing the atrial septum with an inflated balloon at the tip of a catheter. This procedure was relatively easily performed in the catheterization laboratory, and was quickly shown to result in improvement in most patients and to have a much lower mortality (less than 10%) than the

Blalock-Hanlon operation.[90] The Rashkind septostomy results in an adequate systemic arterial oxygen saturation in the majority of patients and short-term palliation, usually 6 to 12 months. The successful short-term palliation of the Rashkind balloon septostomy became the basis for delaying the performance of inflow or atrial procedures to the age of around 6 months.

Now that the arterial switch procedure has replaced the inflow procedures, the operation is usually performed within the first 2 weeks of life before the left ventricle becomes unable to handle systemic pressure.[14] The performance of the Rashkind balloon septostomy is variable at centers peforming the arterial switch procedure.[7,35,61] The cardiologists at our institutions usually perform a Rashkind balloon septostomy in patients who are to undergo an arterial switch procedure. In addition, prostaglandin E_1 is given in the preoperative period.

Choice of Operation

The arterial switch procedure has replaced the atrial procedures because it can be performed with an operative mortality similar to that of the atrial procedures and it is not associated with the long-term complications found with the atrial procedures.[14,47,64] Both the Mustard and Senning operations are associated with late fatal arrhythmias and with late failure of the systemic ventricle, the right ventricle.[53,86,94] In addition the Mustard operation can be complicated by systemic or pulmonary venous obstruction.[85,88]

The arterial switch procedure was first performed in patients with preoperative systemic pressures in their left ventricle caused by the presence of a ventricular septal defect (VSD). Yacoub[96,98] expanded the application of the arterial switch procedure to transposition with intact ventricular septum by preparing the left ventricle for a period of time by pulmonary artery banding. Castaneda[13] then demonstrated in 1984 that the arterial switch procedure could be performed with low operative mortality in newborns with transposition and intact ventricular septum without prior pulmonary artery banding.

Surgical Strategy

Conduct of Cardiopulmonary Bypass

All operations in newborns and infants are performed using profound hypothermia and low flow and very low flow bypass, with brief periods of circulatory arrest if needed. Cold blood cardioplegia is used for myocardial preservation.

Management of Associated Defects

Ventricular Septal Defect
VSD occurs in approximately 20% of patients with transposition of the great arteries.[70] Pulmonary stenosis is also present in approximately 30% of patients with VSDs.[36]

Transposition with VSD and no pulmonary stenosis is associated with very high mortality in infancy: most patients die before 6 months of age. Severe pulmonary vascular disease is common in survivors at 1 year of age. It is our practice to perform the arterial switch procedure and closure of the VSD within the first 2 months of life.[23] Patients with VSD can undergo arterial switch and closure of the VSD with operative mortality as low as that in patients with intact ventricular septum.[14]

Double-Outlet Right Ventricle with Subpulmonary Ventricular Septal Defect (Taussig-Bing Anomaly)
The Taussig-Bing anomaly is repaired by closing the VSD and performing the arterial switch procedure. The aorta is divided somewhat more distally.[40] The

branches of the pulmonary artery are dissected and the ligamentum or ductus is divided, but the Lecompte[44] maneuver (bringing the pulmonary artery anterior to the aorta) is not usually performed, since the Lecompte maneuver can result in excessive tension on the left pulmonary artery.[40,64]

Pulmonary Stenosis
Marked pulmonary stenosis is unusual in transposition with intact ventricular septum, occurring in less than 5% of patients.[76,78] Some anatomic abnormality of the left ventricular outflow tract or small hemodynamic abnormality is common, reported in as many as 33% of patients.[70] The location of the stenosis can be at the valve, below the valve, or both,[6] or it can be due to posterior deviation of the infundibular septum.[93] Wernovsky and colleagues,[93] in a study of 30 children undergoing arterial switch procedure in association with abnormalities of the left ventricular outflow tract, concluded that mild pulmonary valve abnormalities, dynamic or surgically remediable subpulmonary stenosis, or abnormal mitral valve attachments do not preclude a successful arterial switch procedure, but that posterior deviation of the infundibular septum may result in residual obstruction.

Pulmonary stenosis with VSD can be managed by creating an intraventricular baffle directing the left ventricular outflow through the VSD to the aorta and constructing a conduit from the right ventricle to the pulmonary artery (Rastelli operation).[52,66]

Reoperation

Reoperation is sometimes necessary following arterial or atrial repair. The most common cause for reoperation following the arterial switch procedure is the development of pulmonary stenosis, which has been reported in 2%–16% of patients.[47,57,58] The pulmonary stenosis is usually easily repaired by patch arterioplasty.

The Mustard operation can be complicated by venous obstruction (systemic or pulmonary) and patch leaks or dehiscence.[81,84] An area of localized stenosis in the baffle can be repaired with a Dacron patch.[42] Severe diffuse stenosis of the patch or dehiscence may require excision and replacement. Localized areas of detachment may be repaired. Pulmonary venous obstruction can be corrected by patching the pulmonary venous atrium.[67]

Preparation of the Left Ventricle for the Arterial Switch Procedure

Patients may present late for the arterial switch procedure because of sickness, size, or late referral. Jonas and co-workers[39] have described a rapid, two-stage procedure, performed in a group of patients with a mean age of 4.5 months, involving pulmonary artery banding with or without a shunt followed in a very short time (median, 9 days) with the arterial switch procedure. Serial two-dimensional echocardiography showed that left ventricular mass increased by a mean of 85% during this short interval. Yasui and colleagues[100] have studied the cutoff point at which it is safe to perform the arterial switch procedure without preparation of the left ventricle and have concluded that it is safe if the left ventricular mass is larger than 60% of normal as determined by echocardiography.

Arterial Switch Procedure

Surgical Anatomy

An essential component of the arterial switch procedure is transfer of the coronary arteries without kinking, torsion, or tension. This requires knowledge of the anatomic variations present in transposition and the ability to adjust technique to accommodate these variations.

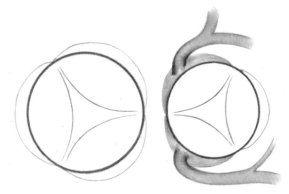

Figure 23–1 Type A.

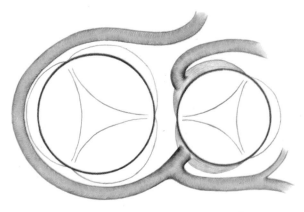

Figure 23–2 Type D.

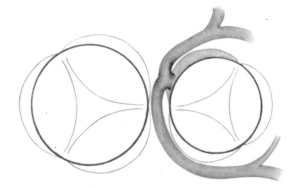

Figure 23–3 Type B.

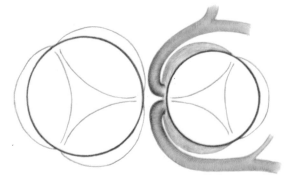

Figure 23–4 Type C.

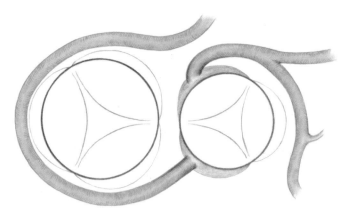

Figure 23–5 Type E.

The classification of coronary anatomy described here is that of Yacoub and Radley-Smith.[97] Other classifications have been described.[30,51,77] The most common anatomy of the coronary arteries is origin from the right and left posterior sinuses of the aorta (type A, Fig. 23–1).[97] The second most common type is D, with the right coronary artery giving rise to the circumflex branch, which passes behind the pulmonary artery to reach the atrioventricular groove (Fig. 23–2). Over 85% of patients have either type A or type D.[61] Both left and right coronary arteries can arise by a common trunk (type B, Fig. 23–3) or by two orifices in close proximity (type C, Fig. 23–4).

A fifth type, E (Fig. 23–5), is associated with the most rightward rotation of the aorta, with the arteries almost side by side. In this type the right coronary artery arises from the left coronary sinus and passes in front of the outflow tract of the right ventricle. Before doing so, it gives rise to the anterior descending coronary artery. The circumflex arises separately from the posterior sinus and curves behind the pulmonary artery to reach the atrioventricular groove.

Types A, D, and E are handled as illustrated in this chapter. Types B and C are managed by suturing the button containing the coronary ostium or ostia to the adjoining edge of the transected pulmonary artery. The distal end of the transected aorta is then fashioned to conform to the remaining circumference of the coronary artery button.

Commissural or intramural coronary arteries have caused the most problems in several series[21,61,99] and have been the reason for changing to an atrial switch procedure rather than proceeding with the arterial switch procedure.[14,51,61] Using the technique described above or using a pericardial hood[21] over the coronary button after it has been sutured to the edge of the transected pulmonary artery can avoid tension, torsion, or kinking.

Surgical Technique

The coronary anatomy is assessed and marking sutures are placed on the pulmonary artery indicating the future positions of the coronary ostia. The aortic cannula is placed as high as possible in the ascending aorta. Cardiopulmonary bypass is begun with systemic cooling. During cooling the ductus is dissected, ligated distally between pledgets, and divided (Fig. 23–6). The pulmonary artery branches are then freed out to their secondary branches (Fig. 23–7).

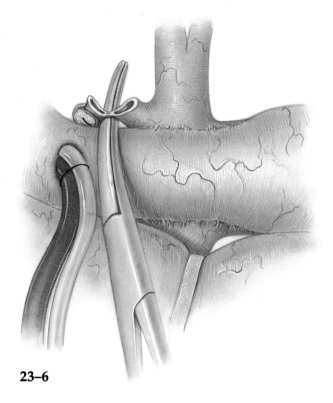

23–6

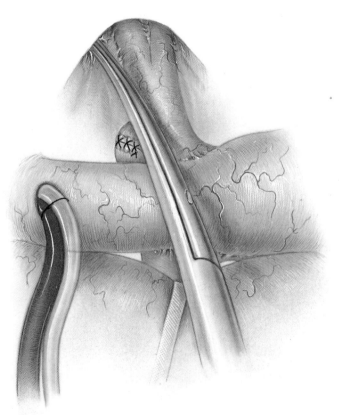

23–7

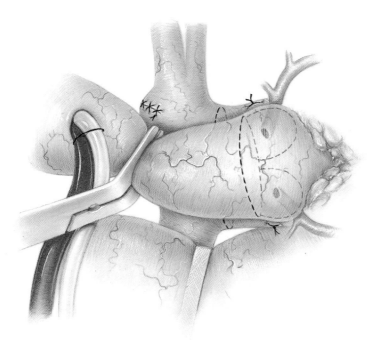

23–8

The aorta is cross-clamped, cold blood cardioplegia solution is administered, the aorta is transected above the top of the commissures, and the pulmonary artery is transected (Fig. 23–8).

The coronary ostia are removed from the aorta, including most of the wall of the sinuses. A short portion of the proximal coronary arteries is dissected to provide mobility without kinking. Oval buttons are then cut from the pulmonary artery at the indicated points. A medially hinged "trapdoor," as described by Brawn and Mee,[11] can be made if necessary to avoid kinking.

The coronary buttons are sutured to the pulmonary artery (neoaorta) with 6-0 absorbable polydioxanone or 6-0 polypropylene (Fig. 23–9). The Le-

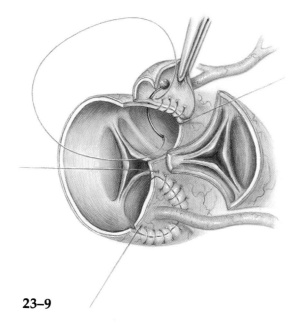

23–9

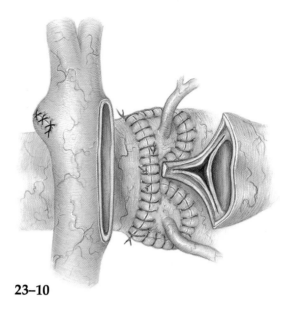

23–10

compte[43,44] maneuver is then performed, bringing the pulmonary artery anterior to the aorta. The distal aorta is then sutured to the neoaorta, with the suture being tied to each coronary anastomosis suture as it is reached (Fig. 23–10) as the patient is rewarmed. The atrial septal defect is closed in standard fashion through a right atriotomy. The aortic clamp is then removed.

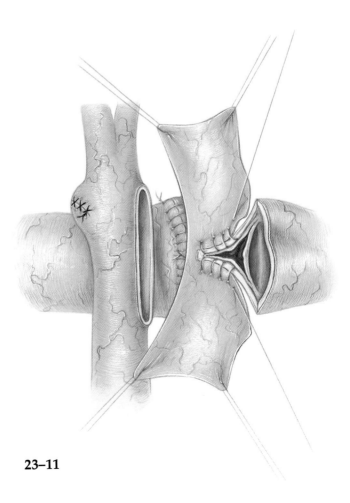

23–11

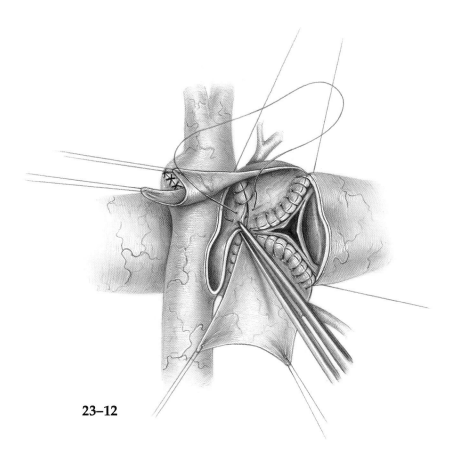

23–12

A pantaloon-shaped patch of fresh autologous pericardium is then sutured to the defects in the sinuses of the neopulmonary artery, beginning in the depth of the left sinus (Fig. 23–11). The pericardial patch is then sutured to the distal pulmonary artery (Figs. 23–12, 23–13). After cardiopulmonary bypass has been discontinued and protamine has been administered, all suture lines are coated with fibrin glue.

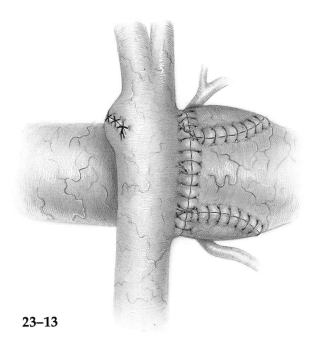

23–13

Special Considerations in Postoperative Care

Patients are supported on the ventilator with hyperventilation and kept heavily sedated with a fentanyl drip for the first 24 to 48 hours or longer as necessary.[3] In addition to inotropes, pulmonary vasodilators are also often used. If primary closure of the sternum is not tolerated, the sternum should be left open and closed secondarily.[50]

Results

Operative Mortality
Operative mortality of less than 5% can be achieved.[11,14,47,64]

Functional Status
Functional status is excellent, with almost all patients having normal growth and development.[47,64]

Electrophysiologic Changes
Sinus rhythm is present in 95%–100% of patients.[47,64] Arrhythmias requiring treatment are extremely rare.[47,49]

Hemodynamics
Colan and colleagues[18] compared myocardial performance in patients after the arterial switch procedure to age-matched normal controls. They found that ventricular size, wall thickness, systolic function, afterload, preload, contractility, and early diastolic function were indistinguishable from control values. Aortic regurgitation, if present, is trivial.[48,92] Coronary and aortic anastomoses grow normally.[4]

Survival
The 2½-year survival rate after arterial switch repair in low-risk institutions for simple transposition was 90% in a study by the Congenital Heart Surgeons Society.[57]

Senning Operation

The theoretical benefits of the Senning operation, compared to the Mustard operation, include (1) the use of atrial wall and interatrial septum, which probably grow; (2) maintenance of atrial contraction; (3) possible decreased incidence of atrial arrhythmias; and (4) a more consistent and reproducible operation, since the dimensions of the baffle are determined by the dimensions of the atrium and interatrial septum and are therefore less variable than when pericardium is used.

Surgical Technique

The technique is essentially that of Senning[45] as modified by Quaegebeur, Brom, and colleagues.[63] The only foreign material is that used to enlarge the septal flap.

The right atrium is incised longitudinally, a few millimeters ventral to the sulcus terminalis (Fig. 23-14). If a large eustachian valve is present, the incision is extended laterally to the base of the valve (*a*). If the eustachian valve is small, the incision is extended more anteriorly (*b*).

The atrial septum is incised to develop a trapezoidal flap based at the interatrial groove (Fig. 23-15). This flap must be small so as to create a degree of rotation of the atrial edge when the flap is sutured over the pulmonary veins. The interatrial groove is dissected and the left atrium is opened by an

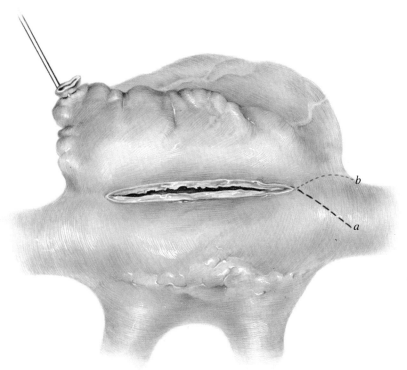

23–14

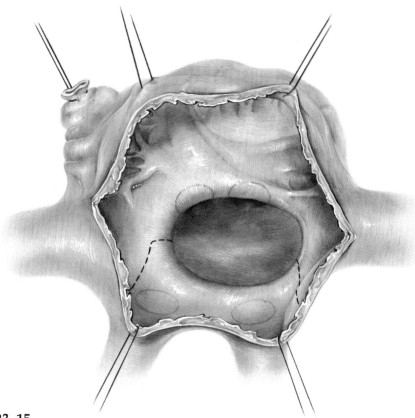

23–15

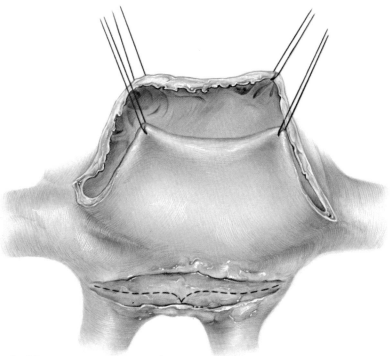

23–16

incision (Fig. 23–16). This incision should not extend under either cava. The left atriotomy is enlarged by a short transverse incision between the right pulmonary veins.

The atrial flap is enlarged, if necessary, in the area of the foramen ovale, using Dacron. The flap is then sutured over the pulmonary veins (Fig. 23–17). The suture line begins between the left superior and inferior pulmonary vein orifices using running suture of 5-0 silk. The superior suture line is carried over the left superior pulmonary vein orifice and laterally and ends 1–2 cm

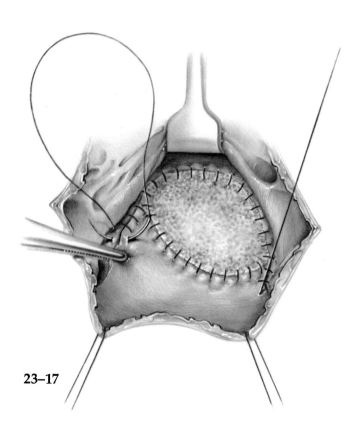

23–17

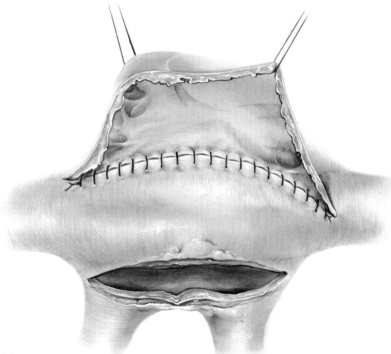

23–18

below the superior vena cava orifice, at the base of the flap. The inferior suture line is also a running suture and proceeds around the inferior pulmonary vein orifice and laterally to the base of the flap, below the inferior vena cava orifice.

The dorsal edge of the right atrium is then sutured to the atrial septum between the tricuspid and mitral valves and over the orifices of the superior and inferior venae cavae, taking very small bites of tissue (Fig. 23–18). If a large eustachian valve is present, the inferior suture line incorporates the edge of the valve. The coronary sinus blood drains with the pulmonary venous blood.

The ventral edge of the right atrium is then sutured to the lateral edge of the left atriotomy and over the superior and inferior caval pathways (Fig. 23–19). Sutures are taken very superficially over the superior vena cava, using interrupted sutures of 6–0 polypropylene to avoid injury to the sinus node. The Senning repair creates overlying channels of venous inflow.

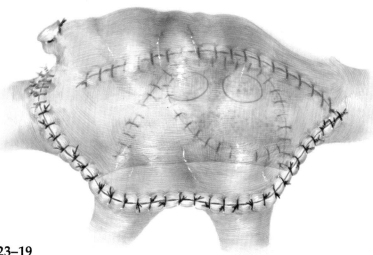

23–19

Results

Operative Mortality

In a recent series, Bender and colleagues[9] reported an operative mortality of 5.4% in 93 consecutive infants.

Functional Status

Parenzan and co-workers[59] reported 24 patients, all of whom were asymptomatic. With the passage of time there is functional deterioration. Turina, Senning, and colleagues[86] reported failure of the systemic ventricle in 8% of patients by 15 years after surgery.

Electrophysiologic Changes

Random electrocardiograms following the Senning operation show sinus rhythm in 83%–100%, junctional rhythm in 0%–17%, and atrioventricular block in 0–%5%.[20,59,63,74] One report[59] of 12 patients undergoing continuous 24-hour electrocardiograms showed constant sinus rhythm in 10 (83%), and 2 patients who had short episodes of junctional rhythm with rates above 80 beats per minute. There is a continuing decrease in stable sinus rhythm after the Senning procedure. Deanfield and colleagues[22] found that at a mean of 7 years after operation only 56% of patients were in stable sinus rhythm. Late dysrhythmias requiring pacemaker implantation occurred in approximately 10% of patients at 10 years.[86]

Hemodynamics

Senning[74] reported 44 patients with late follow-up, with only one case of superior vena caval obstruction and one case of pulmonary venous obstruction. Four reports[8,20,59,63] of postoperative catheterization studies total 40 patients. The incidence of caval obstruction was 0%. The incidence of pulmonary venous obstruction was 5% overall, but it only occurred in one series.[20] The response of right ventricular ejection fraction to afterload stress was abnormal in approximately 85% of patients.[9]

Late Survival

Senning and colleagues[86] found actuarial survival for patients with transposition and intact ventricular septum to be 92% at 10 years.

Mustard Operation

Surgical Technique

The Mustard operation has the most variability of the three operations covered in this chapter. Among the variables are (1) atrial septal excision (amount and location),[46,89] (2) size and shape of the baffle,[1,62] (3) material of the baffle,[12,80,89] (4) position of the suture lines around the pulmonary vein and caval orifices,[89] (5) depth of the suture lines,[24] (6) incision of the coronary sinus,[24] and (7) patching of the new left atrium (pulmonary venous atrium).[24,89] Because of these many variables, the Mustard operation may differ substantially from surgeon to surgeon.

Our technique of performing the Mustard operation is much like the original description by Mustard[56]: (1) the remaining atrial septum is excised; (2) the baffle is rectangular; (3) the baffle is autogenous pericardium; (4) the suture lines are close to the pulmonary venous orifices, but are somewhat away from the caval orifices; (5) the suture bites are relatively shallow, especially near the tricuspid valve; (6) the coronary sinus is left intact; (7) the patch is sutured so the coronary sinus drains with the systemic venous return; and (8) a patch is placed on the new left atrium (this differs from Mustard's original report).

Pericardium is removed from phrenic nerve to phrenic nerve (Fig. 23–20). A rectangle is cut from the pericardium, to be used for the intraatrial baffle, and retraction sutures are placed in each corner. The remaining portion of

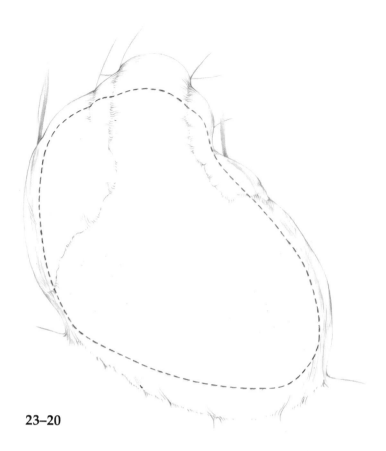

23–20

pericardium is fashioned into a triangle to be used as the patch on the new left atrium (pulmonary venous atrium).

A longitudinal atriotomy is made in the right atrium just ventral to the caval-atrial junction. The edges of the right atrium are suspended.

The remaining atrial septum is excised (Fig. 23–21). The rim posteriorly

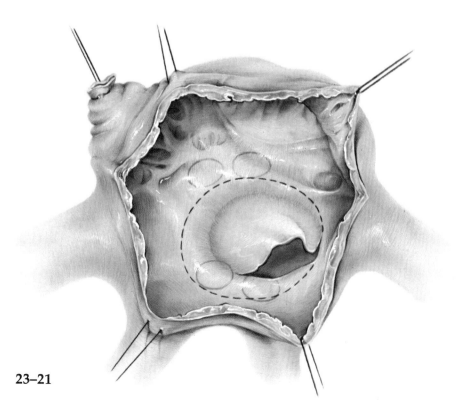

23–21

over the right pulmonary veins, the rim inferiorly above the coronary sinus, the rim between the tricuspid and mitral valves, and the rim superiorly are excised, exercising caution to avoid cutting contiguous structures. The endocardium is reapproximated with interrupted 6-0 polyester sutures.

A retractor is placed over the atrial septum between the mitral and tricuspid valves, exposing the left atrium. The left pulmonary vein orifices and the base of the left atrial appendage are identified.

The first suture is then placed through the baffle and just on the left side of the carina between the left upper and lower pulmonary veins, and the suture is tied (Fig. 23-22). The superior suture line is brought laterally, above the superior pulmonary veins, then below the superior vena cava orifice, 1-2 cm from the caval orifice (Fig. 23-23), around laterally and anteriorly, and tagged (Fig. 23-24).

The other end of the suture is brought inferiorly and laterally just below the inferior pulmonary veins (Fig. 23-25) and then around above the inferior vena cava orifice. This suture line should be parallel to the superior suture line until it reaches the lateral atrial wall.

As the suture line comes around the inferior vena cava orifice and anteriorly, the retractor is moved from over the atrial septum to within the right ventricle, through the tricuspid valve, and retracted anteriorly. This exposes the area of the coronary sinus and anterior atrial septum. The patch is then brought over and the shape is assessed. The suture line proceeds toward the anterior atrial septum, between the coronary sinus and the tricuspid valve

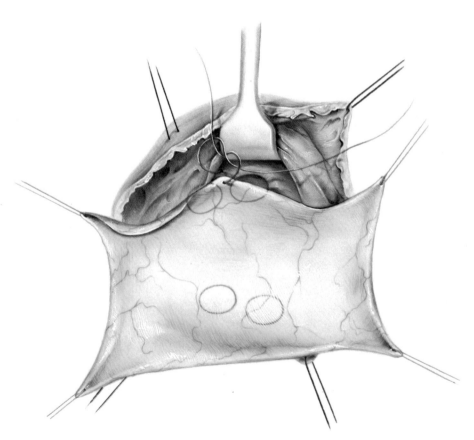

23–22

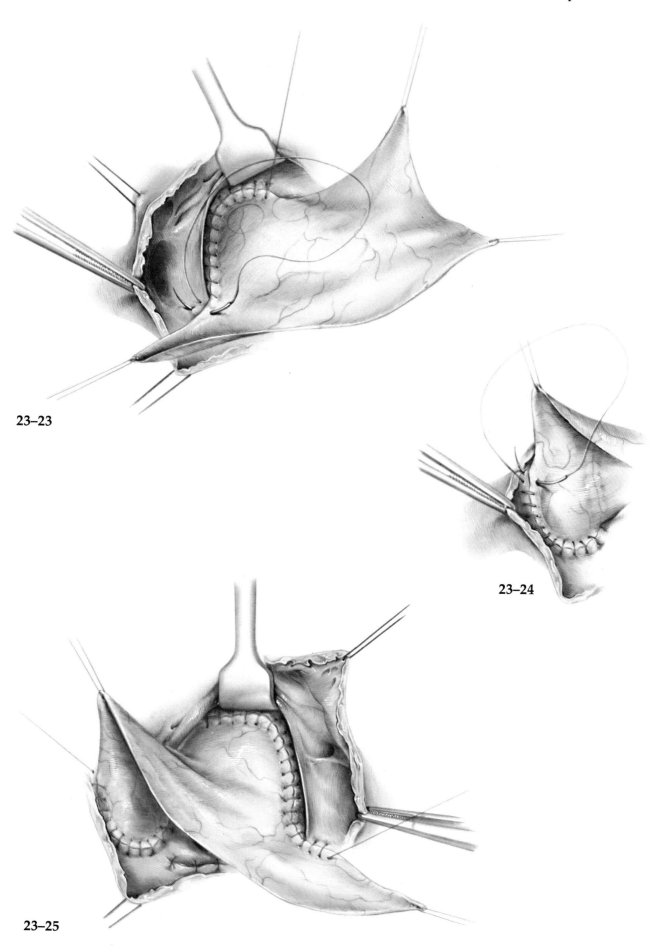

23–23

23–24

23–25

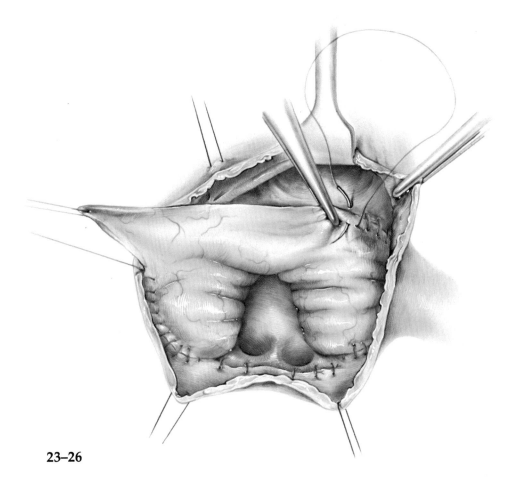

23–26

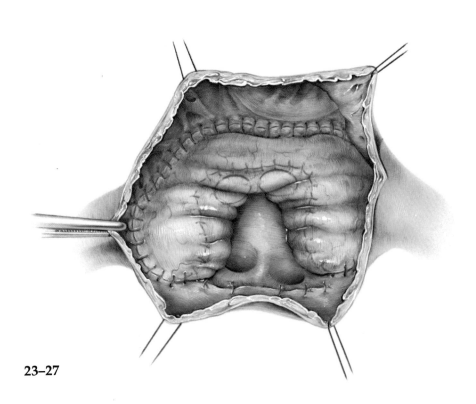

23–27

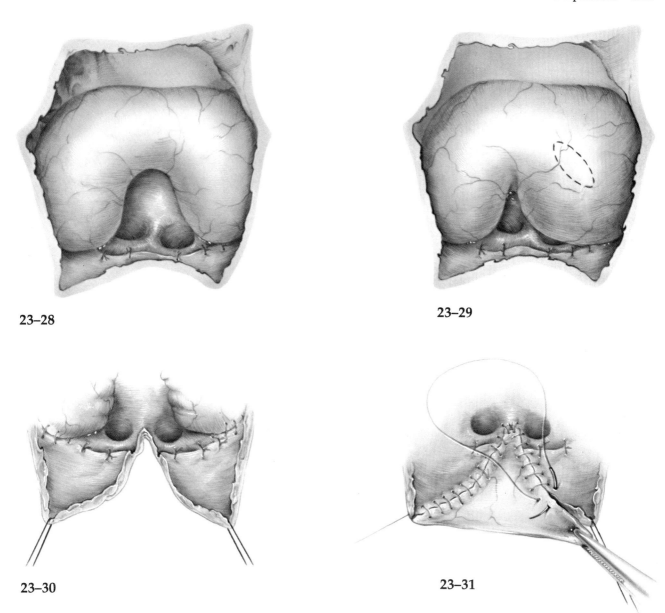

23–28

23–29

23–30

23–31

(Fig. 23–26), and goes across the remnant of atrial septum to complete the baffle suture (Fig. 23–27).

Cardioplegic solution is then injected into the aortic root to distend the baffle and thereby assess its configuration (Fig. 23–28). Any excessively redundant areas can be excised (Fig. 23–29).

The incision to enlarge the new left atrium is then made—down the lateral wall of the right atrium, through the ridge of the remnant of atrial septum, and between the right pulmonary veins (Fig. 23–30). The patch is then sutured from the inside (Fig. 23–31). The closure of the atriotomy incorporates the remaining side of the patch.

Results

Operative Mortality
Operative mortality below 1% has been reported during the 1980s.[85,88]

Functional Status
Most patients, following the Mustard operation, have normal growth and normal physical activity.[15,33,45,83] Champsaur and colleagues[15] from the Hospi-

tal for Sick Children, Toronto, reported 91% of operative survivors were leading a normal life. Mustard's original patient was alive and well 9 years after surgery. Symptoms or growth failure almost always indicates serious hemodynamic abnormalities.[46] Approximately 10% of patients have important right ventricular dysfunction 10 years after surgery. Approximately 90% of patients, essentially all of those who do not have right ventricular dysfunction, are in New York Heart Association class I or II late postoperatively.[94]

Electrophysiologic Changes
The following rhythms can occur following the Mustard[16,25,26,28,32,33,37,69,71,91] operation: (1) sinus rhythm, (2) a regular atrial rhythm appearing to originate in a location other than the sinus node, (3) atrial tachyarrhythmias and bradyarrhythmias, (4) junctional rhythm, and (5) atrioventricular block. There are often combinations of rhythms, usually with one predominating.[69] The incidence of arrhythmias as reported in the literature is influenced by the definition of what constitutes an arrhythmia and whether random electrocardiograms or 24-hour ambulatory monitoring is used for diagnosis. Inclusion of such minor arrhythmias as first-degree block can raise the incidence of arrhythmias to near 100%.[69,89] Holter monitoring for 24 hours also documents a higher incidence of arrhythmias.[69,89]

There is a wide variation in the incidence of arrhythmias reported in the literature: sinus rhythm or a regular atrial rhythm in 63%–97%,[15,69,87,89] junctional rhythm in up to 35%,[15,33,69] atrial flutter in as many as 6%,[15,69] and complete heart block in 0%–3%.[15,69] The difference in the incidence of the various arrhythmias also appears to be related to variations in surgical technique.

There are three possible causes of rhythm disturbance following the Mustard operation: (1) injury to the sinus node or its artery, (2) interruption of atrial pathways, and (3) injury to the atrioventricular (AV) node. Opinions differ as to the relative importance of each factor.

It is clear that injury to the sinus node or its artery can cause arrhythmias.[16,25,26,28,29,71] El-Said and co-workers[25] have documented by histologic examination injury to the SA node, including hemorrhage early after operation and obliteration of the SA nodal artery and replacement of the SA node after longer postoperative periods. They have pointed out the importance of avoiding the area of the SA node during cannulation. The sinus node can also be injured if the suture line is placed too near the superior caval orifice.[46,89]

The importance of the internodal or atrial preferential pathways is the subject of considerable debate. Isaacson and colleagues[37] concluded that extensive disturbance of the atrial septal connections between the sinus and atrioventricular nodes is frequently associated with serious dysrhythmia. This opinion is also held by Waldo[91] and Wittig.[95]

However, the importance of the internodal tracts is called into question by two facts: (1) electrophysiologic studies showing normal atrial conduction postoperatively[28] and (2) the high incidence of sinus rhythm even if no particular attention is paid to preservation of internodal tracts.[16,89] Gillette and co-workers[29] found no intraatrial block between the upper and lower intraatrial electrocardiograms in postoperative studies of patients in whom no special steps were taken to preserve internodal tracts. Ullal, Lincoln, and colleagues[89] report a very high incidence of sinus rhythm following their technique of performing the Mustard operation—a technique that almost certainly interrupts all three internodal tracts.

A disturbing fact is that sinus rhythm does not preclude disease of the sinus node, nor does it preclude the possibility of sudden death. Studies of sinus nodal recovery time have documented the fact that abnormal sinus nodal function can occur in the presence of sinus rhythm.[69] Approximately one-third of patients experiencing sudden death after the Mustard operation are in predominantly sinus rhythm prior to death.[72]

Table 23-1. Late Postoperative Hemodynamic Data After Mustard Operation

Authors	Number of Patients	Date of Report	Average Age at Surgery	Mean Interval Between Operation and Catheterization	Baffle Material	Superior Vena Caval Obstruction (over 5 mm Hg gradient)	Inferior Vena Caval Obstruction (over 5 mm Hg gradient)	Pulmonary Venous Obstruction	Baffle Leak	Tricuspid Insufficiency	Normal Right Ventricular Function
Clarkson et al. 17	42	1976	Not given; range 11 days to 58 months	28 months	Pericardium	7.9%	0%	5.5%	0%	9%	100 % (in patients with an intact septum)
Godman et al. 31	14	1976	Not given; range 1.5 to 4.5 yr	5.5 yr	Pericardium	0%	0%	7.1%	35.7%	14%	93%
Hagler et al. 33	33, all asymptomatic	1979	4.5 yr	4.7 yr	Dacron 73% Pericardium 27%	27.3%	21.2%	12.1%	27.3%	42.4%	97%
Hagler et al. 33	15, all symptomatic	1979	3.1 yr	1.7 yr	Dacron: 53% Pericardium: 47%	Total of 53.3%		33.3%	40%	40%	93%
Morgan et al. 54	16	1972	Not given; range 5 months to 11 yr	10 months	Pericardium	6.3%	0%	Not evaluated	50%	11.1%	93%
Rodriguez-Fernandez et al. 68	11	1972	Not given; range 2 to 7 yr	2.4 yr	Dacron: 55% Pericardium: 45%	9.1%	9.1%	0%	63.6%	Not studied	Not studied
Sunderland et al. 83	11, all asymptomatic	1975	Not given; range 2.5 to 66 months	26 months	Dacron: 36% Pericardium: 64%	54.5%	0%	0%	36.4%	0%	100%

There is a progressive increase in the prevalence of junctional rhythm with the passage of time. Approximately 50% of patients are in junctional rhythm 20 years after operation.[27,94]

Hemodynamics

The physiologic results of the Mustard operation are influenced by the anatomic variations present at the time of operation, the variations in surgical technique, and the thoroughness of postoperative study. Thus, there is a broad range of reported postoperative hemodynamic results.

Table 23–1 lists a number of reports from the 1970s of postoperative catheterization findings in a total of 142 patients. There is wide variation in hemodynamic results: superior vena caval obstruction is present in 0%–55%, inferior vena caval obstruction in 0%–22%, pulmonary venous obstruction in 0%–33%, and baffle leaks in 0%–64%. During the mean intervals between operation and catheterization, which range from 10 months to 5.5 years, tricuspid valve function and right ventricular function were good. Normal right ventricular function is present in over 90% of patients. Although some tricuspid insufficiency may occur in up to 40% of patients, it usually is present in less than 10%, and when present is mild and of no hemodynamic significance.

Late Survival

Williams and colleagues[94] found an actuarial survival of 83% at 10 years and 80% at 20 years.

References

1. Aberdeen E, Waterston DJ, Carr I, Graham G, Bonham-Carter RE, Subramanian S: Successful correction of transposed great arteries by Mustard's operation. Lancet 1:1233,1965.
2. Albert HM: Surgical correction of transposition of the great arteries. Surg Forum 5:74,1954.
3. Anand KJS, Hickey PR: Halothane-morphine compared with high-dose sufentanil for anesthesia and postoperative analgesia in neonatal cardiac surgery. N Engl J Med 326:1,1992.
4. Arensman FW, Sievers HH, Lange P, Radley-Smith R, Bernhard A, Heintzen P, Yacoub MH: Assessment of coronary and aortic anastomoses after anatomic correction of transposition of the great arteries. J Thorac Cardiovasc Surg 90:597,1985.
5. Bailey CP, Cookson BA, Downing DF, Neptune WB: Cardiac surgery under hypothermia. J Thorac Cardiovasc Surg 27:73,1954.
6. Barcia A, Kincaid OW, Davis GD, Kirklin JW, Ongley PA: Transposition of the great arteries: an angiographic study. Am J Roentgenol 100:249,1967.
7. Baylen BG, Grzeszczak M, Gleason ME, Cyran SE, Weber HS, Myers J, Waldhausen J: Role of balloon atrial septostomy before early arterial switch repair of transposition of the great arteries. J Am Coll Cardiol 19:1025,1992.
8. Bender HW, Graham TP, Boucek RJ, Walker WE, Boerth RC: Comparative operative results of the Senning and Mustard procedures for transposition of the great arteries. Circulation 62(Suppl I):I-197,1980.
9. Bender HW, Stewart JR, Merrill WH, Hammon JW Jr, Graham TP: Ten years' experience with the Senning operation for transposition of the great arteries: physiological results and late follow-up. Ann Thorac Surg 47:218,1989.
10. Blalock A, Hanlon CR: The surgical treatment of complete transposition of the aorta and pulmonary artery. Surg Gynecol Obstet 90:1,1950.
11. Brawn WJ, Mee RBB: Early results for anatomic correction of transposition of the great arteries and for double-outlet right venticle with subpulmonary ventricular septal defect. J Thorac Cardiovasc Surg 95:230,1988.
12. Breckenridge IM, Stark J, Bonham-Carter RE, Oelert H, Graham GR, Waterston DJ: Mustard's operation for transposition of the great arteries: review of 200 cases. Lancet 1:1140,1972.

13. Castaneda AR, Norwood WI, Jonas RA, Colon SD, Sanders SP, Lang P: Transposition of the great arteries and intact ventricular septum: an anatomical repair in the neonate. Ann Thorac Surg 38:438,1984.

14. Castaneda AR, Trusler GA, Paul MH, Blackstone EH, Kirklin JW: The early results of treatment of simple transposition in the current era. J Thorac Cardiovasc Surg 95:14,1988.

15. Champsaur GL, Sokol DM, Trusler GA, Mustard WT: Repair of transposition of the great arteries in 123 pediatric patients: early and long-term results. Circulation 47:1032,1973.

16. Clarkson PM, Barratt-Boyes BG, Neutze JM: Late dysrhythmias and disturbances of conduction following Mustard operation for complete transposition of the great arteries. Circulation 52:519,1976.

17. Clarkson PM, Neutze JM, Barratt-Boyes BG, Brandt PWT: Late postoperative hemodynamic results and cineangiographic findings after Mustard atrial baffle repair for transposition of the great arteries. Circulation 53:525,1976.

18. Colan SD, Trowitzsch E, Wernovsky G, Sholler GF, Sanders SP, Castaneda AR: Myocardial performance after arterial switch operation for transposition of the great arteries with intact ventricular septum. Circulation 78:132,1988.

19. Cooley DA, Hallman GL, Bloodwell RD, Leachman RD: Two-stage surgical treatment of complete transposition of the great vessels. Arch Surg 93:704,1966.

20. Coto EO, Norwood WI, Lang PL, Castaneda AR: Modified Senning operation for treatment of transposition of the great arteries. J Thorac Cardiovasc Surg 78:721,1979.

21. Day RW, Laks H, Drinkwater DC: The influence of coronary anatomy on the arterial switch operation in neonates. J Thorac Cardiovasc Surg 104:706,1992.

22. Deanfield J, Camm J, Macartney F, Cartwright T, Douglas J, Drew J, de Leval M, Stark J: Arrhythmia and late mortality after Mustard and Senning operation for transposition of the great arteries: an eight-year prospective study. J Thorac Cardiovasc Surg 96:569,1988.

23. DiDonato RM, Wernovsky G, Walsh EP, Colan SD, Lang P, Wessel DL, Jonas RA, Mayer JE Jr, Castaneda AR: Results of the arterial switch operation for transposition of the great arteries with ventricular septal defect: surgical considerations and midterm follow-up data. Circulation 80:1689,1989.

24. Ebert PA, Gay WA Jr, Engle MA: Correction of transposition of the great arteries: relationship of the coronary sinus and postoperative arrhythmias. Ann Surg 180:433,1974.

25. El-Said GM, Gillette PC, Cooley DA, Mullins CE, Williams RL, McNamara DG: Protection of the sinus node in Mustard's operation. Circulation 53:788,1976.

26. El-Said GM, Rosenberg HS, Mullins CE, Hallman GL, Cooley DA, McNamara DG: Dysrhythmias after Mustard's operation for transposition of the great arteries. Am J Cardiol 30:526,1972.

27. Flinn CJ, Wolff CS, Dick M II, Campbell RM, Borkat G, Casta A, Hordor A, Hougen TJ, Kavey R-E, Kugler J, Liebman J, Greenhouse J, Hees P: Cardiac rhythm after the Mustard operation for complete transposition of the great arteries. N Engl J Med 310:1635,1984.

28. Gillette PC, El-Said GM, Sivarajan N, Mullins CE, Williams RL, McNamara DG: Electrophysiological abnormalities after Mustard's operation for transposition of the great arteries. Br Heart J 36:186,1974.

29. Gillette PC, Kugler JD, Garson A Jr, Gutgesell HP, Duff DF, McNamara DG: Mechanisms of cardiac arrhythmias after the Mustard operation for transposition of the great arteries. Am J Cardiol 45:1225,1980.

30. Gittenberger-de Groot AC, Sauer U, Oppenheimer-Dekker A, Quaegebeur J: Coronary arterial anatomy in transposition of the great arteries: a morphologic study. Pediatr Cardiol 4(Suppl I):15,1983.

31. Godman MJ, Friedli B, Pasternac A, Kidd BSL, Trusler GA, Mustard WT: Hemodynamic studies in children four to ten years after the Mustard operation for transposition of the great arteries. Circulation 53:532,1976.

32. Greenwood RD, Rosenthal A, Sloss LJ, LaCorte M, Nadas AS: Sick sinus syndrome after surgery for congenital heart disease. Circulation 52:532,1976.

33. Hagler DJ, Ritter DG, Mair DD, Tajik AJ, Seward JB, Fulton RE, Ritman EL: Right and left ventricular function after the Mustard procedure in transposition of the great arteries. Am J Cardiol 44:276,1979.

34. Idriss FS, Goldstein IR, Grana L, French D, Potts WH: A new technic for complete correction of transposition of the great vessels. Circulation 24:5,1961.

35. Idriss FS, Ilbawi MN, DeLeon SY, Duffy CE, Muster AJ, Backer CL, Berry TE, Paul MH: Transposition of the great arteries with intact ventricular septum: arterial switch in the first month of life. J Thorac Cardiovasc Surg 95:255,1988.

36. Imamura ES, Morikawa T, Tatsumo K, Konno S, Arai T, Sakakibara S: Surgical considerations of ventricular septal defect associated with complete transposition of the great arteries and pulmonary stenosis: with special reference to the Rastelli operation. Circulation 45:914,1971.

37. Isaacson R, Titus JL, Merideth J, Feldt RH, McGoon DC: Apparent interruption of atrial conduction pathways after surgical repair of transposition of great arteries. Am J Cardiol 30:533,1972.

38. Jatene AD, Fontes VF, Paulista PP, Souza LCB, Neger F, Galantier M, Sousa JEMR: Anatomic correction of transposition of the great vessels. J Thorac Cardiovasc Surg 72:364,1976.

39. Jonas RA, Giglia TM, Sanders SP, Wernovsky G, Nadal-Ginard B, Mayer JE Jr, Castaneda AR: Rapid, two-stage arterial switch for transposition of the great arteries and intact ventricular septum beyond the neonatal period. Circulation 80(Suppl I):I-203,1989.

40. Kanter K, Anderson R, Lincoln C, Firmin R, Rigby M: Anatomic correction of double-outlet right ventricle with subpulmonary ventricular septal defect (the ''Taussig-Bing'' anomaly). Ann Thorac Surg 41:287,1986.

41. Kay EB, Cross FS: Surgical treatment of transposition of the great vessels. Surgery 38:712,1955.

42. Kron IL, Rheuban KS, Joob AW, Jedeiken R, Mentzer RM, Carpenter MA, Nolan SP: Baffle obstruction following the Mustard operation: cause and treatment. Ann Thorac Surg 39:112,1985.

43. Lecompte Y, Neveux JY, Zannini L, Tran-Viet T, Duboys Y, Jarreau MM: Reconstruction of the pulmonary outflow tract without prosthetic conduit. J Thorac Cardiovasc Surg 84:727,1982.

44. Lecompte Y, Zannini L, Hagan E, et al: Anatomic correction of transposition of the great arteries: a new technique without using a prosthetic conduit. J Thorac Cardiovasc Surg 82:629,1981.

45. Levy RJ, Rosenthal A, Castaneda AR, Nadas AS: Growth after surgical repair of simple d-transposition of the great arteries. Ann Thorac Surg 25:225,1978.

46. Lewis AB, Lindesmith GG, Takahashi M, Stanton RE, Tucker BL, Stiles QR, Meyer BW: Cardiac rhythm following the Mustard procedure for transposition of the great vessels. J Thorac Cardiovasc Surg 73:919,1977.

47. Lupinetti FM, Bove EL, Minich LL, Snider AR, Callow LB, Meliones JN, Crowley DC, Beekman RH, Serwer G, Dick M II, Vermilion R, Rosenthal A: Intermediate-term survival and functional results after arterial repair for transposition of the great arteries. J Thorac Cardiovasc Surg 103:421,1992.

48. Martin RP, Ettedgui JA, Qureshi SA, Gibbs JL, Baker EJ, Radley-Smith R, Maisey MN, Tynan M, Yacoub MH: A quantitative evaluation of aortic regurgitation after anatomic correction of transposition of the great arteries. J Am Coll Cardiol 12:1281,1988.

49. Martin RP, Radley-Smith R, Yacoub MH: Arrhythmias before and after anatomic correction of transposition of the great arteries. J Am Coll Cardiol 10:200,1987.

50. Mavroudis C: Anatomical repair of transposition of the great arteries with intact ventricular septum in the neonate: guidelines to avoid complications. Ann Thorac Surg 43:495,1987.

51. Mayer JE Jr, Sanders SP, Jonas RA, Castaneda AR, Wernovsky G: Coronary artery pattern and outcome of arterial switch operation for transposition of the great arteries. Circulation 82(Suppl IV):IV-139,1990.

52. McGoon DC, Wallace RB, Danielson GK: The Rastelli operation. J Thorac Cardiovasc Surg 65:65,1973.

53. Merlo M, De Tommasi SM, Brunelli F, Abbruzzese PA, Crupi G, Ghidoni I, Casari A, Piti A, Mamprin F, Parenzan L: Long-term results after atrial correction of complete transposition of the great arteries. Ann Thorac Surg 51:227,1991.

54. Morgan JR, Miller BL, Daicoff GR, Andrews EJ: Hemodynamic and angiocardiographic evaluation after Mustard procedure for transposition of the great arteries. J Thorac Cardiovasc Surg 64:878,1972.

55. Mustard WT: Successful two-stage correction of transposition of the great vessels. Surgery 55:469,1964.

56. Mustard WT, Chute AL, Keith JD, Sirek A, Rowe RD, Vlad P: A surgical approach to transposition of great vessels with extracorporeal circuit. Surgery 36:39,1954.

57. Norwood WI, Dobell AR, Freed MD, Kirklin JW, Blackstone EH: Intermediate results of the arterial switch repair: a 20-institution study. J Thorac Cardiovasc Surg 96:854,1988.

58. Paillole C, Sidi D, Kachaner J, Planche C, Belot JP, Villain E, Le Bidois J, Piechaud JF, Pedroni E: Fate of pulmonary artery after anatomic correction of simple transposition of great arteries in newborn infants. Circulation 78:870,1988.

59. Parenzan L, Locatelli G, Alfieri O, Villani M, Invernizzi G: The Senning operation for transposition of the great arteries. J Thorac Cardiovasc Surg 76:305,1978.

60. Paul MH: D-transposition of the great arteries. *In* Moss A, Adams F, Emmanouilides G (eds): Heart Diseases in Infants, Children, and Adolescents. Baltimore, Williams & Wilkins, 1978, p 301.

61. Planche C, Bruniaux J, Lacour-Gayet F, Kachaner J, Binet J-P, Sidi D, Villain E: Switch operation for transposition of the great arteries in neonates: a study of 120 patients. J Thorac Cardiovasc Surg 96:354,1988.

62. Quaegebeur JM, Brom AG: The trousers-shaped baffle for use in the Mustard operation. Ann Thorac Surg 25:240,1978.

63. Quaegebeur JM, Rohmer J, Brom AG: Revival of the Senning operation in the treatment of transposition of the great arteries. Thorax 32:517,1977.

64. Quaegebeur JM, Rohmer J, Ottenkamp J, Buis T, Kirklin JW, Blackstone EH, Brom AG: The arterial switch operation: an eight year experience. J Thorac Cardiovasc Surg 92:361,1986.

65. Rashkind WJ, Miller WW: Creation of an atrial septal defect without thoracotomy. JAMA 196:991,1966.

66. Rastelli GC, Wallace RB, Ongley PA: Complete repair of transposition of the great arteries with pulmonary stenosis: a review and report of a case corrected by using a new surgical technique. Circulation 39:83,1969.

67. Reul GJ, Cooley DA, Sandiford FM, Hallman GL: Complications following the contoured Dacron baffle in correction of transposition of the great arteries. Surgery 76:946,1974.

68. Rodriguez-Fernandez HL, Kelly DT, Collado A, Haller A, Krovetz LJ, Rowe RD: Hemodynamic data and angiographic findings after Mustard repair for complete transposition of the great arteries. Circulation 47:799,1972.

69. Saalouke MG, Rios J, Perry LW, Shapiro SR, Scott LP: Electrophysiologic studies after Mustard's operation for d-transposition of the great vessels. Am J Cardiol 41:1104,1978.

70. Sansa M, Tonkin IL, Bargeron LM Jr, Elliott LP: Left ventricular outflow tract obstruction in transposition of the great arteries: an angiographic study of 74 cases. Am J Cardiol 44:88,1979.

71. Schraut W, Lin CY, de la Fuente D, Arcilla R, Replogle RL: Avoiding postoperative dysrhythmias and venous obstruction following Mustard's operation. Ann Thorac Surg 18:142,1974.

72. Scott LP, Saalouke MG, Shapiro SR, Rios JC, Perry LW: Sudden unexpected death following Mustard's procedure for d-transposition of the great vessels (abstr). Circulation 54(Suppl II):II-89,1976.

73. Senning A: Surgical correction of transposition of the great vessels. Surgery 45:966,1959.

74. Senning A: Correction of the transposition of the great arteries. Ann Surg 182:287,1975.

75. Shaher RM: Complete Transposition of the Great Arteries. New York, Academic Press, 1973, p 409.

76. Shaher RM, Moes CAF, Khoury G: Radiologic and angiocardiographic findings in complete transposition of the great vessels with left ventricular outflow tract obstruction. Radiology 88:1092,1967.

77. Shaher RM, Puddu GC: Coronary arterial anatomy in complete transposition of the great vessels. Am J Cardiol 17:355,1966.

78. Shaher RM, Puddu GC, Koury G, Moes CAF, Mustard WT: Complete transposi-

tion of the great vessels with anatomic obstruction of the outflow tract of the left ventricle: surgical implications of anatomic findings. Am J Cardiol 19:658,1967.

79. Shumacker HB Jr: A new operation for transposition of the great vessels. Surgery 50:773,1961.

80. Stafford EG, McGoon DC: The Mustard operation. Mayo Clin Proc 48:119,1973.

81. Stark J, Tynan MJ, Ashcraft KW, Aberdeen E, Waterston DJ: Obstruction of pulmonary veins and superior vena cava after the Mustard operation for transposition of the great arteries. Circulation 45,46(Suppl I):I-116,1972.

82. Starr A, Campbell TJ, Wood J, McCord C, Herr R, Menashe V: Transposition of the great vessels: recent experience with the Blalock-Hanlon procedure. Am J Surg 108:198,1964.

83. Sunderland CO, Henken DP, Nichols GM, Dhindsa DS, Bonchek LI, Menashe VD, Rahimtoola SH, Starr A: Postoperative hemodynamic and electrophysiologic evaluation of the interatrial baffle procedure. Am J Cardiol 35:660,1975.

84. Szarnicki RJ, Stark J, de Leval M: Reoperation for complications after inflow correction of transposition of the great arteries: technical considerations. Ann Thorac Surg 25:150,1978.

85. Trusler GA, Willliams WG, Duncan KF, Hesslein PS, Benson LN, Freedom RM, Izukawa T, Olley PM: Results with the Mustard operation in simple transposition of the great arteries: 1963–1985. Ann Surg 206:251,1987.

86. Turina MI, Siebenmann R, von Segesser L, Schonbeck M, Senning A: Late functional deterioration after atrial correction for transposition of the great arteries. Circulation 80(Suppl I):I-162,1989.

87. Turley K, Ebert PA: Total correction of transposition of the great arteries: conduction disturbances in infants younger than three months of age. J Thorac Cardiovasc Surg 76:312,1978.

88. Turley K, Hanley FL, Verrier ED, Merrick SH, Ebert PA: The Mustard procedure in infants (less than 100 days of age): ten year follow-up. J Thorac Cardiovasc Surg 96:849,1988.

89. Ullal RR, Anderson RH, Lincoln C: Mustard's operation modified to avoid dysrhythmias and systemic venous obstruction. J Thorac Cardiovasc Surg 78:431,1979.

90. Vlad P, Lambert EC: Late results of Rashkind's balloon atrial septostomy in transposition. In Kirklin JW (ed): Advances in Cardiovascular Surgery. New York, Grune & Stratton, 1973, pp 29–36.

91. Waldo AL, Krongrad E, Bowman FO, Kaiser GA, Husson GS, Malm JR: Electrophysiological considerations during total repair of transposition of the great vessels. Circulation 46(Suppl II):II-34,1972.

92. Wernovsky G, Hougen TJ, Walsh EP, Sholler GF, Colan SD, Sanders SP, Parness IA, Keane JF, Mayer JE, Jonas RA, Castaneda AR, Lang P: Midterm results after the arterial switch operation for transposition of the great arteries with intact ventricular septum: clinical, hemodynamic, echocardiographic, and electrophysiologic data. Circulation 77:1333,1988.

93. Wernovsky G, Jonas RA, Colan SD, Sanders SP, Wessel DL, Castaneda AR, Mayer JE Jr: Results of the arterial switch operation in patients with transposition of the great arteries and abnormalities of the mitral valve or left ventricular outflow tract. J Am Coll Cardiol 16:1446,1990.

94. Williams WG, Trusler GA, Kirklin JW, Blackstone EH, Coles JG, Izukawa T, Freedom RM: Early and late results of a protocol for simple transposition leading to an atrial switch (Mustard) repair. J Thorac Cardiovasc Surg 95:717,1988.

95. Wittig JH, de Leval MR, Stark J: Intraoperative mapping of atrial activation before, during, and after the Mustard operation. J Thorac Cardiovasc Surg 73:1,1977.

96. Yacoub MH, Bernhard A, Lange P, Radley-Smith R, Keck E, Stephan E, Heintzen P: Clinical and hemodynamic results of the two-stage anatomic correction of simple transposition of the great arteries. Circulation 62(Suppl I):I-190,1980.

97. Yacoub MH, Radley-Smith R: Anatomy of the coronary arteries in transposition of the great arteries and methods for their transfer in anatomical correction. Thorax 33:418,1978.

98. Yacoub MH, Radley-Smith R, Maclaurin R: Two-stage operation for anatomical correction of transposition of the great arteries with intact interventricular septum. Lancet 1:1275,1977.

99. Yamaguchi M, Hosokawa Y, Imai Y, Kurosawa H, Yasui H, Yagihara T, Okamoto F, Wakaki N: Early and midterm results of the arterial switch operation for transposition of the great arteries in Japan. J Thorac Cardiovasc Surg 100:261,1990.
100. Yasui H, Kado H, Yonenaga K, Hisahara M, Ando H, Iwao H, Fukuda S, Mizoguchi Y, Sunagawa H: Arterial switch operation for transposition of the great arteries, with special reference to left ventricular function. J Thorac Cardiovasc Surg 98:601,1989.

24

Total Anomalous Pulmonary Venous Connection

Total anomalous pulmonary venous connection (TAPVC) can be supracardiac, cardiac, infracardiac, or mixed. A variety of surgical approaches are possible and excellent results can be achieved.

Indications for Surgery

Patients with TAPVC usually present with severe cyanosis and/or pulmonary edema as infants, often within the first days or weeks of life.[2,5,12] The infracardiac type usually presents within the first month of life, the other types usually within the first 3 months. The natural history is death for 80% of symptomatic infants before age 1 year.[2]

The grave prognosis of medical management makes surgery the treatment of choice. Surgery should be performed in symptomatic patients regardless of age or size.[18,36,38] Two-dimensional echocardiography and doppler color flow mapping is extremely accurate in diagnosis of the sites of drainage and the presence or absence of pulmonary venous obstruction.[34,37] Surgical repair can usually be performed on the basis of echocardiographic diagnosis alone.

Preoperative support and stabilization improve surgical results.[27,31] Critically ill infants may require intubation, correction of acidosis, inotropic support, and diuresis. Pulmonary vasodilators may also be beneficial.[31]

Surgical Strategy

Infants are operated upon using profound hypothermia and very low flow bypass with brief periods of circulatory arrest as needed. Cold blood cardioplegia is used for myocardial preservation.

Supracardiac Type

Supracardiac TAPVC is the most common type, accounting for approximately one-half of cases.[36,41]

Surgical Anatomy

The pulmonary veins join a transverse pulmonary venous trunk (Fig. 24–1). The pulmonary venous trunk is usually connected to the innominate vein by

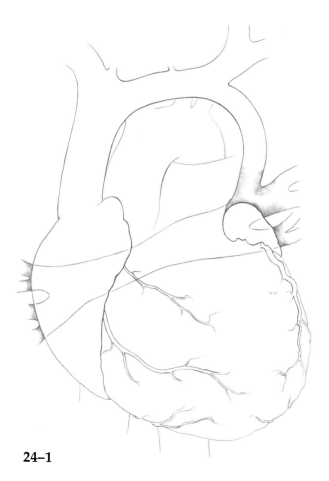

24–1

a left vertical vein. In rare instances, the connection may be to the superior vena cava. There is a foramen ovale atrial septal defect.

The left atrium may be small, although the appendage is usually of normal size.[21] This may limit ventricular filling and cardiac performance in the postoperative period.[25] The left ventricular chamber may also be small.[1,3,4]

Surgical Technique

Muller[22] reported partial correction of supracardiac TAPVC in 1951 using a closed technique for side-to-side anastomosis of the pulmonary venous trunk and left atrium. The first successful complete correction, using cardiopulmonary bypass, was reported by Cooley and Ochsner[7] in 1957. Many approaches to correction have been described, including (1) median sternotomy with repair through the right atrium,[7] (2) left posterolateral thoracotomy,[28,29] (3) median sternotomy with transverse incision through the right atrium into the left atrium and extension of the anastomosis onto the right atrial wall,[32] (4) median sternotomy with elevation and retraction of the cavae to the left and construction of the anastomosis from the right side,[20] (5) median sternotomy with elevation of the apex toward the patient's right shoulder and construction of the anastomosis behind the heart,[6,39] and (6) median sternotomy with anastomosis through the transverse sinus.[35]

Anastomosis with Elevation of the Apex

This is the technique used at the Children's Cardiac Center of Oregon/Portland. The ductus arteriosus is routinely ligated after initiation of cardiopulmo-

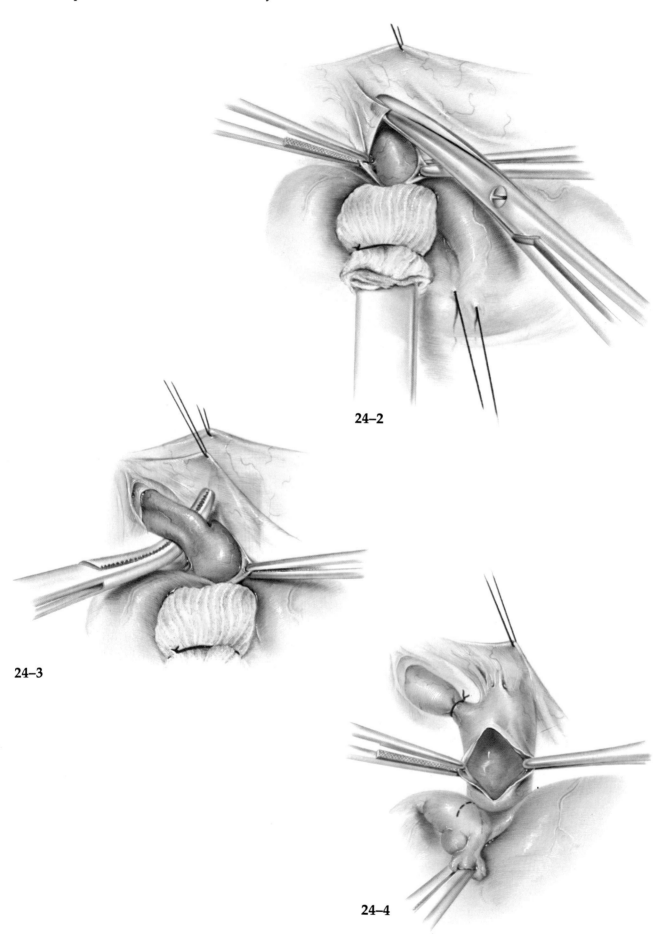

24–2

24–3

24–4

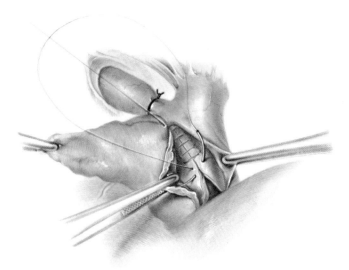

24–5

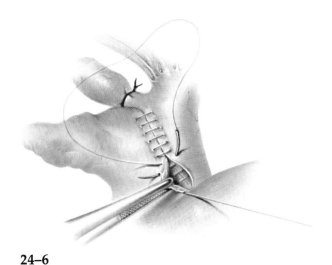

24–6

nary bypass in all infants with TAPVC. Following aortic cross-clamping and administration of cold blood cardioplegic solution, the apex is elevated, exposing the posterior pericardium and the pulmonary venous trunk. The pericardium is incised (Fig. 24–2), exposing the venous trunk and the connection of the left vertical vein. The left vertical vein is encircled and tied (Fig. 24–3) with careful identification of and avoidance of the phrenic nerve, which is in close approximation. The superior and inferior pulmonary veins should be identified so the ligature is definitely above the superior pulmonary vein. Incisions are made in the venous trunk and the left atrium (Fig. 24–4). If the left atrium is very small, the incision is extended onto the appendage.

The posterior suture line is performed from inside, using running suture of 6–0 or 7–0 polypropylene (Fig. 24–5). The anterior row is then performed (Fig. 24–6). The atrial septal defect is closed through the right atrium.

Right Atrial Approach

Cooley and Ochsner[7] in their original report in 1957 described repair through the right atrium with anastomosis between the posterior left atrium and the

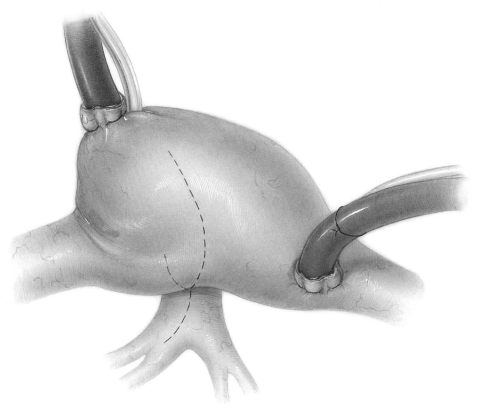

24–7

common pulmonary venous trunk. Shumacker and King[32] modified this technique by extending the anastomosis onto the right atrium and patching the atrial septal defect (ASD). This technique provides excellent exposure, results in a large anastomosis, creates the anastomosis in the anatomically natural position, and may result in a lower incidence of postoperative pulmonary venous stenosis.[8,15,17,40] This technique is used at Sutter/Sacramento.

The ductus arteriosus is ligated after initiation of cardiopulmonary bypass in all infants. The left vertical vein is dissected during cooling, with care to avoid the phrenic nerve. After aortic cross-clamping and administration of cold blood cardioplegia, the patient is placed on total cardiopulmonary bypass and a right atriotomy is performed, taking care to stay well away from the sinus node (Fig. 24-7). This incision is carried through the back of the foramen ovale onto the left atrium to the base of the left atrial appendage. The left vertical vein is ligated after the superior and inferior pulmonary veins are identified. An incision is made in the common pulmonary venous trunk from the base of the right superior pulmonary vein to the base of the left superior pulmonary vein. The anastomosis of the common pulmonary venous trunk to the atrium is started at the base of the left atrial appendage and proceeds to the right, using 6–0 absorbable polydioxanone suture, carrying the suture line across the atrial septum onto the right atrium (Fig. 24-8). The superior suture line is performed in a similar fashion (Fig. 24-9).

A pericardial patch is used to close the atrial septal defect, with the patch often extending onto the right superior pulmonary vein, using the same

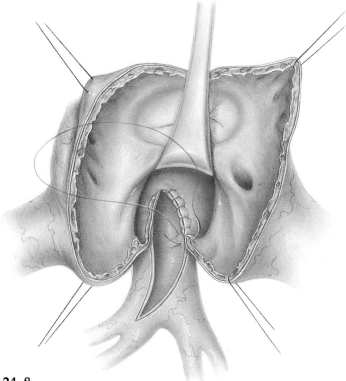

24–8

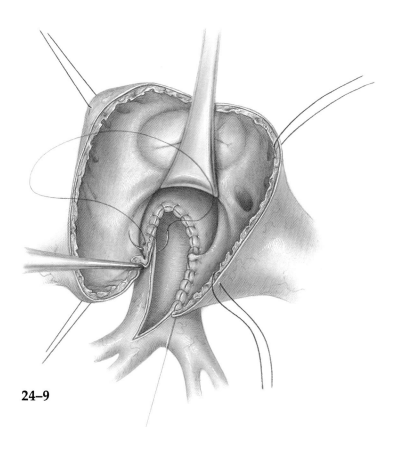

24–9

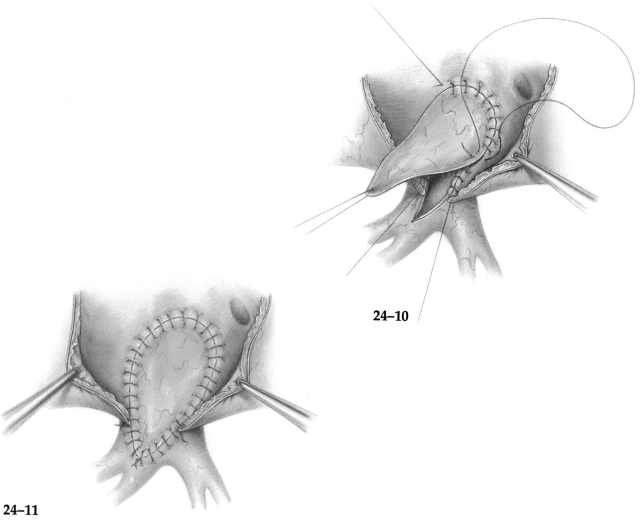

24–10

24–11

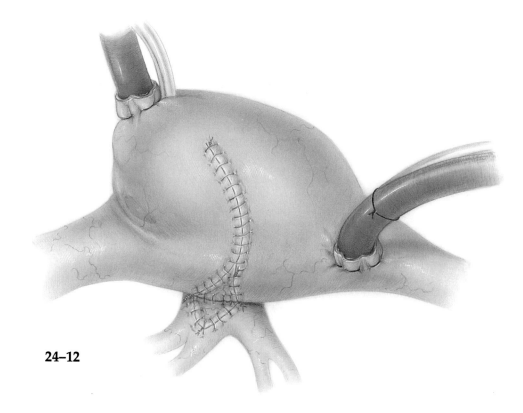

24–12

suture material (Fig. 24–10). The pericardial patch sutures are tied to the previously placed sutures when they meet (Fig. 24–11). A triangular patch of pericardium is often used to augment the closure of the right atrium (Fig. 24–12).

Cardiac Type

Surgical Anatomy

The pulmonary veins empty into a greatly enlarged coronary sinus (Fig. 24–13). A foramen ovale defect is present. Mixed types usually have a cardiac component.[9]

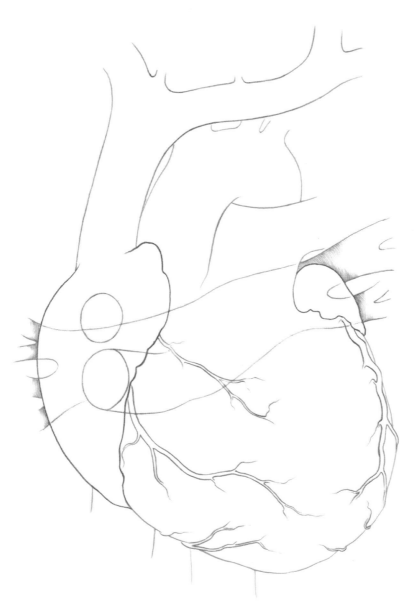

24–13

Surgical Technique

The wall between the coronary sinus and the left atrium is excised (Fig. 24–14). Endocardium is reapproximated to minimize the exposure of atrial muscle. A pericardial patch is then sutured over the atrial septal defect and the coronary sinus with running suture of polypropylene (Fig. 24–15), staying just below the upper rim of the coronary sinus to avoid injury to the conduction system. Figure 24–16 shows the completed repair.

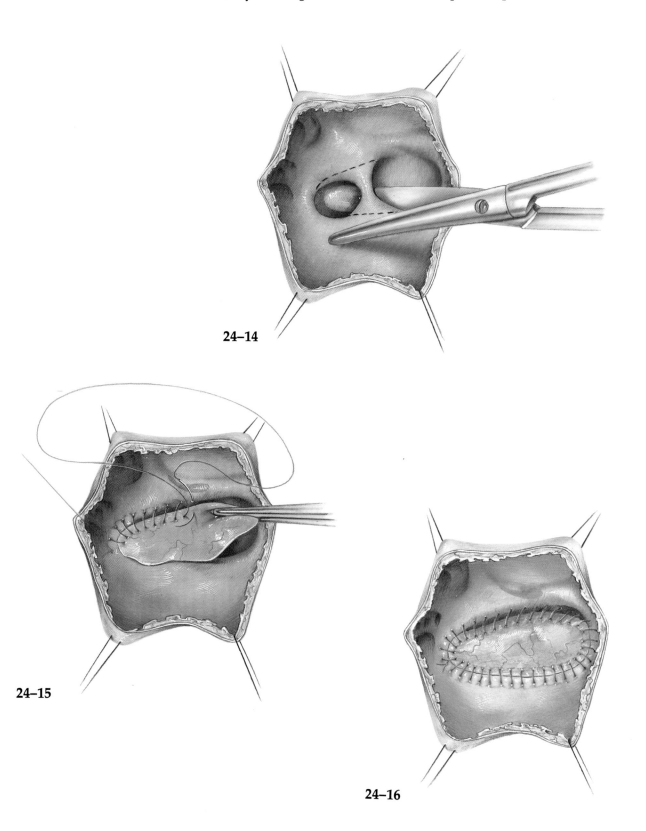

24–14

24–15

24–16

Infracardiac Type

Surgical Anatomy

Infracardiac TAPVC connects below the diaphragm (Fig. 24–17). Approximately 70% connect to the portal vein; other connections are to the inferior vena cava, ductus venosus, or hepatic vein.[10] In some instances the common pulmonary venous trunk can be quite small,[19] and when associated with hypoplasia of the pulmonary veins it is uncorrectable.

Surgical Technique

The vertical vein is dissected, ligated distally, and divided. Incisions are made in the common pulmonary trunk and the posterior left atrium (Fig. 24–18). A "T" incision with an extension into the pulmonary veins can also be performed,[26] if additional opening is necessary for a large anastomosis. The anastomosis is then performed with running polypropylene or absorbable polydioxanone suture (Fig. 24–19). The atrial defect is closed through the right atrium.

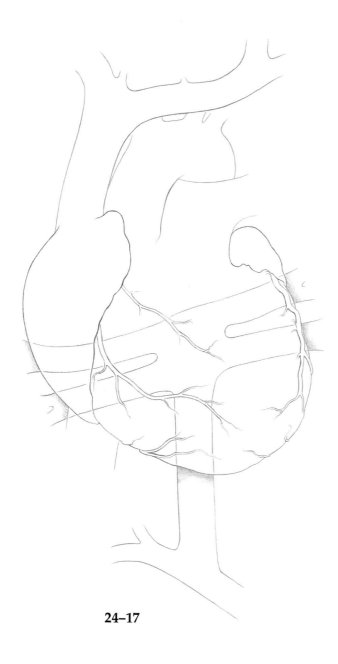

24–17

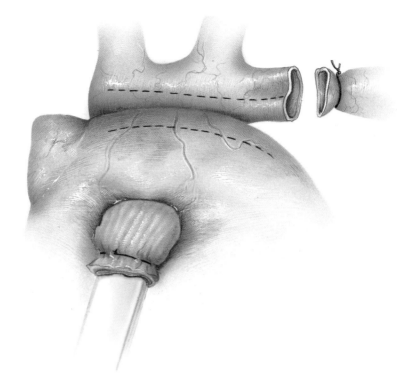

24–18

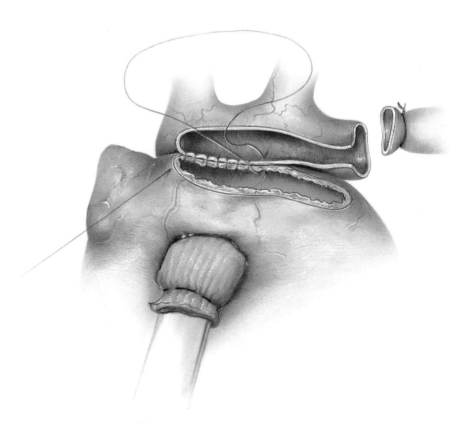

24–19

Special Aspects of Postoperative Care

All critically ill infants have continuous pulmonary artery pressure monitoring with a line placed in the pulmonary artery through the right ventricle. This makes the diagnosis and management of pulmonary hypertensive crises much easier.[31] Pulmonary hypertensive crises are managed with prostaglandin E$_1$ or other pulmonary vasodilators. In addition, for the first 24 hours or more the patients are kept on ventilatory support with hyperventilation and are kept heavily sedated. Inotropic support is used as needed. Some patients may not tolerate closing of the sternum and should be managed with delayed closure.

Results

Operative mortalities reported in the 1960s and early 1970s were frequently high, from 50% to 65% for patients less than 1 year of age[6,41] and as high as 89% for patients less than 6 months of age.[23] With improvements in perioperative support and surgical technique, some reports of operative mortality from the late 1970s were below 20%.[18,36,38] Reports of operative mortality below 10% have appeared recently.[27,30] The infracardiac type is usually associated with a higher operative mortality.[10,31,36] Risk factors that were previously associated with operative death, such as anatomical type, degree of pulmonary venous obstruction, severity of pulmonary hypertension, and young age[18,24] appear to have been neutralized in some recent series.[27,30]

Late survival and functional result in patients repaired in childhood are excellent.[5,14] Postoperative hemodynamics are frequently normal following repair in infancy.[21] Hammon and colleagues[16] have reported that left ventricular size and function which were markedly depressed preoperatively rose to normal levels in postoperative survivors. The presence of severe depression of left ventricular size and function preoperatively does not predict a higher operative risk.

Late death following repair in infancy is unusual,[13] but when it occurs a common cause is intimal fibroplasia of the pulmonary veins away from the anastomosis, a syndrome occurring more commonly in the infracardiac type.[11,36,38] Pulmonary venous obstruction usually occurs within 6 months of surgery.[30] Doppler echocardiography is an extremely accurate method of identifying and localizing postoperative pulmonary venous obstruction.[33,37]

References

1. Bharati S, Lev M: Congenital anomalies of the pulmonary veins. Cardiovasc Clin 5:23,1973.
2. Bonham-Carter RE, Capriles M, Noe Y: Total anomalous pulmonary venous drainage: a clinical and anatomical study of 75 children. Br Heart J 31:45,1969.
3. Bove KE, Geiser EA, Meyer RA: The left ventricle in anomalous pulmonary venous return. Arch Pathol Lab Med 99:522,1975.
4. Burroughs JT, Edwards JE: Total anomalous pulmonary venous connection. Am Heart J 59:913,1960.
5. Clarke DR, Stark J, de Laval M, Pincott JR, Taylor JFN: Total anomalous pulmonary venous drainage in infancy. Br Heart J 39:436,1977.
6. Cooley DA, Hallman GL: Surgical Treatment of Congenital Heart Disease. Philadelphia, Lea & Febiger, 1966, p 143.
7. Cooley DA, Ochsner A Jr: Correction of total anomalous pulmonary venous drainage: technical considerations. Surgery 42:1014,1957.
8. Corno A, Giamberti A, Carotti A, Giannico S, Marino B, Marcelletti C: Total anomalous pulmonary venous connection: surgical repair with a double-patch technique. Ann Thorac Surg 49:492,1990.

9. de Laval M, Stark J, Waterston DJ: Mixed type of total anomalous pulmonary venous drainage. Ann Thorac Surg 16:464,1973.

10. Duff DF, Nihill MR, McNamara DG: Infradiaphragmatic total anomalous pulmonary venous return: review of clinical and pathological findings and results of operation in 28 cases. Br Heart J 39:619,1977.

11. Fleming WH, Clark EB, Dooley KJ, Hofschire PJ, Ruckman RN, Hopeman AR, Sarafian L, Mooring PK: Late complications following surgical repair of total anomalous pulmonary venous return below the diaphragm. Ann Thorac Surg 27:435,1979.

12. Gathman GE, Nadas AS: Total anomalous pulmonary venous connection: clinical and physiologic observations of 75 pediatric patients. Circulation 42:143,1970.

13. Gersony WM, Bowman FO, Steeg CN, Hayes CJ, Jesse MJ, Malm JR: Management of total anomalous pulmonary venous drainage in early infancy. Circulation 43(Suppl I):I-19,1971.

14. Gomes MMR, Feldt RH, McGoon DC, Danielson GK: Long-term results following correction of total anomalous pulmonary venous connection. J Thorac Cardiovasc Surg 61:253,1971.

15. Goor DA, Yellin A, Frand M, Smolinsky A, Neufeld HN: The operative problem of small left atrium in total anomalous pulmonary venous connection. Ann Thorac Surg 22:244,1976.

16. Hammon JW Jr, Bender HW, Graham TP, Boucek RJ, Smith CW, Erath HG Jr: Total anomalous pulmonary venous connection: ten years' experience including studies of postoperative ventricular function. J Thorac Cardiovasc Surg 80:544,1980.

17. Hawkins JA, Clark EB, Doty DB: Total anomalous pulmonary venous connection. Ann Thorac Surg 36:548,1983.

18. Katz NM, Kirklin JW, Pacifico AD: Concepts and practices in surgery for total anomalous pulmonary venous connection. Ann Thorac Surg 25:479,1978.

19. Kawashima Y, Matsuda H, Nakano S, Miyamoto K, Fujino M, Kozuka T, Manabe H: Tree-shaped pulmonary veins in infracardiac total anomalous pulmonary venous drainage. Ann Thorac Surg 23:436,1977.

20. Kirklin JW: Surgical treatment of total anomalous pulmonary venous connection in infancy. In Barratt-Boyes BG, Neutze JM, Harris EA (eds): Heart Disease in Infancy, Diagnosis and Surgical Treatment. Edinburgh and London, Churchill/Livingstone, 1973, p 89.

21. Mathew R, Thilenius OG, Replogle RL, Arcilla RA: Cardiac function in total anomalous pulmonary venous return before and after surgery. Circulation 55:361,1977.

22. Muller WH: The surgical treatment of transposition of the pulmonary veins. Ann Surg 134:683,1951.

23. Mustard WT, Keon WJ, Trusler GA: Transposition of the lesser veins (total anomalous pulmonary venous drainage). Prog Cardiovasc Dis 11:145,1968.

24. Oelert H, Schafers H-J, Stegmann T, Kallfelz H-C, Borst HG: Complete correction of total anomalous pulmonary venous drainage: experience with 53 patients. Ann Thorac Surg 41:392,1986.

25. Parr GVS, Kirklin JW, Pacifico AD, Blackstone EH, Lauridsen P: Cardiac performance in infants after repair of total anomalous pulmonary venous connection. Ann Thorac Surg 17:561,1974.

26. Phillips SJ, Kongtahworn C, Zeff RH, Skinner JR, Chandramouli B, Gay JH: Correction of total anomalous pulmonary venous connection below the diaphragm. Ann Thorac Surg 49:734,1990.

27. Raisher BD, Grant JW, Martin TC, Strauss AW, Spray TL: Complete repair of total anomalous pulmonary venous connection in infancy. J Thorac Cardiovasc Surg 104:443,1992.

28. Roe BB: Total anomalous pulmonary venous drainage: technical and physiological considerations. Ann Surg 160:1,1964.

29. Roe BB: Posterior approach to correction of total anomalous pulmonary venous return: further experience. J Thorac Cardiovasc Surg 59:748,1970.

30. Sano S, Brawn WJ, Mee RBB: Total anomalous pulmonary venous drainage. J Thorac Cardiovasc Surg 97:886,1989.

31. Serraf A, Bruniaux J, Lacour-Gayet F, Chambran P, Binet J-P, Lecronier G,

Demontoux S, Planche C: Obstructed total anomalous pulmonary venous return: toward neutralization of a major risk factor. J Thorac Cardiovasc Surg 101: 601,1991.

32. Shumacker HB Jr, King H: A modified procedure for complete repair of total anomalous pulmonary venous drainage. Surg Gynecol Obstet 112:763,1961.

33. Smallhorn JF, Burrows P, Wilson G, Coles J, Gilday DL, Freedom RM: Two-dimensional and pulsed Doppler echocardiography in the postoperative evaluation of total anomalous pulmonary venous connection. Circulation 76:298,1987.

34. Sreeram N, Walsh K: Diagnosis of total anomalous pulmonary venous drainage by Doppler color flow imaging. J Am Coll Cardiol 19:1577,1992.

35. Tucker BL, Lindesmith GG, Stiles QR, Meyer BW: The superior approach for correction of the supracardiac type of total anomalous pulmonary venous return. Ann Thorac Surg 22:374,1976.

36. Turley K, Tucker WY, Ullyot DJ, Ebert PA: Total anomalous pulmonary venous connection in infancy: influence of age and type of lesion. Am J Cardiol 45: 92,1980.

37. van der Velde ME, Parness IA, Colan SD, Spevak PJ, Lock JE, Mayer JE, Sanders SP: Two-dimensional echocardiography in the pre- and postoperative management of totally anomalous pulmonary venous connection. J Am Coll Cardiol 18: 1746,1991.

38. Whight CM, Barratt-Boyes BG, Calder AL, Neutze JM, Brandt PWT: Total anomalous pulmonary venous connection: long-term results following repair in infancy. J Thorac Cardiovasc Surg 75:52,1978.

39. Williams GR, Richardson WR, Campbell GS: Repair of total anomalous pulmonary venous drainage in infancy. J Thorac Cardiovasc Surg 47:199,1964.

40. Wilson WR, Ilbawi MN, DeLeon SY, Quinones JA, Arcilia RA, Sulayman RF, Idriss FS: Technical modifications for improved results in total anomalous pulmonary venous drainage. J Thorac Cardiovasc Surg 103:861,1992.

41. Wukasch DC, Deutsch M, Reul GJ, Hallman GL, Cooley DA: Total anomalous pulmonary venous return: review of 125 patients treated surgically. Ann Thorac Surg 19:622,1975.

Index

357

in coarctation of the aorta, 229
infected teeth as a source of, 2
destruction of anulus in, 187–88
and homograft aortic valve replacement, 186
indications for surgery with, 185
prosthetic valve, 73
tricuspid valve replacement in, after tricuspid valve excision, 215
Endotracheal tube, monitoring of, 67
Endoventricular repair, of a left ventricular aneurysm, 137
Enflurane, for anesthesia, 8
Epicardial topical hypothermia, 48–49
Epicardium, incision of, 13
Epigastric artery, inferior, as conduit, coronary artery bypass, 98
Epinephrine, 79
Esmolol
for myocardial oxygen demand reduction, 7
for postoperative hypertension, 244
for preinduction tachycardia, 7
European Coronary Surgery Study Group (ECSS), survival after coronary artery bypass, 123
Exercise capacity, after coronary artery bypass, and angina relief, 123
Exercise stress test
for diagnosis of coronary artery disease, 92
and prognosis in coronary artery disease, 96
Extubation, postoperative, guidelines, 68

Failure to thrive, in ventricular septal defects, 288
Fallot's tetralogy. See Tetralogy of Fallot
Femoral artery
cannulation of, 27–28, 29
for insertion of an intraaortic balloon, 80–81
Femorofemoral bypass, preparation for
in patent ductus arteriosus, 219
in repeat sternotomy, 25
Fentanyl
for anesthesia, 8, 9
in postoperative care, after the arterial switch procedure, 324
Fever, postoperative, 69
Fiberoptic lighting, 21
Fiber shortening, mean velocity of
after aortic valve replacement, 200
circumferential, 182

Fibrillating heart, mitral valve replacement in a, 41
Fibrillation. See Atrial fibrillation; Ventricular fibrillation
Fibrin glue, coating for suture lines, 323
Fibrosis, mitral subvalvular, and commissurotomy versus valve replacement, 149
Fibrous body, central. See Central fibrous body
Filling pressures, mean left ventricular, 138
Filtration, of cardiotomy sucker return, 34
Flow rates
in cardiopulmonary bypass, infants, 38
in coronary perfusion, for aortic valve replacement, 42
and high-energy phosphate preservation, 37
in standard cardiopulmonary bypass, 33
monitoring, 35
Fluids
overload of, and respiratory failure, 71
postoperative, glucose in water, 67
Fontan procedure, 261
Foramen ovale
atrial septal defect, in supracardiac TAPVC, 343
defect of, in cardiac type TAPVC, 349
management of, with pulmonary valvotomy, 262
patent
management of, with tetralogy of Fallot repair, 304
and pulmonary valvotomy, 261
Frank-Starling mechanism, in aortic stenosis, 182
Free radicals, scavenging of, by blood, 52
Functional regurgitation, and tricuspid valve insufficiency, 210–11
Functional status. See also Cardiac performance; Hemodynamics; Pulmonary function; Ventricular function
after the arterial switch procedure, 324
after the Mustard operation, 333–34
after the Senning operation, 328
Fungi, endocarditis from, indication for surgery, 185
Furosemide, to improve urine output, 36

Gastroepiploic artery, as conduit, coronary artery bypass, 98
Gastrointestinal complications, postoperative, 74
bowel infarction, from paradoxical hypertension, 244
Glucose
in cardioplegic arrest solutions, 53
replenishing, in cold cardioplegic solution, 55
Glucose-6-phosphate, production of, in ischemia, 45
Glutamate, modification of warm blood induction of cardioplegia, 56, 95
Glutaraldehyde, treatment of autologous pericardial patches with, 188
Glycogen, and irreversible ischemia, 46
Glycolytic pathway, in ischemia, 45–46
Grafts/grafting. See also Bioprostheses, porcine; Dacron; Homografts; Polytetrafluoroethylene graft; Teflon
angina relief, after coronary bypass, 123
autograft, pulmonary valve replacement, 186
bypass
for coarctation of the aorta, 230, 242–43
for coarctation of the aorta, recurrence of, 233
in coronary artery disease, ventricular septal defect repair, 143
patency of, after coronary bypass, 93, 123
perfusion of, 56
tube
for coarctation of the aorta, 230
for repair in absent pulmonary valve, 304
Growth, normal
after Blalock-Taussig shunt, 250
after subclavian flap repair, 230
after ventricular septal defect repair, 298

Halothane, for anesthesia, 8, 9
with morphine, 8
Hancock porcine bioprosthesis, 201
Handedness, and basic surgical technique, 21
Heart. See Cardi- entries; Coronary entries; Ischemia; Myocard- entries

in balloon angioplasty, in children, 228
in balloon atrial septostomy, 315–16
in coarctation of the aorta
   with associated congenital defects, 245
   unrepaired, 229
in coronary bypass surgery, 93
in emergency coronary bypass, for failed PTCA, 95–96
in the Mustard operation, 333
operative
   in aortic valve replacement, 200
   in the arterial switch procedure, 324
   in atrioventricular canal correction, 280
   in coarctation of the aorta repair, 244, 245
   in complete atrioventricular canal, 285
   in left ventricular aneurysm repair, 137
   in left ventricular aneurysm resection, 133
   in mitral valve replacement, 166
   in mitral valve replacement, by functional class, 174
   in the Modified Blalock-Taussig shunt, 254
   in open mitral commissurotomy, 153
   in ostium primum defect repair, 277
   in ostium secundum defect repair, 271
   in patent ductus arteriosus, 219, 220
   in pulmonary valvotomy in neonates, 264
   in the Senning operation, 328
   in total anomalous pulmonary venous connection surgery, 353
   in tricuspid valve anuloplasty, 214
   in tricuspid valve replacement, 216
   in unstable angina, 94
   in valvotomy for children, 181
   in valvuloplasty/anuloplasty, 163
   in ventricular septal defect repair, 298
   in ventricular septal defect repair, postinfarction, 145–46
   in ventricular septal defect repair, with coarctation of the aorta, 245
in patent ductus arteriosus, 218–19
   with coarctation, 244–45
after percutaneous balloon valvuloplasty for aortic stenosis, 183

in potassium cardioplegic arrest, 50
in total anomalous pulmonary venous connection, 342
in total primary correction, tetralogy of Fallot, 301
in transposition of the great arteries, untreated, 315
in valve replacements
   due to anticoagulants, 175
   with coronary artery disease, 185
   with coronary perfusion, 44
   with normothermic ischemic arrest, 45
   prediction of, 166
   in the presence of, 96
in valvotomy in neonates, 181
in ventricular septal defect, 289
   postinfarction, 142
Mural chordae, 150
Mural leaflet, in mitral valve replacement, 169
Muscles. *See also Myo-* entries; Papillary muscles
   cardiac, degeneration of, 184
   defective, with ventricular septal defects, 291, 297
Mustard procedure, 315, 328–36
   complications of, 316, 317
Myectomy, transaortic, for idiopathic hypertrophic subaortic stenosis, 202
Myocardial contractility
   defined, 77–78
   factor in stroke volume, 77
   manipulation of, 79–80
Myocardial infarction
   acute
      coronary artery bypass for, 94–95
      diagnosis with radioactive pyrophosphate, 92
      as an indication for coronary arteriography, 88
   left ventricular aneurysm following, 132
   mitral regurgitation secondary to, 166
   and myocardial preservation method, aortic valve replacement, 49
   perioperative
      and coronary anatomy, 43
      in coronary bypass surgery, 93, 94
   ventricular septal defect following, 142–46
Myocardial ischemia. *See* Ischemia, myocardial
Myocardial necrosis. *See* Necrosis, myocardial

Myocardial oxygen demand. *See* Oxygen, supply/demand balance
Myocardium
   akinetic, differentiating from ventricular aneurysm, 132
   blood flow in
      after coronary artery bypass, 123
      diastolic pressure-time index (DPTI) to measure, 79–80
   edema of
      from hypoosmolar solutions in cold cardioplegic arrest, 52
      from infusion pressure, in cold cardioplegic arrest, 54
   factors affecting aerobic metabolism in, 43
   perfusion of, after coronary artery bypass, 123
   preservation of, 41–57
      and anesthesia, 6–8
      in coronary artery bypass, 99
      in left ventricular aneurysm resection, 134
Myofibrils, loss of, in aortic regurgitation, 184
Myosin filaments, loss of, in aortic regurgitation, 184
Myxomatous degeneration, tricuspid regurgitation associated with, 210–11

Nadolol, preoperative management of, 2
^{13}N ammonia for PET, 92
National Cooperative Study Group on Unstable Angina Pectoris, on unstable angina
   definition of, 93
   randomized study of treatment, 94
Necrosis, myocardial
   in acute myocardial infarction, 95
   in aortic valve replacement, 49
   after continuous coronary perfusion, 44
   after ischemic arrest, 45
   after potassium cardioplegic arrest, 50
   during precardiopulmonary bypass, 6, 8
Necrotizing arteritis, in coarctation of the aorta repair, 244
Neonates
   arterial switch procedure for, 316
   blood versus crystalloid cardioplegia for, 53
   cardiopulmonary bypass in, 37–38
   coarctation of the aorta repair in choice of operation, 229–30

ISBN 0-387-94220-3

EAN

9 780387 942209 >